Machine Learning and Generative AI in Smart Healthcare

Swarnalatha Purushotham
Vellore Institute of Technology, India

S. Prabu
Pondicherry University, India

A volume in the Advances in Medical Technologies and Clinical Practice (AMTCP) Book Series

Published in the United States of America by
IGI Global
Medical Information Science Reference (an imprint of IGI Global)
701 E. Chocolate Avenue
Hershey PA, USA 17033
Tel: 717-533-8845
Fax: 717-533-8661
E-mail: cust@igi-global.com
Web site: http://www.igi-global.com

Copyright © 2024 by IGI Global. All rights reserved. No part of this publication may be reproduced, stored or distributed in any form or by any means, electronic or mechanical, including photocopying, without written permission from the publisher.
Product or company names used in this set are for identification purposes only. Inclusion of the names of the products or companies does not indicate a claim of ownership by IGI Global of the trademark or registered trademark.

Library of Congress Cataloging-in-Publication Data

CIP DATA PENDING

ISBN13: 9798369337196
EISBN13: 9798369337202

British Cataloguing in Publication Data
A Cataloguing in Publication record for this book is available from the British Library.

All work contributed to this book is new, previously-unpublished material.
The views expressed in this book are those of the authors, but not necessarily of the publisher.

For electronic access to this publication, please contact: eresources@igi-global.com.

Table of Contents

Foreword xviii

Preface xx

Chapter 1
Advances in AI and Machine Learning for Healthcare Informatics 1
    K. Maithili, Vel Tech Rangarajan Dr. Sagunthala R&D Institute of
        Science and Technology, India
    A. Ponmalar, R.M.K. Engineering College, India
    B. Yamini, SRM Institute of Science and Technology, India
    M. Karthikeyan, R.M.K. College of Engineering and Technology, India
    T. P. Anish, R.M.K. College of Engineering and Technology, India
    B. Maheswari, R M K. Engineering College, India
    R. Siva Subramanian, R M K. College of Engineering and Technology,
        India

Chapter 2
Data Mining and Knowledge Discovery: Transforming Healthcare Through
Biomedical Intelligence 23
    Akshat Shree Mishra, International Institute of Information Technology,
        Naya, India
    J. Vijaya, International Institute of Information Technology, Naya, India

Chapter 3
Design and Development of AI-Powered Healthcare System 41
    A. K. P. Kovendan, Vellore Institute of Technology, India
    G. N. Balaji, Vellore Institute of Technology, India
    Srijita Khatua, Vellore Institute of Technology, India
    Harmanpreet Singh, Vellore Institute of Technology, India
    Dibyani Chatterjee, Vellore Institute of Technology, India

Chapter 4
Applications of AI Techniques in Healthcare and Wellbeing 61
    S. C. Vetrivel, Kongu Engineering College, India
    V. P. Arun, JKKN College of Engineering and Technology, India
    R Maheswari, Kongu Engineering College, India
    T. P. Saravanan, Kongu Engineering College, India

Chapter 5
Artificial Intelligence in Records Structures Research: A Systematic Literature Review and Research Agenda 93

    P. Immaculate Rexi Jenifer, SASTRA University (Deemed), India
    M. Rajakumaran, SASTRA University (Deemed), India
    A. Dennis Ananth, SASTRA University (Deemed), India
    S. Markkandeyan, SASTRA University (Deemed), India
    R. G. Gokila, SASTRA University (Deemed), India

Chapter 6
The Use of Artificial Intelligence in Health Communication: A Research on ChatGPT 117

    Nural Imik Tanyildizi, Fırat University, Turkey
    Ilkay Yıldız, Bingöl Üniversitesi, Turkey

Chapter 7
Federated Learning for Securing Glomeruli Detection in Digital Pathology ... 139

    Shiva Chaithanya Goud Bollipelly, Vellore Institute of Technology, India

Chapter 8
Advances and Strategies in Addressing Plant Health Challenges: Insights from Recent Research 157

    Sameera Kuppam, Vellore Institute of Technology, India
    R. Venkatesan, SASTRA University (Deemed), India
    Vuppala Balaji, Vardhaman College of Engineering, India

Chapter 9
Early Detection of Skin Cancer Using Convolutional Neural Networks 169

    Shukraditya Bose, Vellore Institute of Technology, India
    G. Megala, Vellore Institute of Technology, India
    Raghupathyraj Valluvan, University of Jaffna, Sri Lanka

Chapter 10
Automatic Screening of Skin Cancer 185

    Singaravelan Shanmugasundaram, PSR Engineering College, India
    P. Alwin John, PSR Engineering College, India
    M. Vargheese, PSN College of Engineering and Technology, India
    P. Gopalsamy, PSR Engineering College, India
    D. Pavunraj, Vel Tech Multi Tech Dr. Rangarajan Dr. Sakunthala Engineering College, India
    V. Selvakumar, PSR Engineering College, India
    D. Arun Shunmugam, PSR Engineering College, India

Chapter 11
Usage of Machine Learning and Deep Learning for Lung Cancer Detection: Current Scenario, Challenges and Futuristic Direction 223
    Ishaan Dawar, DIT University, India
    Sumedha Bhardwaj, DIT University, India

Chapter 12
Efficient Brain Tumor Classification With Optimized Hybrid Deep Neural Networks 253
    V. Sanjay, Vellore Institute of Technology, India
    G. Megala, Vellore Institute of Technology, India
    Vuppala Balaji, Vardhaman College of Engineering, India

Chapter 13
Enhancing Brain Cancer Detection and Localization Using YOLOv8 Object Detection: A Deep Learning Approach 261
    Seetharam Nagesh Appe, CVR College of Engineering, India
    G. Arulselvi, Annamalai University, India
    G. N. Balaji, Vellore Institute of Technology, India

Chapter 14
Multi-Cancer Detection Using Deep Learning Techniques 281
    G. N. Balaji, Vellore Institute of technology, India
    A. K. P. Kovendan, Vellore Institute of Technology, India
    Kirti Nayak, Vellore Institute of Technology, India
    R. Venkatesan, SASTRA University (Deemed), India
    D. Yuvaraj, Cihan University, Iraq

Chapter 15
A Multimodal Deep Learning Approach for Early Detection of Alzheimer's Disease 305
    V. Sanjay, Vellore Institute of Technology, India
    P. Swarnalatha, Vellore Institute of Technology, India
    Ragupathyraj Valluvan, University of Jaffna, Sri Lanka

Chapter 16
Generative Adversarial Networks for Advanced EEG Data Analysis 321
    Evin Şahin Sadık, Kütahya Dumlupınar University, Turkey

Chapter 17
Confluence of Deep Learning Using Watershed Segmentation GAN for
Advancing Endoscopy Surgery Imaging 345
    G. Megala, Vellore Institute of Technology, India
    P. Swarnalatha, Vellore Institute of Technology, India
    S. Prabu, Pondicherry University, India
    R. Venkatesan, SASTRA University (Deemed), India
    Anantharajah Kaneswaran, University of Jaffna, Sri Lanka

Chapter 18
Review on Facial Emotion Recognition Using Deep Learning With Multiple
Databases 369
    Hari Prasad Mal, Vellore Institute of Technology, India
    P. Swarnalatha, Vellore Institute of Technology, India
    Anantharajah Kaneswaran, University of Jaffna, Sri Lanka
    S. Prabu, Pondicherry University, India

Compilation of References 383

About the Contributors 431

Index 441

Detailed Table of Contents

Foreword xviii

Preface xx

Chapter 1
Advances in AI and Machine Learning for Healthcare Informatics 1
    K. Maithili, Vel Tech Rangarajan Dr. Sagunthala R&D Institute of
        Science and Technology, India
    A. Ponmalar, R.M.K. Engineering College, India
    B. Yamini, SRM Institute of Science and Technology, India
    M. Karthikeyan, R.M.K. College of Engineering and Technology, India
    T. P. Anish, R.M.K. College of Engineering and Technology, India
    B. Maheswari, R M K. Engineering College, India
    R. Siva Subramanian, R M K. College of Engineering and Technology,
        India

This study focuses on how medical informatics, bioinformatics and health records are getting rejuvenated by AI and ML, which is leading to a new paradigm in healthcare. It drives home the significance of data-driven methods to address the health problems and enhancing the patient outcomes in healthcare. The study begins with a highlight of AI and ML technologies being used in healthcare. Then it delves deep into the machine learning approaches, appropriate optimisation techniques, methods of disease prediction, and signal processing advances. Besides that, this paper obtains new technological developments such as the improvement of healthcare information systems and the application of artificial intelligence and machine learning to medical signal and image processing. By means of this purpose, one aims to teach scholars, specialists, and decision-makers concerning the transformative capacity of AI and ML in healthcare. Ethical surrounding matters and the future pathways of research and innovation are also discussed.

Chapter 2
Data Mining and Knowledge Discovery: Transforming Healthcare Through
Biomedical Intelligence 23
> Akshat Shree Mishra, International Institute of Information Technology, Naya, India
> J. Vijaya, International Institute of Information Technology, Naya, India

This chapter proposal aims to explore the transformative potential of data mining and knowledge discovery in healthcare, focusing on optimizing healthcare computing systems, integrating technologies like AI and IoT, and emphasizing patient-centric care. It delves into precision medicine, disease pathways, and current trends in health and disease, while addressing concerns around privacy, biases, and responsible data use. The methodology includes a systematic review of healthcare computing systems and real-world case studies. The chapter advocates for interdisciplinary collaboration and ethical frameworks, concluding with a discussion on future directions and challenges to inspire a future of data-driven, patient-centered healthcare.

Chapter 3
Design and Development of AI-Powered Healthcare System 41
> A. K. P. Kovendan, Vellore Institute of Technology, India
> G. N. Balaji, Vellore Institute of Technology, India
> Srijita Khatua, Vellore Institute of Technology, India
> Harmanpreet Singh, Vellore Institute of Technology, India
> Dibyani Chatterjee, Vellore Institute of Technology, India

Cancer patient survival is an integral part of the healthcare sector, with researchers offering clinicians snipping information as they consider treatment options that have a big impact on patients' lifestyle decisions. Evidently, no study of predicting survival or death from breast cancer using XGBoost method has been attempted. The goal of this project is to design a prediction system that can forecast both the survival rate and the death rate from breast cancer at an early stage by examining the most limited collection of clinical dataset variables. The potential of the XGBoost method is determined using mainly age at the time of diagnosis along with other clinical characteristics, assessed for its relative significance. The project findings show that the XGBoost model fits the testing dataset more effectively, with outcome of accuracy 82.72% approximately.

Chapter 4

Applications of AI Techniques in Healthcare and Wellbeing 61

    S. C. Vetrivel, Kongu Engineering College, India
    V. P. Arun, JKKN College of Engineering and Technology, India
    R Maheswari, Kongu Engineering College, India
    T. P. Saravanan, Kongu Engineering College, India

The integration of Artificial Intelligence (AI) techniques in healthcare and wellbeing systems has witnessed significant advancements, offering transformative solutions to traditional healthcare paradigms. This chapter provides a comprehensive overview of the diverse applications of AI in the healthcare sector, highlighting its potential to enhance diagnostics, treatment planning, personalized medicine, and overall patient outcomes. AI techniques, including machine learning and deep learning algorithms, have demonstrated remarkable capabilities in analyzing large datasets such as medical images, genetic information, and electronic health records. These technologies enable more accurate and timely disease detection, improving diagnostic accuracy and aiding healthcare professionals in making informed decisions. In treatment planning, AI-driven systems contribute to the development of personalized therapeutic strategies. By leveraging patient-specific data, AI models can predict treatment responses, optimize drug regimens, and minimize adverse effects.

Chapter 5

Artificial Intelligence in Records Structures Research: A Systematic
Literature Review and Research Agenda 93

    P. Immaculate Rexi Jenifer, SASTRA University (Deemed), India
    M. Rajakumaran, SASTRA University (Deemed), India
    A. Dennis Ananth, SASTRA University (Deemed), India
    S. Markkandeyan, SASTRA University (Deemed), India
    R. G. Gokila, SASTRA University (Deemed), India

AI has received expanded interest from the data systems (IS) studies network in recent years. There is, however, a developing difficulty that studies on AI should enjoy a loss of cumulative building of information, which has overshadowed IS research formerly. This look at addresses this subject, by way of engaging in a scientific literature overview of AI studies in IS between 2005 and 2020. The seek approach ended in 1877 research, of which 98 had been diagnosed as primary research and a synthesise of key issues which might be pertinent to this take a look at is presented. In doing so, this has a look at makes important contributions, namely (i) an identification of the modern mentioned enterprise price and contributions of AI, (ii) research and sensible implications on the use of AI and (iii) opportunities for destiny AI studies inside the shape of the AI research.

Chapter 6
The Use of Artificial Intelligence in Health Communication: A Research on
ChatGPT 117
    Nural Imik Tanyildizi, Fırat University, Turkey
    Ilkay Yıldız, Bingöl Üniversitesi, Turkey

Communication is of great importance in health services. Nowadays, new media, especially the internet, are frequently used in health communication. Artificial intelligence has also begun to be used in healthcare. Artificial intelligence studies generally aim to develop artificial methods that imitate human ways of thinking. In addition, it is predicted that some programs produced based on artificial intelligence will affect health communication processes in daily use. The most important of these programs is the ChatGPT (Chatbot Generative Pre-trained Transformer) program. The purpose of this study is to reveal the benefits and drawbacks of using the ChatGPT program in health communication by providing a qualitative framework. For this purpose, a semi-structured interview was conducted with 30 people over the age of 18, determined by a purposeful sampling method. In line with the data obtained, the use of Chat GPT in health communication was tried to be explained.

Chapter 7
Federated Learning for Securing Glomeruli Detection in Digital Pathology ... 139
    Shiva Chaithanya Goud Bollipelly, Vellore Institute of Technology, India

This chapter addresses the imperative for secure and precise glomeruli detection in histopathological images, crucial for diagnosing renal conditions. Using the YOLOv3 object detection algorithm, it integrates federated learning to ensure data security. A custom dataset, annotated with XML labels from histopathological images of sclerosed and normal glomeruli, is created. Initially, a traditional YOLOv3 model achieved 98.55% accuracy but posed privacy risks with centralized data storage. Federated learning decentralizes data across clients, preserving privacy and achieving 98.79% accuracy. Employing cryptographic techniques for data transmission security, this chapter demonstrates federated learning's robustness in medical image analysis. A comparative analysis with traditional methods highlights federated learning's advantages in data security and collaborative learning, showcasing its transformative potential in digital pathology.

Chapter 8
Advances and Strategies in Addressing Plant Health Challenges: Insights
from Recent Research 157
    Sameera Kuppam, Vellore Institute of Technology, India
    R. Venkatesan, SASTRA University (Deemed), India
    Vuppala Balaji, Vardhaman College of Engineering, India

This chapter explores the complex issues that contemporary agriculture and natural ecosystems face when it comes to plant health. It starts by going over the several biotic variables that endanger plant productivity and vigor, like pests, invasive species, and diseases. The dynamic aspect of these threats is emphasized, which is made worse by climate change and global trade, which promote the spread and evolution of dangerous species. The chapter also looks at abiotic stresses, such as pollution, soil deterioration, and drought, emphasizing how these factors interact to reduce plant resilience. Sustainable agriculture methods and integrated pest management (IPM) techniques are highlighted as essential solutions to these problems. The chapter also emphasizes the value of sophisticated biotechnology instruments, early detection methods, and the protection of plant health through legislation and education.

Chapter 9
Early Detection of Skin Cancer Using Convolutional Neural Networks 169
    Shukraditya Bose, Vellore Institute of Technology, India
    G. Megala, Vellore Institute of Technology, India
    Raghupathyraj Valluvan, University of Jaffna, Sri Lanka

The substantial health risks associated with skin cancer make early detection techniques imperative. In this work, we investigate using convolutional neural networks (CNNs) to identify skin cancer. By utilizing the vast HAM10000 dataset comprising various skin lesion images, we aim to create a robust artificial intelligence model to classify pictures accurately. Our approach preprocesses image data, adjusts the Xception architecture, and uses data augmentation techniques to improve model performance. The model's efficacy is evaluated using accuracy, precision, recall, and F1-score metrics. With possible benefits for bettering patient outcomes and healthcare delivery, this research advances automated diagnostic tools for skin cancer detection.

Chapter 10
Automatic Screening of Skin Cancer 185
Singaravelan Shanmugasundaram, PSR Engineering College, India
P. Alwin John, PSR Engineering College, India
M. Vargheese, PSN College of Engineering and Technology, India
P. Gopalsamy, PSR Engineering College, India
D. Pavunraj, Vel Tech Multi Tech Dr. Rangarajan Dr. Sakunthala Engineering College, India
V. Selvakumar, PSR Engineering College, India
D. Arun Shunmugam, PSR Engineering College, India

The segmentation of skin lesions plays a crucial role in the prompt and precise detection of skin cancer through computerized systems. Automating the segmentation of skin lesions in dermoscopic images presents a formidable challenge due to obstacles such as artifacts (hairs, gel bubbles, ruler markers), unclear boundaries, poor contrast, and the diverse sizes and shapes of lesion images. Our study introduces an innovative and efficient approach for skin lesion segmentation in dermoscopic images by integrating a deep convolutional neural network with the active contour segmentation algorithm. The technique involves segmenting lesions in dermoscopic images through a five-step process: Pre-processing, identifying lesion location, separating lesion area from the background, ResNet-CNN classification, and Sending automatic notifications via Arduino controller and GSM technology. The proposed approach is expected to yield results similar to existing methods in terms of accuracy, specificity, Dice coefficient, and Jaccard index.

Chapter 11
Usage of Machine Learning and Deep Learning for Lung Cancer Detection:
Current Scenario, Challenges and Futuristic Direction 223
    Ishaan Dawar, DIT University, India
    Sumedha Bhardwaj, DIT University, India

Cancer is a dangerous disease and has been a cause of substantial morbidity and fatality in the world. This chapter provides an exploration of ML and DL techniques used for lung cancer detection between 2019 and 2023. It provides a complete overview of the current methodology, the language used for model implementation, and the results of these models along with the advantages and disadvantages of the studies. It also provides information on the many datasets used to diagnose lung cancer and highlights the unresolved research gaps in the field which can inspire additional research. Furthermore, the chapter outlines futuristic directions, envisioning the integration of emerging technologies such as federated learning, explainable AI, and multimodal data fusion to address existing limitations and enhance the efficacy of lung cancer detection systems. By synthesizing current research findings and identifying key areas for advancement, this chapter serves as a valuable resource for researchers, clinicians, and stakeholders invested in leveraging ML and DL for combating lung cancer.

Chapter 12
Efficient Brain Tumor Classification With Optimized Hybrid Deep Neural
Networks 253
    V. Sanjay, Vellore Institute of Technology, India
    G. Megala, Vellore Institute of Technology, India
    Vuppala Balaji, Vardhaman College of Engineering, India

Segmentation is an important stage in the processing of images. Following preprocessing, segmentation methods are used to isolate the tumor region from the MRI images. It's one of the most crucial CAD procedures from the perspective of medical imaging. The challenges in segmenting the tumor area is overcome by using the semantic segmentation method, in which each pixel in an image receives a name or classification. It is used to recognize collections of pixels that stand in for different categories. Semantic Segmentation is proposed which is used to separate the tumor region and then the deep learning classification is done using Augmented Radial Basis Function Network (ARBFNs) based deep learning, Long Short Term Based Recurrent Neural Network (LSTM-RNN) methodology and Regularized Convolutional Neural Network with Dimensionally Reduction Module (RCNN-DRM) architecture. The proposed algorithm providing 95% accuracy on training data.

Chapter 13
Enhancing Brain Cancer Detection and Localization Using YOLOv8 Object
Detection: A Deep Learning Approach 261
    Seetharam Nagesh Appe, CVR College of Engineering, India
    G. Arulselvi, Annamalai University, India
    G. N. Balaji, Vellore Institute of Technology, India

Brain cancer poses a significant challenge to patient survival, necessitating early detection. Recent advancements in computer-aided diagnosis systems, leveraging magnetic resonance imaging (MRI), offer promising solutions for detecting brain tumors. This study introduces a transfer learning approach using deep learning to detect malignant brain tumors from MRI scans. Leveraging the YOLO (You Only Look Once) object detection framework, specifically YOLOv8, known for its efficiency in computational architecture, we present a deep learning-based approach for brain tumor identification and classification. By leveraging MRI analysis, our method aims to enhance detection and precise localization to improve patient prognosis and treatment outcomes. Employing the YOLOv8 model, we achieve a precision of 0.894 and a recall of 0.915 in brain cancer detection and an mAP_0.5 of 0.938 in brain cancer localization, demonstrating the effectiveness of the proposed model.

Chapter 14
Multi-Cancer Detection Using Deep Learning Techniques 281
    G. N. Balaji, Vellore Institute of technology, India
    A. K. P. Kovendan, Vellore Institute of Technology, India
    Kirti Nayak, Vellore Institute of Technology, India
    R. Venkatesan, SASTRA University (Deemed), India
    D. Yuvaraj, Cihan University, Iraq

Cancer is one of the main causes of death for people worldwide. Breast, lung, colon, brain and lymphoma are some of the most common types of cancer. Successful treatment can significantly increase the chances of survival. Enhancing the probability of a successful cancer treatment requires initial identification and treatment. In this paper a model is proposed using denset121 pretrained model with modified dense net block and softmax function as output layer. There are two subgroups of the total number of diseases: task 1 and task 2. Task1 include breast, kidney, cervical, leukemia while task2 include lung, oral, lymphoma, brain.A person suffering from the disease of task 1 may also suffer from a disease belonging to task 2. This model is examined using a dataset with multiple cancers, which is publicly available on Kaggle. The suggested method performs with an accuracy of 99.31% for task 1 as well as 97.02% for task 2, respectively, when analyzed alongside the most recent techniques.

Chapter 15
A Multimodal Deep Learning Approach for Early Detection of Alzheimer's
Disease 305
    V. Sanjay, Vellore Institute of Technology, India
    P. Swarnalatha, Vellore Institute of Technology, India
    Ragupathyraj Valluvan, University of Jaffna, Sri Lanka

Artificial Neural Networks (ANNs) optimized with Particle Swarm Optimization (PSO) for predicting Alzheimer's disease have demonstrated reliability in estimating mild cognitive impairment (LSM). Traditional ANN training faces challenges such as slow learning rates and difficulty overcoming local minima. Integrating PSO, a Resquare Optimization Algorithm (ROA), enhances ANN performance. In our study, using a dataset of 12,130 preparation records and 51,642 test records, we trained ICA-ANN and ICA-PSO-ROA-ANN models. PSO parameters were optimized to maximize accuracy while minimizing computational load. Evaluation using Root-Mean-Squared Error (RMSE) showed that the ROA-PSO-ANN model consistently outperformed traditional ANN and hybrid models, highlighting its effectiveness in complex medical diagnostics for Alzheimer's disease prediction.

Chapter 16
Generative Adversarial Networks for Advanced EEG Data Analysis 321
    Evin Şahin Sadık, Kütahya Dumlupınar University, Turkey

This chapter examines the use of Generative Adversarial Networks (GANs) in analyzing electroencephalogram (EEG) data. EEG is an electrophysiological method that records brain activity. EEG is used to diagnose neurological disorders and is also very important for brain-computer interface (BCI) systems. Although EEG data processing and analysis is widely used, it faces some difficulties, which reveals the necessity of advanced signal processing techniques. GANs, on the other hand, are advanced machine learning techniques and play an essential role in EEG data analysis. GANs are known for their ability to produce synthetic data similar to actual data, and this feature provides significant advantages in the analysis of EEG data. In particular, GANs are effective at filtering noise, improving data quality, and generating synthetic data. Given the complexity and diversity of EEG data, caution must be exercised in training GAN models and the accuracy of synthetic data. Current limitations of GANs in EEG data analysis and ongoing research to overcome these limitations are also examined.

Chapter 17
Confluence of Deep Learning Using Watershed Segmentation GAN for
Advancing Endoscopy Surgery Imaging 345
    G. Megala, Vellore Institute of Technology, India
    P. Swarnalatha, Vellore Institute of Technology, India
    S. Prabu, Pondicherry University, India
    R. Venkatesan, SASTRA University (Deemed), India
    Anantharajah Kaneswaran, University of Jaffna, Sri Lanka

Accurate segmentation in medical images is critical for effective diagnosis and treatment. This study presents a novel approach using a watershed-segmented Generative Adversarial Network (GAN) for segmentation in the Cholec80 laparoscopic cholecystectomy videos. Initially, a watershed algorithm preprocesses the images, providing robust initial segmentation that highlights potential lesion boundaries. This segmented output trains a GAN, which refines and improves segmentation accuracy. The GAN comprises a generator producing segmentation masks and a discriminator evaluating their realism against ground truth. Evaluated on the Cholec80 dataset, our approach demonstrates significant improvements in segmentation accuracy over existing methods. Quantitative results indicate superior performance in dice coefficient, intersection over union (IoU), and other metrics. Qualitative analysis supports the efficacy of our method in accurately delineating boundaries in complex surgical scenes. This integration presents a promising direction for enhancing medical image analysis.

Chapter 18
Review on Facial Emotion Recognition Using Deep Learning With Multiple
Databases 369
    Hari Prasad Mal, Vellore Institute of Technology, India
    P. Swarnalatha, Vellore Institute of Technology, India
    Anantharajah Kaneswaran, University of Jaffna, Sri Lanka
    S. Prabu, Pondicherry University, India

Facial expression-based automatic emotion recognition is an intriguing field of study that has been presented and used in a variety of contexts, including human-machine interfaces, safety, and health. In order to improve computer predictions, researchers in this field are interested in creating methods for interpreting, coding, and extracting facial expressions. Deep learning has been incredibly successful, and as a result, its various architectures are being used to improve performance. This paper aims to investigate recent advances in deep learning-based automatic facial emotion recognition (FER). We highlight the contributions addressed, the architecture, and the databases employed. We also demonstrate the advancement by contrasting the suggested approaches with the outcomes attained. This paper aims to assist and direct researchers by reviewing current literature and offering perspectives to advance this field.

Compilation of References 383

About the Contributors 431

Index 441

Foreword

When I was invited to write a foreword for this book "Machine Learning and Generative AI in Smart Healthcare", I felt glad to note the varied tools, challenges, methods are applied in Artificial Intelligence for Smart Technology

The convergence of technology and healthcare is one of the most transformative phenomena of our time. As we stand on the brink of a new era, artificial intelligence (AI) and machine learning (ML) are not merely tools of convenience but essential drivers of progress in the medical field. These technologies have the potential to revolutionize every facet of healthcare, from diagnosis and treatment to patient care and management.

"Machine Learning and Generative AI in Smart Healthcare" comes at a pivotal moment, offering a comprehensive exploration of how these advanced technologies are reshaping the healthcare landscape. This book is a testament to the incredible strides being made, providing insights into the current state of AI and ML in healthcare and peering into the promising future these innovations herald.

Throughout history, healthcare has seen numerous advancements, each significantly improving patient outcomes and the efficiency of medical practice. However, the advent of AI and ML represents a leap unlike any other. These technologies have the capacity to analyze vast amounts of data with unparalleled speed and accuracy, uncovering patterns and insights that would be impossible for humans to discern. This ability is particularly crucial in medical diagnostics, where early detection of diseases can save lives and improve the quality of care.

Generative AI, a subset of artificial intelligence, is also making remarkable contributions. By creating new data from existing datasets, generative AI can simulate medical scenarios, predict potential outcomes, and assist in the development of new treatments and drugs. Its applications in medical imaging, personalized medicine, and predictive analytics are already proving to be game-changers.

This book meticulously examines these applications, providing a detailed understanding of how machine learning and generative AI are being employed to tackle some of the most pressing challenges in healthcare. Each chapter delves into specific areas, from AI-powered diagnostics and personalized treatment plans to smart medical imaging and wearable technology. The discussions are enriched with real-world examples and case studies, illustrating the tangible benefits of these technologies.

Moreover, the book does not shy away from addressing the ethical considerations and challenges that accompany the integration of AI and ML in healthcare. Issues such as data privacy, algorithmic bias, and the need for robust AI governance are critically examined, underscoring the importance of ethical frameworks in the deployment of these technologies.

The authors of this book, experts in their respective fields, bring a wealth of knowledge and experience, making this a valuable resource for healthcare professionals, researchers, and anyone interested in the intersection of technology and medicine. Their insights provide a roadmap for navigating the complexities and harnessing the potential of AI and ML in healthcare.

As we look to the future, the role of machine learning and generative AI in healthcare will only grow in significance. This book not only captures the current state of these technologies but also inspires innovation and encourages the ongoing pursuit of excellence in healthcare.

"Machine Learning and Generative AI in Smart Healthcare" is an essential read for those who wish to understand and contribute to the ongoing transformation of healthcare. It is a clarion call to embrace the future, armed with knowledge, curiosity, and a commitment to improving patient outcomes through the power of artificial intelligence.

I am happy to commend the editors and authors on their accomplishment, and to inform the readers that they are looking at a major piece in the development of computational intelligence on healthcare. I am familiar with your research interests and expertise in the related research areas of Machine Learning and Generative AI in Smart Healthcare which would make an excellent addition to this publication. This book is a main step in this field's maturation and will serve to challenge the academic, research and scientific community in various significant ways.

S. Arunkumar Sangaiah
National Yunlin University of Science and Technology, Taiwan

Preface

The landscape of healthcare is undergoing a transformative shift, driven by rapid advancements in technology and the burgeoning field of artificial intelligence. Among the myriad AI applications, machine learning and generative AI have emerged as pivotal forces, reshaping how healthcare is delivered, managed, and experienced. This book, "Machine Learning and Generative AI in Smart Healthcare," delves into these cutting-edge technologies, exploring their profound impact on modern healthcare systems.

Integrating machine learning and generative AI in healthcare promises to enhance diagnostic accuracy, personalize treatment plans, streamline operations, and ultimately improve patient outcomes. This book is a comprehensive guide to understanding how these technologies revolutionize healthcare, providing theoretical insights and practical applications.

This book would not have been possible without the contributions of numerous individuals and organizations. We extend our gratitude to the researchers, practitioners, and thought leaders who have generously shared their insights and expertise. Special thanks to our reviewers for their invaluable feedback and to the publishing team for their support and dedication.

Machine Learning and Generative AI in Smart Healthcare intends to be both an instructional resource and a catalyst for future innovation. Whether you are a healthcare practitioner, researcher, student, or enthusiast, we hope this book will help you gain a better grasp of how AI is altering healthcare and motivate you to contribute to this exciting subject.

We invite you to embark on this journey through the chapters that follow, exploring the intersection of technology and healthcare, and discovering the endless possibilities that machine learning and generative AI hold for the future of medicine.

NEED FOR A BOOK ON THE PROPOSED TOPICS

The healthcare industry is undergoing a profound transformation fuelled by advancements in artificial intelligence (AI) and machine learning (ML). These technologies are revolutionizing how we diagnose, treat, and manage diseases, offering unprecedented accuracy, efficiency, and personalization. Despite the vast potential and ongoing integration of AI and ML in healthcare, there is a significant knowledge gap among healthcare professionals, researchers, and policymakers regarding these complex technologies. A comprehensive book dedicated to "Machine Learning and Generative AI in Smart Healthcare" is essential to bridge this gap, providing a structured and detailed exploration of these innovations and their applications.

This book will serve as an invaluable resource, demystifying advanced concepts and showcasing practical applications through real-world examples and case studies. It will address current challenges and anticipate future trends, ensuring that readers are well-equipped to leverage AI and ML in their practice. Additionally, the book will delve into critical ethical and regulatory considerations, promoting responsible AI deployment in healthcare. By fostering interdisciplinary collaboration and empowering innovation, this book will not only enhance understanding but also drive forward the integration of AI and ML in healthcare, ultimately improving patient outcomes and healthcare efficiency.

ORGANIZATION OF THE BOOK

The book is organized into 18 chapters. A brief description of each chapter is given as follows:

1. Advances in AI and Machine Learning for Healthcare Informatics

This study focuses on how medical informatics, bioinformatics and health records are getting rejuvenated by AI and ML, which is leading to a new paradigm in healthcare. It drives home the significance of data-driven methods to address the health problems and enhancing the patient outcomes in healthcare. The study begins with a highlight of AI and ML technologies being used in healthcare. Then it delves deep into the machine learning approaches, appropriate optimisation techniques, methods of disease prediction, and signal processing advances. Besides that, this paper obtains new technological developments such as the improvement of healthcare information systems and the application of artificial intelligence and machine learning to medical signal and image processing. By means of this purpose, one aims to teach scholars, specialists, and decision-makers concerning the transformative capacity of AI and ML in healthcare. Ethical surrounding matters and the future pathways of research and innovation are also discussed.

2. Data Mining and Knowledge Discovery: Transforming Healthcare Through Biomedical Intelligence

This chapter proposal aims to explore the transformative potential of data mining and knowledge discovery in healthcare, focusing on optimizing healthcare computing systems, integrating technologies like AI and IoT, and emphasizing patient-centric care. It delves into precision medicine, disease pathways, and current trends in health and disease, while addressing concerns around privacy, biases, and responsible data use. The methodology includes a systematic review of healthcare computing systems and real-world case studies. The chapter advocates for interdisciplinary collaboration and ethical frameworks, concluding with a discussion on future directions and challenges to inspire a future of data-driven, patient-centered healthcare.

3. Design and Development of AI-Powered Healthcare System

Cancer patient survival is an integral part of the healthcare sector, with researchers offering clinicians snipping information as they consider treatment options that have a big impact on patients' lifestyle decisions. Evidently, no study of predicting survival or death from breast cancer using XGBoost method has been attempted. The goal of this research is to design a prediction system that can forecast both the survival rate and the death rate from breast cancer at an early stage by examining the most limited collection of clinical dataset variables. The potential of the XGBoost method is determined using mainly age at the time of diagnosis along with other clinical characteristics, assessed for its relative significance. The project findings show that the XGBoost model fits the testing dataset more effectively, with outcome of accuracy 82.72% approximately.

4. Applications of AI Techniques in Healthcare and Wellbeing

The integration of Artificial Intelligence (AI) techniques in healthcare and wellbeing systems has witnessed significant advancements, offering transformative solutions to traditional healthcare paradigms. This chapter provides a comprehensive overview of the diverse applications of AI in the healthcare sector, highlighting its potential to enhance diagnostics, treatment planning, personalized medicine, and overall patient outcomes. AI techniques, including machine learning and deep learning algorithms, have demonstrated remarkable capabilities in analyzing large datasets such as medical images, genetic information, and electronic health records. These technologies enable more accurate and timely disease detection, improving diagnostic accuracy and aiding healthcare professionals in making informed decisions. In treatment planning, AI-driven systems contribute to the development of personalized therapeutic strategies. By leveraging patient-specific data, AI models can predict treatment responses, optimize drug regimens, and minimize adverse effects.

5. Artificial Intelligence in Information Systems Research: A Systematic Literature Review and Research Agenda

AI has received expanded interest from the data systems studies network in recent years. There is, however, a developing difficulty that studies on AI should enjoy a loss of cumulative building of information, which has overshadowed IS research formerly. This chapter addresses this issue by conducting a scientific literature review of AI experiments in information systems from 2005 to 2020. The seek approach ended in 1877 research, of which 98 had been diagnosed as primary research and a synthesise of key issues which might be pertinent to this take a look at is presented. In doing so, this has a look at makes important contributions, namely (i) an identification of the modern mentioned enterprise price and contributions of AI, (ii) research and sensible implications on the use of AI and (iii) opportunities for destiny AI studies inside the shape of the AI research.

6. The Use of Artificial Intelligence in Health Communication: A Research on ChatGPT

Communication is of great importance in health services. Nowadays, new media, especially the internet, are frequently used in health communication. Artificial intelligence has also begun to be used in healthcare. Artificial intelligence studies generally aim to develop artificial methods that imitate human ways of thinking. In addition, it is predicted that some programs produced based on artificial intelligence will affect health communication processes in daily use. The most important of these programs is the ChatGPT (Chatbot Generative Pre-trained Transformer) program. The purpose of this study is to reveal the benefits and drawbacks of using the ChatGPT program in health communication by providing a qualitative framework. For this purpose, a semi-structured interview was conducted with 30 people over the age of 18, determined by a purposeful sampling method. In line with the data obtained, the use of Chat GPT in health communication was tried to be explained.

7. Federated Learning for Securing Glomeruli Detection in Digital Pathology

This chapter focuses on a novel approach to glomeruli detection in histopathological images, aiming to address concerns regarding data security in medical image analysis. By integrating YOLOv3 object detection with federated learning, the study explores the effectiveness of federated learning in preserving data privacy while maintaining high detection accuracy. A comparative analysis is conducted between traditional model training methods and federated learning, demonstrating the superior performance of the latter in safeguarding sensitive medical data. The experimental results highlight the significance of prioritizing data security in AI-driven pathology and underscore the potential of federated learning to advance the integration of artificial intelligence with pathology.

8. Advances and Strategies in Addressing Plant Health Challenges: Insights From Recent Research

This chapter explores the complex issues that contemporary agriculture and natural ecosystems face when it comes to plant health. It starts by going over the several biotic variables that endanger plant productivity and vigor, like pests, invasive species, and diseases. The dynamic aspect of these threats is emphasized, which is made worse by climate change and global trade, which promote the spread and evolution of dangerous species. The chapter also looks at abiotic stresses, such as pollution, soil deterioration, and drought, emphasizing how these factors interact to reduce plant resilience. Sustainable agriculture methods and integrated pest management (IPM) techniques are highlighted as essential solutions to these problems. The chapter also emphasizes the value of sophisticated biotechnology instruments, early detection methods, and the protection of plant health through legislation and education.

9. Early Detection of Skin Cancer Using Convolutional Neural Networks

The substantial health risks associated with skin cancer make early detection techniques imperative. In this work, we investigate using convolutional neural networks (CNNs) to identify skin cancer. By utilizing the vast HAM10000 dataset comprising various skin lesion images, we aim to create a robust artificial intelligence model to classify pictures accurately. Our approach preprocesses image data, adjusts the Xception architecture, and uses data augmentation techniques to improve model performance. The model's efficacy is evaluated using accuracy, precision, recall, and F1-score metrics. With possible benefits for bettering patient outcomes and healthcare delivery, this research advances automated diagnostic tools for skin cancer detection.

10. Automatic Screening of Skin Cancer

Skin lesion segmentation has a critical role in the early and accurate diagnosis of skin cancer by computerised systems. A automatic segmentation of skin lesions in dermoscopic images is a challenging task owing to difficulties including artifacts (hairs, gel bubbles, ruler markers), indistinct boundaries, low contrast and varying sizes and shapes of the lesion images. In our work proposes a novel and effective method for skin lesion segmentation in dermoscopic images combining a deep convolution neural network and the active contour segmentation algorithm. This method performs lesion segmentation using a dermoscopic image in five steps: Pre-processing, Detection of the lesion location, Segmentation of the lesion area from the background, ResNet-CNN classification and Automatic notification through the Arduino controller and GSM technology. Proposed method will obtain close results compared with previous methods of accuracy, specificity, Dice coefficient, and Jaccard index.

11. Usage of Machine Learning and Deep Learning for Lung Cancer Detection: Current Scenario, Challenges, and Futuristic Direction

Cancer is a dangerous disease and has been a cause of substantial morbidity and fatality in the world. This chapter provides an exploration of ML and DL techniques used for lung cancer detection between 2019 and 2023. It provides a complete overview of the current methodology, the language used for model implementation, and the results of these models along with the advantages and disadvantages of the studies. It also provides information on the many datasets used to diagnose lung cancer and highlights the unresolved research gaps in the field which can inspire additional research. Furthermore, the chapter outlines futuristic directions, envisioning the integration of emerging technologies such as federated learning, explainable AI, and multimodal data fusion to address existing limitations and enhance the efficacy of lung cancer detection systems. By synthesizing current research findings and identifying key areas for advancement, this chapter serves as a valuable resource for researchers, clinicians, and stakeholders invested in leveraging ML and DL for combating lung cancer.

12. Efficient Brain Tumor Classification With Optimized Hybrid Deep Neural Networks

Segmentation is an important stage in the processing of images. Following pre-processing, segmentation methods are used to isolate the tumor region from the MRI images. It's one of the most crucial CAD procedures from the perspective of medical imaging. The challenges in segmenting the tumor area is overcome by using the semantic segmentation method, in which each pixel in an image receives a name or classification. It is used to recognize collections of pixels that stand in for different categories. Semantic Segmentation is proposed which is used to separate the tumor region and then the deep learning classification is done using Augmented Radial Basis Function Network (ARBFNs) based deep learning, Long Short Term Based Recurrent Neural Network (LSTM-RNN) methodology and Regularized Convolutional Neural Network with Dimensionally Reduction Module (RCNN-DRM) architecture. The proposed algorithm providing 95% accuracy on training data.

13. Enhancing Brain Cancer Detection and Localization Using YOLOv8 Object Detection: A Deep Learning Approach

Brain cancer poses a significant challenge to patient survival, necessitating early detection. Recent advancements in computer-aided diagnosis systems, leveraging magnetic resonance imaging (MRI), offer promising solutions for detecting brain tumors. This study introduces a transfer learning approach using deep learning to detect malignant brain tumors from MRI scans. Leveraging the YOLO (You Only Look Once) object detection framework, specifically YOLOv8, known for its efficiency in computational architecture, we present a deep learning-based approach for brain tumor identification and classification. By leveraging MRI analysis, our method aims to enhance detection and precise localization to improve patient prognosis and treatment outcomes. Employing the YOLOv8 model, we achieve a precision of 0.894 and a recall of 0.915 in brain cancer detection and an mAP_0.5 of 0.938 in brain cancer localization, demonstrating the effectiveness of the proposed model.

14. Multi-Cancer Detection Using Deep Learning Techniques

Cancer is one of the main causes of death for people worldwide. Breast, lung, colon, brain and lymphoma are some of the most common types of cancer. Successful treatment can significantly increase the chances of survival. Enhancing the probability of a successful cancer treatment requires initial identification and treatment. In this paper a model is proposed using denset121 pretrained model with modified dense net block and softmax function as output layer. There are two subgroups of the total number of diseases: task 1 and task 2. Task1 include breast, kidney, cervical, leukemia while task2 include lung, oral, lymphoma, brain. A person suffering from the disease of task 1 may also suffer from a disease belonging to task 2. This model is examined using a dataset with multiple cancers, which is publicly available on Kaggle. The suggested method performs with an accuracy of 99.31% for task 1 as well as 97.02% for task 2, respectively, when analyzed alongside the most recent techniques.

15. A Multimodal Deep Learning Approach for Early Detection of Alzheimer's Disease

Artificial Neural Networks (ANNs) optimized with Particle Swarm Optimization (PSO) for predicting Alzheimer's disease have demonstrated reliability in estimating mild cognitive impairment (LSM). Traditional ANN training faces challenges such as slow learning rates and difficulty overcoming local minima. Integrating PSO, a Resquare Optimization Algorithm (ROA), enhances ANN performance. In our study, using a dataset of 12,130 preparation records and 51,642 test records, we trained ICA-ANN and ICA-PSO-ROA-ANN models. PSO parameters were optimized to maximize accuracy while minimizing computational load. Evaluation using Root-Mean-Squared Error (RMSE) showed that the ROA-PSO-ANN model consistently outperformed traditional ANN and hybrid models, highlighting its effectiveness in complex medical diagnostics for Alzheimer's disease prediction.

16. Generative Adversarial Networks for Advanced EEG Data Analysis

This chapter examines the use of Generative Adversarial Networks (GANs) in analyzing electroencephalogram (EEG) data. EEG is an electrophysiological method that records brain activity. EEG is used to diagnose neurological disorders and is also very important for brain-computer interface (BCI) systems. Although EEG data processing and analysis is widely used, it faces some difficulties, which reveals the necessity of advanced signal processing techniques. GANs, on the other hand, are advanced machine learning techniques and play an essential role in EEG data analysis. GANs are known for their ability to produce synthetic data similar to actual data, and this feature provides significant advantages in the analysis of EEG data. In particular, GANs are effective at filtering noise, improving data quality, and generating synthetic data. Given the complexity and diversity of EEG data, caution must be exercised in training GAN models and the accuracy of synthetic data. Current limitations of GANs in EEG data analysis and ongoing research to overcome these limitations are also examined.

17. Confluence of Deep Learning Using Watershed Segmentation GAN for Advancing Endoscopy Surgery Imaging

Accurate segmentation in medical images is critical for effective diagnosis and treatment. This chapter presents a novel approach using a watershed-segmented Generative Adversarial Network (GAN) for segmentation in the Cholec80 laparoscopic cholecystectomy videos. Initially, a watershed algorithm preprocesses the images, providing robust initial segmentation that highlights potential lesion boundaries. This segmented output trains a GAN, which refines and improves segmentation accuracy. The GAN comprises a generator producing segmentation masks and a discriminator evaluating their realism against ground truth. Evaluated on the Cholec80 dataset, our approach demonstrates significant improvements in segmentation accuracy over existing methods. Quantitative results indicate superior performance in dice coefficient, intersection over union (IoU), and other metrics. Qualitative analysis supports the efficacy of our method in accurately delineating boundaries in complex surgical scenes. This integration presents a promising direction for enhancing medical image analysis.

18. Review on Facial Emotion Recognition Using Deep Learning With Multiple Databases

Facial expression-based automatic emotion recognition is an intriguing field of study that has been presented and used in a variety of contexts, including human-machine interfaces, safety, and health. In order to improve computer predictions, researchers in this field are interested in creating methods for interpreting, coding, and extracting facial expressions. Deep learning has been incredibly successful, and as a result, its various architectures are being used to improve performance. This paper aims to investigate recent advances in deep learning-based automatic facial emotion recognition (FER). We highlight the contributions addressed, the architecture, and the databases employed. We also demonstrate the advancement by contrasting the suggested approaches with the outcomes attained. This paper aims to assist and direct researchers by reviewing current literature and offering perspectives to advance this field.

ACKNOWLEDGMENT

It is obvious that the development of a book of this scope needs the support of many people. We must thank Ms. Kaylee Renfrew, Assistant Development Editor and the editorial team, IGI Global for their encouragement and support enabled the book publication project to materialize and contributed to its success.

We would like to express our sincere gratitude to all the contributors, who have submitted their high-quality chapters, and to the experts for their supports in providing insightful review comments and suggestions on time.

    Gopinath Ganapathy, *Bharathidasan University, India*
    V. Susheela Devi, *Department of Computer Science and Automation, Indian Institute of Science, Bangalore, India*
    Anantharajah Kaneswaran, *Department of Computer Engineering, Faculty of Engineering, University of Jaffna, Srilanka*

    Editors:

Swarnalatha Purushotham
Vellore Institute of Technology, India

S. Prabu
Pondicherry University, India

Chapter 1
Advances in AI and Machine Learning for Healthcare Informatics

K. Maithili
https://orcid.org/0000-0003-0755-907X
Vel Tech Rangarajan Dr. Sagunthala R&D Institute of Science and Technology, India

A. Ponmalar
R.M.K. Engineering College, India

B. Yamini
https://orcid.org/0000-0003-3531-108X
SRM Institute of Science and Technology, India

M. Karthikeyan
R.M.K. College of Engineering and Technology, India

T. P. Anish
R.M.K. College of Engineering and Technology, India

B. Maheswari
R M K. Engineering College, India

R. Siva Subramanian
https://orcid.org/0000-0002-7509-9223
R M K. College of Engineering and Technology, India

ABSTRACT

This study focuses on how medical informatics, bioinformatics and health records are getting rejuvenated by AI and ML, which is leading to a new paradigm in healthcare. It drives home the significance of data-driven methods to address the health problems and enhancing the patient outcomes in healthcare. The study begins with a highlight of AI and ML technologies being used in healthcare. Then it delves deep into the machine learning approaches, appropriate optimisation techniques, methods of disease prediction, and signal processing advances. Besides that, this paper obtains new technological developments such as the improvement of health-

DOI: 10.4018/979-8-3693-3719-6.ch001

care information systems and the application of artificial intelligence and machine learning to medical signal and image processing. By means of this purpose, one aims to teach scholars, specialists, and decision-makers concerning the transformative capacity of AI and ML in healthcare. Ethical surrounding matters and the future pathways of research and innovation are also discussed.

1. INTRODUCTION

Healthcare is changing in the wake of AI and machine learning (ML) as those technologies bring previously unimagined opportunities to better patient care, optimize operations, and change how treatments are prescribed(Panesar A 2019). Utilization of AI and ML technologies in healthcare systems indicates the start of the era of data-driven strategies that can considerably speed up clinical workflow and accelerate medical innovations.

1.1 AI and ML's Significance in Healthcare:

It can be emphasized that AI and ML are indispensable in healthcare. The quantity of data produced by wearable sensors, medical imaging, genetics, electronic health records, and other sources is growing at an alarming rate so that existing data analysis techniques become less and less useful. Large and complex datasets can be analysed through AI and ML algorithms which may also find patterns and provide useful insights that may be used for clinical decision-making(Garg et al 2022).

1.2 The Study's Objectives:

This research has two goals in consideration:

1.2.1 Comprehensive Overview of AI and ML Applications in Healthcare:

The main objective of this essay is to show how AI and ML technologies are used in healthcare today:

Diagnostic Imaging: Image analysis AI solutions are raising the accuracy and precision of medical imaging interpretation, thus allowing for the medical issues to be detected in an early stage.

Clinical Decision Support: With the real-time insights and recommendations provided by AI-based systems that use a patient's data, along with doctors' experience and clinical guidelines, the accuracy of diagnoses and effectiveness of treatment are increased.

Personalised Medicine: Lately, more exact and more effective therapies are being developed using ML algorithms to design individualized treatment plans for each patient taking into account the specific features of a patient, his/her genetic characteristics, and the course of the condition.

Population Health Management: To improve the population health outcomes, healthcare organisations are now using AI-powered predictive analytics to identify the groups at-risk, forecast disease outbreaks, and so on allocate resources in a much more efficient way(Nithya, T et al 2023).

1.2.2 Determining Current Advancements and Innovations:

Our second goal is to consider AI systems and ML models in healthcare critically and to bring out the latest developments and progress. Nevertheless, although using AI and ML to better treat patients improved greatly, there are yet many opportunities and challenges to overcome. undefined

Data Privacy and Security: Patient trust and regulatory compliance rely on the confidentiality and integrity of healthcare data.

Algorithmic prejudice and Fairness: Privacy and fairness are considered to guarantee the equal delivery and decision-making in healthcare technology.

Healthcare System Interoperability: Leveraging different data sources and healthcare systems with seamless communication and cooperation.

Ethical Implications of AI-powered Decision-making: Addressing the ethical issues of AI in healthcare decisions, looking at the aspects of patients autonomy, accountability, and transparency.

The goal is to inform policymakers, healthcare professionals, and scholars about the pros and cons of using AI and ML in healthcare by discussing these problems and outlining some of the possible solutions.

In conclusion, the paper aims to provide a general and systematic understanding about AI and ML in healthcare and present the latest advancements in this area. And indeed, we are capable of revolutionizing how care continues, improving patient experiences, and in the long run, improving the wellbeing of individuals across the globe with the help of AI and ML technology.

2. STRATEGIES AND METHODS FOR DISEASE PREDICTION:

Another function of healthcare services is disease prevention which involves the early and accurate prognosis of diseases in individuals or groups. Data mining, knowledge discovery and predictive modelling techniques have advanced disease prediction as a theme, according to Kohli et al (2018). This has been helpful most specially to the health care workers in identifying and managing health threats most efficiently.

Figure 1. Strategies and Methods for Disease Prediction

| Predictive Modeling | ←──Strategies and Methods for Disease Prediction──→ | Healthcare Data Mining and Knowledge Discovery |

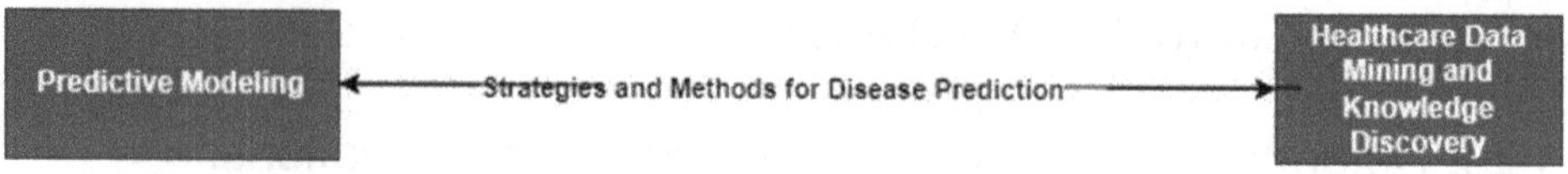

2.1 Predictive Modeling

The technique of formulating statistical models or mathematical algorithms that determine the likelihood of future events or outcomes by applying past data is what we mean by predictive modeling. Predictive models are employed to estimate the chance that a disease will either develop or worsen(Gracious et al 2023). They do this through the analysis of a range of healthcare information, which include patient demographics, clinical characteristics, genetic data as well as environmental factors. These models include the simple regression models and more advanced machine learning techniques such as decision trees, support vector machines, and neural networks.

Healthcare practitioners can discover such patterns and trends that help identify a patient's increased risk of suffering from particular diseases when they feed massive datasets comprising the symptoms, medical history, lab test results, and treatment outcomes to predictive models for training. For example, predictive models can help spot the highly vulnerable people who might be prone to chronic diseases such as diabetes, heart disease or cancer. It gives opportunity for early intervention and prevention.

2.2 Healthcare Data Mining and Knowledge Discovery:

Data mining approaches are critical because they yield relevant patterns, trends, and relationships from the huge mass of healthcare data that, in turn, are essential for illness prediction. Healthcare professionals can discover hidden connections and more sophisticated insights in really complex datasets through data mining methods such as clustering, anomaly detection, and association rule mining (Yamini et al 2023). Data mining can detect risk factors, disease biomarkers and predictive markers by examining health data from different sources which include genomic data, medical imaging data, wearable sensor data and electronic health records.

Data mining is strengthened by knowledge discovery techniques which offer an opportunity of converting raw data into valuable information that informs clinical decisions. Steps such as data preprocessing, feature selection, model training, and model validation are the actions that make predictive models accurate and reliable. Medical professional, in combination with domain knowledge, clinical skill, and data-driven wisdom, can create reliable illness prediction models that are operational and clinically relevant using knowledge discovery methodologies.

Eventually, a number of approaches, like information discovery, data mining, and predictive modeling, are being used in the process. By applying those techniques, healthcare professionals have chances to take advantages from the use of healthcare data such as predicting diseases, at the early stage, detecting patients with high risk and executing focused therapies that improve patient outcomes and reduce cost. Besides that, illness prediction in healthcare will work better if the problems like data quality, interoperability, and ethics are resolved.

3. DEEP LEARNING AND MACHINE LEARNING TECHNIQUES:

DL and ML are the formidable tools that have immensely altered the human healthcare by introducing innovative ways of diseases diagnosis, prognosis and treatment scheduling(Kamala et al 2023). ML and DL methodologies aid healthcare practitioners arrive at objective medical decisions by enabling them to obtain useful information from complex healthcare data through the assistance of large data sets and sophisticated algorithms(Subramanian, R. S et al 2024). ML and DL applications in healthcare is extensively reviewed and compared with some leading algorithms in this section in order to lay out a clear picture about their effectiveness and metrics of performance.

3.1 Healthcare Machine Learning:

Computer systems may learn from data and develop capacity to make predictions and decisions through machine learning algorithms without many programming requirements for explicit programming. Machine learning is used in various activities of healthcare field such as outcome prediction, treatment planning, risk assessment and illness diagnosis(Shailaja et al 2018). Among the machine learning (ML) methods, logistic regression, decision trees, random forests, support vector machines, and k-nearest neighbours are most frequently applied in healthcare(Bhardwaj et al 2017).

These algorithms have got tendency to look for patterns and correlations that show up in health data of patients like genetic material, medical pictures, electronic health records and sensor data(K., Lakshmipriya, et al2024). Health professionals by building predictive models may achieve a proper allocation of the patients into specific risk categories or they may predict upcoming health events by using ML models trained on the labelled datasets where the outcomes are known to them(Siva, S. R et al 2024).

3.2 Deep Learning in the Medical Field:

This form of machine learning using deep learning models with multiple layers of linked nodes, named also neurones, contributes to the model's ability to represent and learn very complex data. CNNs and RNNs, the two types of deep learning architecture, have been particularly successful in high-dimensional data processing, such as time series data, genetic sequences or medical images(Bakator, M, & Radosav, D. 2018).

Deep learning programs have proven high achievement in healthcare in tasks such as drug development, diagnostics of illness, medical image analysis and genomics. Such as, CNNs are commonly applied in medical imaging for classification, segmentation, and feature extraction. In contrast, RNNs are used in the analysis of sequences of data which are applied to electrocardiogram or electronic health records.

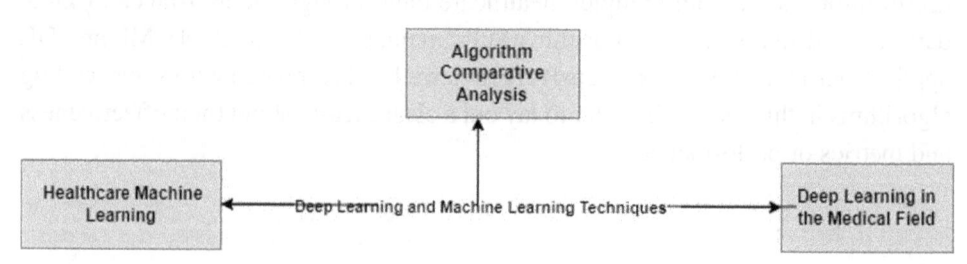

Figure 2. Deep Learning and Machine Learning Techniques

3.3 Algorithm Comparative Analysis:

Understanding the performance metrics of these algorithms, their pros and cons is essential to compare them for their applications to healthcare. Professionals in healthcare can also establish the dependability and efficacy of diverse algorithms by performance metrics such as accuracy, sensitivity, specificity, precision, and area under the receiver operating characteristic curve (AUC-ROC). Such metrics are ones that have numerical values which show the performance of the algorithms(Rajendran et al 2023).

Health practitioners can arrive at an algorithm that is specifically suited for a particular work or application by examining algorithms processing benchmark datasets or actual clinical data to evaluate their suitability. Furthermore, trade-off analysis may highlight the trade-offs between the computing resources, interpretability, generalizability, and algorithm complexity, making it easier for healthcare professionals to pick the appropriate method for their respective needs.

Summarily, methods of machine learning and deep learning are in existence that are applicable in health care, for example disease diagnosis, prediction and planning therapy. Healthcare providers can help modifying patient outcomes and advancing healthcare informatics by applying the method of comparison and contrast of the different algorithms in order to assess their efficacy and performance measures.

4. OPTIMIZATION FOR HEALTHCARE PROBLEMS:

Strategies of optimization are needed to deal with complex problems in health care as it increases productivity, reduces costs and, improves patient outcomes. This part of the discussion reveals the importance of including case studies that explain the unique applications of the optimization algorithms in healthcare and, thus, broadens the ideas of the successful implementations.

4.1 Application of Optimisation Techniques in Practice:

Optimization techniques include a variety of mathematical methods and algorithms allowing to find, within a set of restrictions, the best way to address the task under consideration. That is, optimization techniques are used in the healthcare industry to tackle different problems, among them scheduling, decision-making, treatment planning, etc.

Optimization of healthcare resource allocation is the case which shows an area where optimization is usually used. Efficient management of hospital beds, operating rooms, medical personnel, and equipment is crucial in order to cope with the patient burden and keep down the costs of hospitalization. The optimisation techniques allow healthcare organizations take into account of such factors as patient flow, service demand, capacity limits and resource options, in order to ensure efficient resource utilization.

The goal is to enhance therapy effectiveness, improve patient satisfaction and the treatment process at the same time, reducing undesirable side effects and healthcare costs. This is usually achieved by means of optimisation models that can be used to personalise treatment plans, optimise medication dosages, or schedule patients' appointments. This is only one major field of improvement in which optimisation is used in the health care business.

Figure 3. Optimization for Healthcare Problems

```
┌─────────────────┐                                              ┌─────────────────┐
│  Application of │                                              │                 │
│   Optimisation  │◄────── Optimization for Healthcare Problems ─►│ Optimisation Case│
│Techniques in Practice│                                         │     Studies     │
└─────────────────┘                                              └─────────────────┘
```

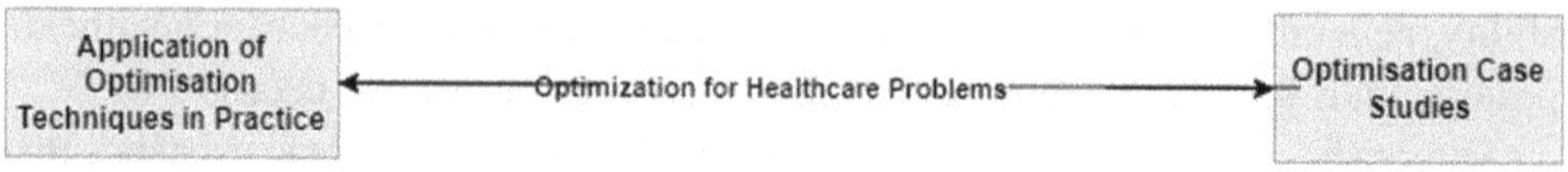

4.2 Optimisation Case Studies:

Integrating case studies on the matter of optimisation for healthcare issues is one of the most important factors of improving the way of thinking about the efficient application of the optimisation methods and of practical outcomes of these methods in terms of implementation. Case studies demonstrate those concrete examples of using optimization models and algorithms in healthcare with the intention of achieving a solution to a certain problem and a significant outcome.

After all, a case study could depict how an optimisation model would help a large healthcare system allocate the bed in a way that the wait time for patients would be shorter, the resources would be used better and the satisfaction of patients would be bigger. Another paper might demonstrate the use of an optimization model to obtain the best scheduling plan of chemotherapy for cancer participants, resulting in less delays, better success and lower expenses.

case studies demonstrate how the optimisation tools and methods can be implemented in practice in healthcare and how they can result in enormous benefits for patient care, operational efficiency and the delivery of health care.

I think it is safe to say that optimisation methods are handy instruments applied to solve complicated healthcare problems and improve patients outcomes. Optimisation is a common practice in healthcare organisations which they use to make intelligent decisions, optimal resource distribution, and individually tailored treatment plans, by installing and giving examples of successful implementations using a wide variety of optimisation mechanisms.

5. MEDICAL SIGNAL FORECASTING AND REGRESSION:

The purpose of this study is to determine whether a disease is there, how it is evolving over time, and if therapy is working. To that end, we use several sources of medical information such as physiological data, patient vitals, and diagnostic test results. Regression and forecasting is the stage. For the purpose of advancement of patient care and clinical decisions making in healthcare sector, this part of speech stresses the importance of signal processing in healthcare and analyses the contribution of recent development in this area.

Figure 4. Medical Signal Forecasting and Regression

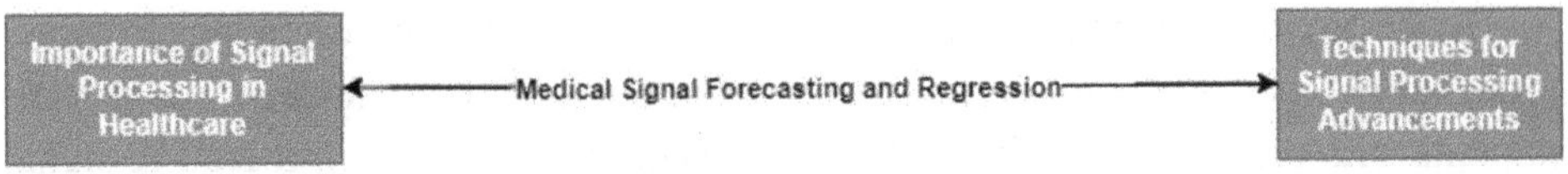

5.1 Importance of Signal Processing in Healthcare:

A major factor in medical signals processing is its use in the healthcare industry, where the extraction of useful information from complicated and chaotic signals is key. Medical signals are essentially all the information related to the physiology or anatomy of the patient and their health status including ECG, EEG, and data from vital signs monitoring. Medical staff can scrutinise and interpret these signals in a bid to arrive at diagnoses of illnesses, follow patient states and formulate treatment options. Signal processing methods, such as filtering, feature extrication, and pattern recognition, are some of the examples.

Note that, for example, arrhythmias, ischemia, heart rate variation and other cardiac diseases are diagnosed by means of signal processing of ECG data in cardiology. Neurology analyses EEG signals to detect epileptic seizures, track brain activity and diagnose neurological conditions(Berkaya et al 2018). In the critical care settings, the health condition of patients is monitored by their vital signs as heart rate, blood pressure, and oxygen saturation. These parameters are examined to help early detecting of deterioration, so that the appropriate treatments can be initiated in a timely way.

5.2 Techniques for Signal Processing Advancements:

Signal processing techniques have introduced great improvements in patient care and in the healthcare outcomes(Khatri, K, & Sharma, A. 2020). Medical signal processing has increasingly found a place for the machine learning methods, such as deep learning architectures or neural networks including the support vector machines. The algorithms are enabling automated analyses, diagnoses, and foreseeing of the medical disorders.

The examples of such models are deep learning models that process medical data, like MRI and CT scans, to reach the required diagnostic complemented with prognostic conclusions, as convolutional neural networks (CNNs) and recurrent neural networks (RNNs) demonstrate good results(Miao, K. H., & Miao, J. H 2018). Additionally, besides improving the accuracy of diagnosis and the extraction of important clues from medical signal data, some complicated and efficient signal processing methods have been developed, such as wavelet analysis, time-frequency analysis and empirical mode decomposition.

Healthcare professionals may see to passage of the diseases, come up with customized treatment plans for patients, and get better view of the health state of their patients with the use of new breakthroughs. There is a scope for integrating signal processing with wearable sensors, electronic health records to run real-time monitoring that further expands the early diagnosis of conditions and thereby reduces healthcare costs.

In general, the medical signal regression and forecasting algorithms are the special tools of the healthcare sector which enable the analysis of the complex physiological data and provide information about diseases and its development as well as the state of health of patients. Healthcare professionals can use signal processing methods to advance clinical decision-making, research in medicine, and patient care by directing their focus to the importance of such techniques and sharing information on modern innovations.

6. INFORMATION SYSTEMS FOR HEALTHCARE:

Healthcare decision-making, hot running healthcare operations, as well quality patient service are all can be carried out with the help of healthcare information systems. In the ensuing part of the essay, a description of information systems development in the healthcare is given, as well as the discussion of the imperfections in the software development in the area.

Figure 5. Information Systems for Healthcare

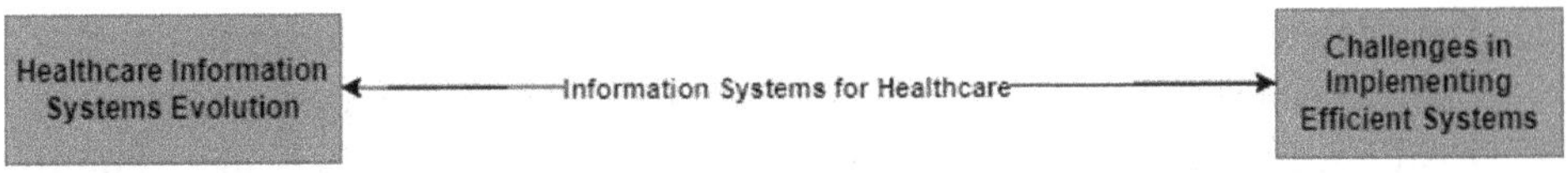

6.1 Healthcare Information Systems Evolution:

The first implementation of the HIS or the EMR took place in the 70s but most of them arrived in the 80s; and this is how the medical information systems began in health care. So a major aim of these systems was that they were meant to automate especially the administrative procedures such as appointment placing and billing, and also inventory management at the same time, digitise patients information away from the hectic paper work.

This trend of HIS has centered and expanded into more interconnected, interoperable, and patient-oriented systems, which have been propelled by technology innovations, legal laws, and deformation of care delivery. EHRs or electronic health records have been one of the most important tools to reduce doctors' time consumption for paper work and the errors from the flow of information from one clinic to another. Through the platforms, coordination of patient's treatment and information sharing among practitioners can be enhanced. Moreover, patients can also have access for their health data.

Remote patient monitoring Virtual care and personalised medicine have been further enhanced by progressing HIEs platform, telemedicine and mHealth apps. Besides, HIS has benefits of recording patient data to apply data-driven insights in population health management, precision medicine transformation, and predictive analytics because of using artificial intelligence, cloud computing, and data analytics technologies(Sudha, K. et al 2023).

6.2 Challenges in Implementing Efficient Systems:

Healthcare information systems have advanced significantly, however there are still a number of obstacles to overcome before having effective and efficient systems in place:

1. Interoperability: One of the biggest challenges in healthcare continues to be ensuring interoperability between various systems and data sources. Data silos and fragmented care result from proprietary software solutions, incompatible

data formats, and a lack of standardisation that impedes the easy interchange of information across healthcare providers.
2. Data Security and Privacy: It is critical for the healthcare industry to safeguard patient health information from cyberthreats, unauthorised access, and breaches. Health information of patients should meet legal requirements including the Health Insurance Portability and Accountability Act (HIPAA) and should be secured by the use of tools like encryption and restricted access.
3. Usability and User Experience: The extent to which HIS are adopted and utilised depends on whether they are developed to be easy to comprehend and use, and tailored to the needs of users in healthcare facilities. Some of the impacts of poor usability are among the following: data input and documentation error, low productivity, and end users' resistance.
4. Cost and Resource Constraints: The implementation and management of healthcare information systems require capital investment, many resources, and expertise. It may also present a challenge to healthcare organisations in terms of funding and sustaining complex HIS systems especially in small practices and distant centres.
5. Change Management: The effective deployment of HIS depends on controlling organisational change and promoting an innovative and continuous improvement culture. A new system's adoption and use may be hampered by stakeholder buy-in, resistance to change, and insufficient support and training.

Sharing the burden between legislators, technology vendors, regulators and industry players in the healthcare is fundamental for dealing with the issues. To develop powerful healthcare information systems, it is necessary to apply stringent cybersecurity measures, develop interoperable platforms, standardise data interchange formats, and besides, provide appropriate training and help to end users.

Besides that, the delivery, provision, and nature of healthcare have all undergone a drastic change following the technological revolution of healthcare information systems. Although this progress has been made, the issues of interoperability, data security, usability, cost, and change management are still present and need to be solved with collaborative efforts form all involved parties.

7. SIGNAL AND IMAGE PROCESSING IN MEDICINE:

Medical signal and image processing are the key elements of the modern healthcare system that are essential for access and analysis of the medical data used for patients' supervision, treatment planning, and diagnosis. The following part provides a detailed account of medical image processing applications with emphasis on our effectiveness in determining diagnosis and therapy planning.

7.1 Medical Applications of Image Processing:

A graphical analysis of a myriad of medical imaging modalities such as computed tomography (CT), magnetic resonance imaging (MRI), ultrasound, and positron emission tomography (PET), requires several image processing approaches. These methods have a broad spectrum of the techniques through which image quality is enhanced, abnormal structures are detected, anatomical structures are segmented and quantitative data are extracted(Rani et al 2020).

Example of such techniques of image processing is that a 3D CT scan image is reconstructed, the contrast and resolution of an X-ray pictures is heightened and superior visualization of soft tissues in an MRI scan is effected. Digital image analysis strategy incorporated in pathology enables the classification of tissue type by excluding histology images, identification of biomarkers, and automatic counting of cellular structure.

Figure 6. Signal and Image Processing in Medicine

Medical Applications of Image Processing	←——Signal and Image Processing in Medicine——→	Impact on Treatment Planning and Diagnostics

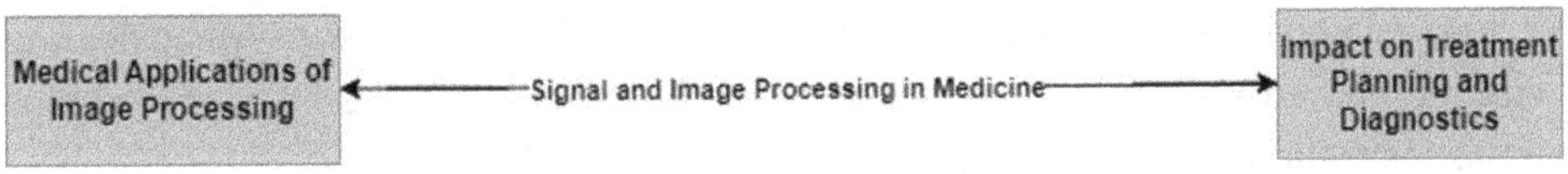

7.2 Impact on Treatment Planning and Diagnostics:

The application of image processing techniques in medicine has dramatically affected the process of making treatment plans and diagnosis that patients are now more accurately diagnosed, have their treatment customized into specific needs and that their outcomes are improved.

In the field of oncology, image processing algorithms are applied to analyse medical imaging data that include CT, MRI and PEG scans to determine the location and size of tumors, their progress rate, and revert to see whether the treatment is effective. Digital image processing techniques able cancer to be detected in its early stages, help in disease staging, and the choice of the most suitable treatment options by quantifying tumour features like volume, density, and metabolic activity, like radiation therapy, chemotherapy, and surgery (Kumar, N., & Kumar, D 2021).

In this way, imaging processing algorithms, especially in cardiology, are applied with echocardiograms and cardiac MRI to measure myocardial perfusion, discover anatomical anomalies and evaluate heart function. Beginning from the measurement of determinants of cardiac disorders as ejection fraction, irregularity in the heart wall motion, and myocardial viability, image processing algorithms act as a tool for cardiologists, to identify cardiac problems, forecast cardiovascular events, and schedule treatment procedures like bypass or angioplasty.

To conclude, medical signal and image processing techniques are vital to the delivery of healthcare because they help medical practitioners to obtain significant information on monitoring, treatment, and diagnose patients from their medical data. The presented review on the impact of image processing applications on medicine reveals that these approaches are crucial for better diagnosis and treatment planning, aiding physicians to make the best decisions, care for patients more effectively, and further medical studies.

8. APPLICATIONS IN BIOMEDICINE:

With the aim to deal with a range of health care problems, biomedical applications are the ones, that utilize the achievements in biology, medicine and engineering and various related technologies and approaches. With this segment, we will be dealing with the numerous applications of the biomedical field and stress the importance of the case studies in improving the understanding and relevance.

8.1 Diverse Range of Applications:

These biomedical applications comprise of broad range and diverse technologies and approaches that help human beings and contain ill prevention, diagnosis and treatment. In fact, they are utilized across numerous fields ranging from bioinformatics, wearable technology, biotechnology, biomaterials, and medical imaging and regenerative medicine.

Perhaps a good example is in biotechnology where recent innovations in gene editing procedures like CRISPR-Cas9 have really taken genetic engineering and gene therapy to another level, making it possible for scientists to precisely modify the human genome for curing infectious diseases like cancer and genetic mutations. Developments of medical imaging technologies, like MRI, CT, PET, and ultrasound, enable us to clearly scan anatomical structures and physiological processes at a high resolution level. This state of affairs has revolutionized medical diagnostics and therapy, as it has enabled physicians to diagnose patients correctly and promptly, and also to identify diseases early.

The principle idea of tissue engineering is the replacement or repair of the diseased or damaged tissues and organs by harnessing the renewal ability of the organism. Prospective therapies of the future for a diverse range of illnesses, including neurological disorders, injuries of the musculoskeletal system, cardiovascular diseases, and more, are a few of the important examples that include tissue scaffolding, organ transplantation, and cell therapy.

Besides, in addition to biomedical uses, wearable technology and digital health solutions are getting more and more important since they facilitate the real-time healthcare services, personal health monitoring and remote patients observation as well.

Figure 7. Applications in Biomedicine

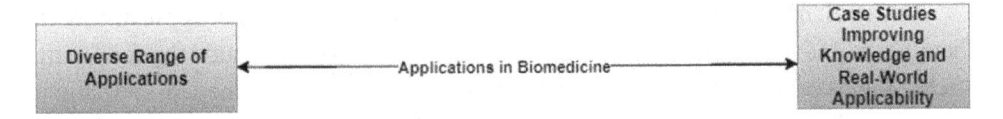

8.2 Case Studies Improving Knowledge and Real-World Applicability:

The importance of case studies in fundamental and conceptual understanding of organic chemistry and practical applications of biological systems cannot be overemphasized. Case examples show to the students how various biomedical methods and technologies give solutions to healthcare problems and bring about desired results. A case study may depict for instance a new biomaterial scaffold, which is constructed and applied to patients with spinal cord injuries to help in tissue regeneration, thus, elevating the quality of life and motor and functions of the patients. Another possible case study will be based on the role of mobile health applications and wearable biosensors in the observation of patients with long-term conditions such as diabetes or hypertension. This will enable doctors to discover health issues at their early stages and make corrective treatment before the problems worsen. Biomedical researchers, physicians, and elected officials may harness cutting-edge scientific technology in medicine through the observation of the case studies. Moreover, case studies are instrumental in knowledge-sharing within the biomedical community and thus they provide a platform for sharing success stories, lessons learned, and best practices which further improves teamwork and boosts innovation.

In general, biomedical applications diversity of techniques and technologies which are aimed at improving humans' health and living conditions. The next segment of this section presents a vivid picture of the conversion aspect of biomedical research and innovation in healthcare by including almost all the applications in the biomedical sector while highlighting the imperative of case studies in dissemination information and practical skills.

9. UTILISING AI METHODS IN HEALTH AND WELLNESS SYSTEMS:

Artificial intelligence (AI) approaches have a wide range of applications in healthcare and wellness systems. Some of these applications include the following technologies designed to enhance clinical decision-making, overall health, and patient treatment. This section discusses the ethical concerns as well as the real-world challenges of applying the wide range of AI techniques in health and well-being systems.

9.1 Wide Range of AI Techniques:

The major AI techniques applied in healthcare and wellness systems include ML, natural language processing, computer vision, robotics, and expert systems(Jiang et al 2017). The duties conducted by the machine algorithms involved include disease identification, images analysis, prediction, and the development of individualized treatment plans(Kavitha et al 2023). Natural language processing techniques facilitate the extraction of interesting and useful information from clinical text like Electronic Health Records and other forms of documentations thereby making clinical decision support as well as medical research more refined. Computer vision systems are employed in the segmentation of distinct features to assist in surgery planning as well as in the detection of abnormalities in the images obtained through radiology. Expert systems and robotics provide patient monitoring, virtual healthcare assistants, and surgical support, all of which improve patient care and provider productivity.

9.2 Ethical Considerations:

It is common for ethical issues to emerge when AI is used in healthcare and wellness systems which among others include patient privacy, cyber security, algorithmic bias, accountability and transparency. Strict adherence to privacy laws by European Union such as the General Data Protection Regulation (GDPR) and the

Health Insurance Portability and Accountability Act (HIPAA) in USA whenever sensitive health information is used for AI-driven application and decision making. To privatize data against cyber threats, unauthorized access, and data breach, make security measures are really necessary. Algorithms may be able to contribute to the precondition and aggravation of the existing disparities in healthcare. It is attributed to the fact that the data that is fed to these systems to learn from or the faulty algorithms in these systems. To achieve trust in supervisory institutions, clinicians, and patients, transparency and accountability are crucial tools in the implementation of AI-enhanced systems.

Figure 8. Utilising AI Methods in Health and Wellness Systems

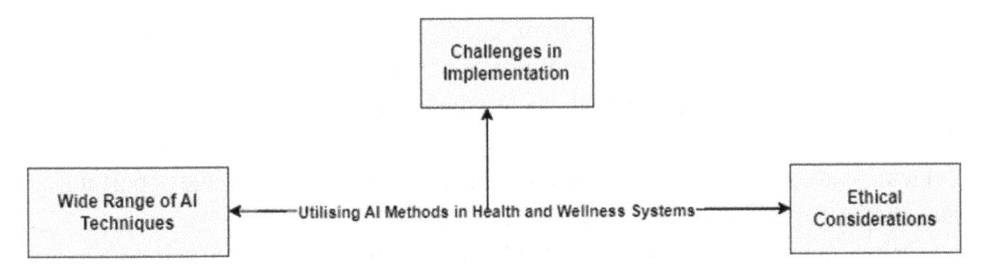

9.3 Challenges in Implementation:

The application of AI approaches in health and wellness systems presents various challenges such as workforce readiness, legal concerns, data quality and accessibility, and compatibility despite the opportunities. The nature of data in the healthcare field is distributed over many formats and systems which makes their analysis and utilization by AI-based technologies precise. It also might be not standardised, contain some mistakes, omit necessary information, and have some contradictions. Lack of integrated communication hinders the effectiveness of AI solutions since it deals with the proper coordination of various health care systems and gadgets. There are a number of norms and restrictions that are mandatory to follow in case of AI driven health care solutions, the compliance to which may include privacy laws or regulations pertaining to health care data or medical devices. Also, when it comes to AI approaches, specific training and qualifications of the healthcare personnel are needed to ensure that they provide sufficient knowledge and skills for effective implementation of AI in clinical practice.

In conclusion, it can be noted that the introduction of artificial intelligence approaches into the healthcare and wellness solutions has potential for the development of clinical decisions, augmentation of patient care, and enhancement of overall well-being for all individuals. However, for AI-based healthcare solutions to yield the benefits intended and for patients' safety, privacy and trust in their care to be upheld, ethical challenges need to be met and implementation barriers dealt with.

10.CONCLUSION:

To sum up, existing studies examining the application of AI & ML in providing healthcare have revealed the possibilities of paradigm shift for providing patients' treatment, clinicians' decision making and the healthcare organizations as a whole. The valuable conclusions from this profound review regard the significance of the evidence-based approaches, pros and cons of different AI methods, and opportunities and challenges in the usage of AI in health care.

On the same note, the use of predictive modelling, data mining, and knowledge discovery tools made it easier to predict illnesses, plan treatment, and improve patient outcomes. When it comes to the illness diagnosis, prediction, and decision support systems, machine learning and deep learning have provided higher level of efficiency in the clinical processes and provided faster and accurate treatments. In managing hospitals operations, utilisation of healthcare resource, appointment, and treatment has been enhanced through optimisation problems investing more efficiency and cost.

Despite these advances, challenges such as workforce readiness, algorithm bias, data privacy, and compatibility persist and require collective action from all stakeholders. It is crucial to address the ethical matters that accompany patient data protection, AI system security, and credibility to ensure the proper and ethical use of AI solutions in healthcare.

Some of the important considerations for the future of AI research include the continuous need for the development of novel AI methods, the development of guidelines and best practices regarding the application of AI in healthcare, as well as promoting collaboration between members of the healthcare domain and data science community, policymakers, and regulatory bodies. To ensure that AI is adopted widely in the health sector and incorporated into practice, research activities must focus on addressing the core challenges concerning data and people within the domain.

In conclusion, this survey provides valuable information about the disruptive potential of AI and ML in the healthcare context and highlights opportunities for innovation, collaboration, and improved patient care and health care organization. With the help of AI and taking into account the potential economic and other obstacles to the use of such innovations, the sphere of healthcare may help to introduce a new paradigm of personalized, efficient, and high-quality treatment for all people.

REFERENCES:

Bakator, M., & Radosav, D. (2018). Deep learning and medical diagnosis: A review of literature. *Multimodal Technologies and Interaction*, 2(3), 47. 10.3390/mti2030047

Berkaya, S. K., Uysal, A. K., Gunal, E. S., Ergin, S., Gunal, S., & Gulmezoglu, M. B. (2018). A survey on ECG analysis. *Biomedical Signal Processing and Control*, 43, 216–235. 10.1016/j.bspc.2018.03.003

Bhardwaj, R., Nambiar, A. R., & Dutta, D. (2017, July). A study of machine learning in healthcare. In 2017 IEEE 41st annual computer software and applications conference (COMPSAC) (Vol. 2, pp. 236-241). IEEE. 10.1109/COMPSAC.2017.164

Garg, A., Venkataramani, V. V., Karthikeyan, A., & Priyakumar, U. D. (2022, January). Modern AI/ML methods for healthcare: Opportunities and challenges. In *International Conference on Distributed Computing and Internet Technology* (pp. 3-25). Cham: Springer International Publishing. 10.1007/978-3-030-94876-4_1

Gracious, L. A., Jasmine, R. M., Pooja, E., Anish, T. P., Johncy, G., & Subramanian, R. S. (2023, October). Machine Learning and Deep Learning Transforming Healthcare: An Extensive Exploration of Applications, Algorithms, and Prospects. In 2023 4th IEEE Global Conference for Advancement in Technology (GCAT) (pp. 1-6). IEEE.

Jiang, F., Jiang, Y., Zhi, H., Dong, Y., Li, H., Ma, S., Wang, Y., Dong, Q., Shen, H., & Wang, Y. (2017). Artificial intelligence in healthcare: Past, present and future. *Stroke and Vascular Neurology*, 2(4), 230–243. 10.1136/svn-2017-00010129507784

Sudha, K., Lakshmipriya, C., Pajila, P. B., Venitha, E., & Anita, M. (2024, January). Enhancing Diabetes Prediction and Management through Machine Learning: A Comparative Study. In *2024 Fourth International Conference on Advances in Electrical, Computing, Communication and Sustainable Technologies (ICAECT)* (pp. 1-6). IEEE.

Kamala, S. P. R., Gayathri, S., Pillai, N. M., Gracious, L. A., Varun, C. M., & Subramanian, R. S. (2023, July). Predictive Analytics for Heart Disease Detection: A Machine Learning Approach. In 2023 4th International Conference on Electronics and Sustainable Communication Systems (ICESC) (pp. 1583-1589). IEEE.

Kavitha, G., Sudha, K., Jayasutha, D., Sivaraman, V., Nalini, M., & Subramanian, R. S. (2023, November). Accelerating Alzheimer's Research with Machine Learning Models for Improved Detection. In 2023 7th International Conference on Electronics, Communication and Aerospace Technology (ICECA) (pp. 855-862). IEEE.

Khatri, K., & Sharma, A. (2020). ECG Signal Analysis for Heart Disease Detection Based on Sensor Data Analysis with Signal Processing by Deep Learning Architectures. Research Journal of Computer Systems and Engineering, 1(1), 06-10.

Kohli, P. S., & Arora, S. (2018, December). Application of machine learning in disease prediction. In 2018 4th International conference on computing communication and automation (ICCCA) (pp. 1-4). IEEE. 10.1109/CCAA.2018.8777449

Kumar, N., & Kumar, D. (2021, August). Machine learning based heart disease diagnosis using non-invasive methods: A review. [). IOP Publishing.]. *Journal of Physics: Conference Series*, 1950(1), 012081. 10.1088/1742-6596/1950/1/012081

Miao, K. H., & Miao, J. H. (2018). Coronary heart disease diagnosis using deep neural networks. international journal of advanced computer science and applications, 9(10).

Nithya, T., Kumar, V. N., Gayathri, S., Deepa, S., Varun, C. M., & Subramanian, R. S. (2023, August). A comprehensive survey of machine learning: Advancements, applications, and challenges. In *2023 Second International Conference on Augmented Intelligence and Sustainable Systems (ICAISS)* (pp. 354-361). IEEE. 10.1109/ICAISS58487.2023.10250547

Panesar, A. (2019). *Machine learning and AI for healthcare*. Apress. 10.1007/978-1-4842-3799-1

Rajendran, T., Rajathi, S. A., Balakrishnan, C., Aswini, J., Prakash, R. B., & Subramanian, R. S. (2023, December). Risk Prediction Modeling for Breast Cancer using Supervised Machine Learning Approaches. In 2023 2nd International Conference on Automation, Computing and Renewable Systems (ICACRS) (pp. 702-708). IEEE. 10.1109/ICACRS58579.2023.10404482

Rani, M., Bakshi, A., & Gupta, A. (2020, March). Prediction of Heart Disease Using Naïve bayes and Image Processing. In *2020 International Conference on Emerging Smart Computing and Informatics (ESCI)* (pp. 215-219). IEEE. 10.1109/ESCI48226.2020.9167537

Shailaja, K., Seetharamulu, B., & Jabbar, M. A. (2018, March). Machine learning in healthcare: A review. In 2018 Second international conference on electronics, communication and aerospace technology (ICECA) (pp. 910-914). IEEE. 10.1109/ICECA.2018.8474918

Siva, S. R., Sudha, K., Pooja, E., Maheswari, B., & Girija, P. (2024). Revolutionizing Healthcare Delivery: Applications and Impact of Cutting-Edge Technologies. AI and IoT Technology and Applications for Smart Healthcare Systems, 75-91.

Subramanian, R. S., Yamini, B., Sudha, K., & Sivakumar, S. (2024). Ensemble-based deep learning techniques for customer churn prediction model. *Kybernetes*. Advance online publication. 10.1108/K-08-2023-1516

Sudha, K., Ambhika, C., Maheswari, B., Girija, P., & Nalini, M. (2023). AI and IoT Applications in Medical Domain Enhancing Healthcare Through Technology Integration. In AI and IoT-Based Technologies for Precision Medicine (pp. 280-294). IGI Global.

Yamini, B., Kaneti, V. R., Nalini, M., & Subramanian, S. (2023). Machine Learning-driven PCOS prediction for early detection and tailored interventions. *SSRG International Journal of Electrical and Electronics Engineering*, 10(9), 61–75. 10.14445/23488379/IJEEE-V10I9P106

Chapter 2
Data Mining and Knowledge Discovery:
Transforming Healthcare Through Biomedical Intelligence

Akshat Shree Mishra
International Institute of Information Technology, Naya, India

J. Vijaya
International Institute of Information Technology, Naya, India

ABSTRACT

This chapter proposal aims to explore the transformative potential of data mining and knowledge discovery in healthcare, focusing on optimizing healthcare computing systems, integrating technologies like AI and IoT, and emphasizing patient-centric care. It delves into precision medicine, disease pathways, and current trends in health and disease, while addressing concerns around privacy, biases, and responsible data use. The methodology includes a systematic review of healthcare computing systems and real-world case studies. The chapter advocates for interdisciplinary collaboration and ethical frameworks, concluding with a discussion on future directions and challenges to inspire a future of data-driven, patient-centered healthcare.

1. INTRODUCTION

The healthcare landscape is undergoing a paradigm shift, driven by an unprecedented explosion of data. From electronic health records (EHRs) to wearable devices and genomic sequencing, the amount of information generated about human health is growing exponentially (Li et al., 2021). However, harnessing this vast data ocean

DOI: 10.4018/979-8-3693-3719-6.ch002

effectively remains a significant challenge. Thankfully, data mining and knowledge discovery (KDD) emerge as powerful tools to navigate this information deluge and unlock hidden patterns with the potential to revolutionize healthcare (Fayyad et al., 1996).

This chapter delves into how data mining and KDD are transforming healthcare through the lens of "biomedical intelligence," a concept that emphasizes the application of data-driven insights to optimize healthcare systems, personalize patient care, and ultimately improve health outcomes.

1.1 Healthcare Computing Systems and Data Integration

The foundation for data-driven healthcare lies in the complex ecosystem of healthcare computing systems. These systems, ranging from EHRs and imaging platforms to clinical decision support tools, act as data capture and storage mechanisms (Raghupathi & Raghupathi, 2014). However, the true power of data mining lies in its ability to synthesize information from diverse sources (Fayyad et al., 1996). Imagine a patient's journey through the healthcare system, leaving behind a trail of data in each interaction. This might include EHR entries capturing diagnoses, medications, and lab results; wearable data monitoring vital signs and activity levels; and even genomic data revealing unique genetic predispositions (Hersh et al., 2002). Data mining bridges these isolated data silos, enabling a holistic view of the individual and facilitating comprehensive analysis (Park et al., 2015). Figure 1 depicts this concept, illustrating various healthcare data sources converging into a central platform for data mining and analysis.

Figure 1. Integration of Healthcare Data Sources

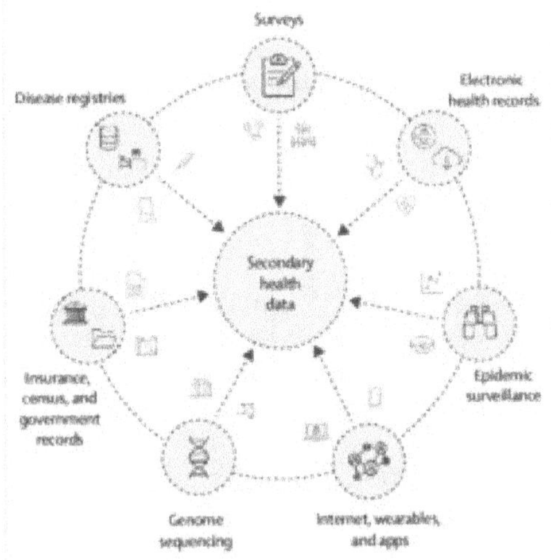

1.1.1. Data Mining and Knowledge Discovery for Patient-Centric Care

At the heart of this transformation lies the concept of patient-centric care, an approach that prioritizes the individual needs and preferences of each patient. Data mining plays a crucial role in driving this shift by enabling personalized medicine and treatment plans. Imagine a patient diagnosed with cancer. By analyzing their genetic data in conjunction with clinical history and other relevant information, data mining can identify specific genetic mutations driving their disease (Aye et al., 2020). This information can then be used to select targeted therapies with higher efficacy and reduced side effects, offering a more personalized approach compared to traditional, "one-size-fits-all" treatments.

1.1.2. Precision Medicine

Precision medicine, a cornerstone of patient-centric care, utilizes individual genetic and molecular data to tailor treatment strategies. Data mining plays a critical role in this process by identifying genetic markers associated with specific diseases or treatment responses. Figure 2 demonstrates this concept, showcasing a hypothetical bar chart representing the varying cancer risks individuals might have based on specific gene variants. Such insights empower clinicians to make informed decisions about targeted therapies with higher success rates and fewer side effects for each patient.

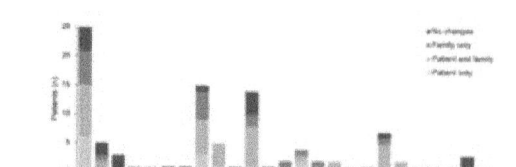

Figure 2. Example of Using Genetic Data to Predict Cancer Risk

1.1.3. Disease Pathway Analysis

Beyond individual genetic markers, data mining unlocks the secrets hidden within complex biological pathways. By analyzing vast datasets of gene expression, protein interactions, and other molecular data, researchers can uncover hidden relationships between genes, proteins, and diseases. This "pathway analysis" has the potential to revolutionize how we understand and treat diseases. Imagine a researcher analyzing gene expression data from thousands of cancer patients. Data mining might reveal a previously unknown pathway that plays a crucial role in tumor growth (Raghupathi, 2011). This knowledge can then be used to develop new drugs targeting that specific pathway, offering a more effective approach than traditional treatments that target individual genes in isolation.

1.1.4. Emerging Trends in Health and Disease

The power of data mining extends beyond individual patients, allowing researchers to analyze population-level health data and identify emerging trends in health and disease. Imagine tracking patterns of disease outbreaks across social media platforms and healthcare systems. Data mining can analyze this data in real time, identifying geographical hotspots, predicting the spread of the disease, and facilitating targeted interventions to contain outbreaks before they become widespread (Nsoesie et al., 2015). Similarly, analyzing data from wearable devices can provide insights into population-level trends in physical activity, sleep patterns, and other health indicators, guiding public health initiatives and preventive measures.

2. CASE STUDIES AND REAL-WORLD EXAMPLES

2.1. Personalized Medicine in Action:
Optimizing Cancer Treatment

The Dana-Farber Cancer Institute, in collaboration with IBM Watson, implemented a data mining platform that analyzes patient genomic data alongside clinical history and other relevant information. This platform identified a rare genetic mutation in a patient with metastatic melanoma, previously considered untreatable. By analyzing vast datasets of cancer patients with similar mutations, the platform identified a targeted therapy that had shown efficacy in those cases. This personalized approach led to a remarkable remission in the patient, highlighting the potential of data mining in precision medicine (Chan et al, 2017).

2.2. Predicting Disease Outbreaks: The Case of Ebola

During the 2014 Ebola outbreak in West Africa, researchers utilized data mining techniques to analyze real-time data from social media, news reports, and travel records. Imagine a map of West Africa, with hotspots highlighted based on social media sentiment analysis, allowing healthcare workers to prioritize resource allocation and containment efforts.

This analysis identified emerging hotspots of the disease and predicted its spread with remarkable accuracy, leading to targeted interventions that helped contain the outbreak (Hossain et al., 2016).

2.3. Optimizing Healthcare Systems:
Reducing Hospital Readmissions

A study published in the Journal of the American Medical Informatics Association analyzed EHR data of hospitalized patients to identify factors associated with readmission within 30 days. By applying data mining techniques, the researchers developed a predictive model that could accurately identify high-risk patients. Imagine a risk score displayed on a patient's chart, alerting healthcare professionals to potential readmission risks and triggering targeted interventions like medication reconciliation and post-discharge support programs. This model was then used to implement targeted interventions, resulting in a significant reduction in readmission rates, saving lives and healthcare costs. (Helm et al., 2016).

3. DATA MINING IN ARES OF HEALTHCARE

Beyond these individual cases, data mining is also making waves in other areas of healthcare such as Transforming Drug Discovery, Clinical Trials, and Public Health Surveillance.

3.1. Drug Discovery: Unlocking Hidden Targets

Imagine a vast network of molecular interactions, where proteins, genes, and other molecules connect in intricate pathways crucial to disease development. Data mining acts as a powerful microscope, analyzing massive datasets of these interactions to identify potential drug targets as represented in Figure 3. This approach, known as **computational drug discovery**, offers several advantages:

> **Speed and Efficiency:** Compared to traditional trial-and-error methods, data mining can rapidly screen millions of potential drug candidates, significantly accelerating the discovery process.
> **Precision:** By focusing on specific targets within disease pathways, data mining can lead to the development of more targeted and effective treatments with fewer side effects.
> **Reduced Costs:** By streamlining the drug development pipeline, data mining can potentially save billions of dollars in research and development costs (Weth et al., 2024).
> Examples:

- Researchers used data mining to identify a protein target associated with Alzheimer's disease, leading to the development of promising new drug candidates currently in clinical trials.
- By analyzing genetic data from cancer patients, scientists discovered mutations linked to tumor growth, enabling them to design drugs targeting those specific mutations.

Figure 3. Unveiling Drug Targets through Data Mining

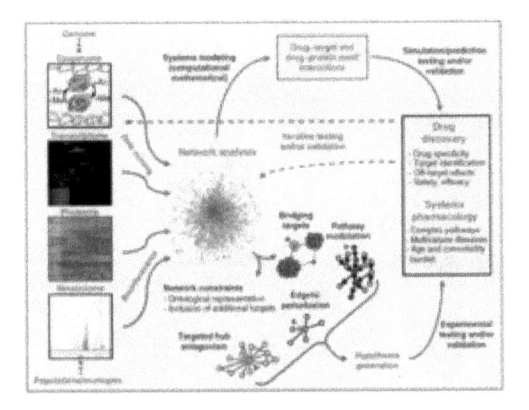

3.2. Clinical Trial Design: Optimizing Success

Clinical trials are crucial for evaluating the safety and efficacy of new drugs, but designing them effectively can be challenging as represented in Figure 4. Data mining steps in to optimize trial design in several ways:

> **Identifying Patient Populations:** Data mining can analyze patient data to identify individuals with specific characteristics most likely to benefit from the new drug, ensuring trials recruit the right participants.
> **Selecting Treatment Combinations:** By analyzing past clinical trial data and patient information, data mining can suggest promising drug combinations for testing, potentially leading to more effective therapies.
> **Predicting Trial Outcomes:** By analyzing vast datasets of past trials, data mining can predict the potential success or failure of new trials, informing resource allocation and decision-making (El-Hagrassy et al, 2018).
> Examples:

- Data mining helped identify specific genetic markers in patients with a certain type of cancer, allowing researchers to recruit only those most likely to respond to a new therapy in a clinical trial.
- By analyzing data from past trials of different cancer drugs, researchers were able to select a combination of drugs with synergistic effects, leading to improved patient outcomes

Figure 4. Data Mining for Smarter Clinical Trials

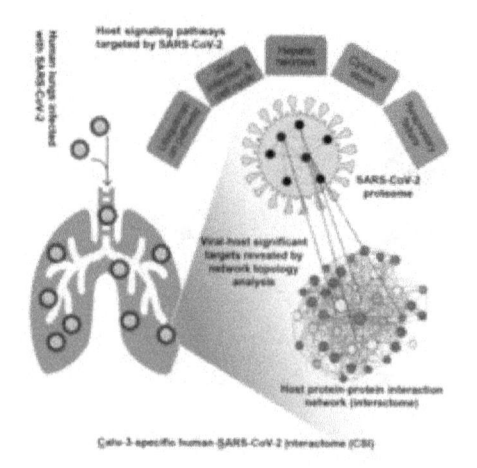

3.3. Public Health Surveillance: Proactive Disease Prevention

Public health surveillance traditionally relies on reported cases, but often by the time these are identified, outbreaks have already spread significantly as represented in Figure 5. Data mining offers proactive solutions by analyzing data from various sources in real time:

Healthcare Systems: Analyzing data from electronic health records and patient visits can identify early signs and symptoms of outbreaks, allowing for quicker intervention.

Social Media: By analyzing trends and keywords on social media platforms, data mining can detect discussions of potential outbreaks before they reach official channels.

Environmental Monitoring: Analyzing data from environmental sensors can identify changes in air quality, water quality, or other factors linked to disease outbreaks (Aiyar et al, 2020).

Examples:

- During the 2014 Ebola outbreak, data mining of social media data helped identify hotspots of the disease earlier than traditional methods, enabling targeted interventions and containment efforts.

- By analyzing data from airline travel and disease cases, researchers can predict the spread of emerging infectious diseases and allocate resources proactively.

Figure 5. Data Mining for Early Disease Outbreak Detection

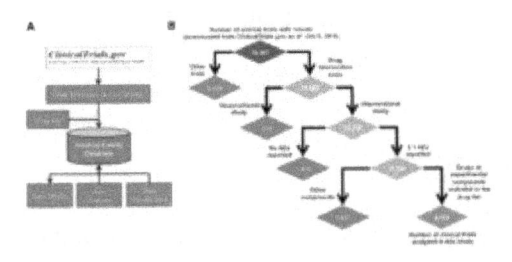

4. DATA MINING IN HEALTH CARE CHALLENGES CASE STUDY

4.1. Patient Privacy and Data Security

Imagine A bustling hospital, bustling with activity. Yet, within its secure confines lies a hidden vault: the data sanctuary. Here, patients' medical records reside, protected by multiple layers of digital defense.

Encryption safeguards their information, while access control ensures that only authorized personnel can enter. Regular audits act as vigilant sentinels, guarding against any breaches or unauthorized attempts (Bani Issa et al., 2020).

Beyond the Vault: Data travels, too. Imagine couriers carrying sensitive information, cloaked in a digital shield. Secure communication protocols ensure its safe passage, from one authorized user to another.

De-identification: But what about the data itself? Imagine transforming patient records, and removing names, addresses, and other direct identifiers. This process, like k-anonymity, grants anonymity while preserving valuable statistical insights. Think of it as creating a masked version of the data, still useful for analysis, but unrecognizable as belonging to any specific individual.

Challenges and Considerations

- **Access Control:** Implementing granular access controls can be complex, requiring careful planning and ongoing maintenance.
- **Encryption:** Choosing the right encryption algorithms and managing encryption keys requires expertise and secure storage solutions.
- **Auditing:** Regular audits demand resources and expertise to effectively identify and address vulnerabilities.
- **De-identification Techniques:** Balancing anonymity with utility can be tricky, and different techniques offer varying levels of protection and information retention.

4.2. Informed Consent

Imagine: A patient, empowered by knowledge. They hold a consent form, translated into their native language, clearly explaining the data mining project at hand. It outlines the purpose, potential benefits and risks, and most importantly, their right to choose (Bazzano et al., 2021). They ask questions, understand the implications, and ultimately decide whether to participate.

Transparency is Key: Imagine the consent form as a window into the research project. It should explain:

- **The specific data being collected and used:** What information will be gathered, and how will it be processed and analyzed?
- **The intended purpose of the project:** What are the researchers hoping to achieve with this data?
- **Potential risks and benefits:** Are there any privacy concerns, and what potential advantages could result from participation?
- **Right to withdraw:** The patient should have a clear understanding that they are free to decline or withdraw consent at any time.

Accessibility and Comprehension: Consent forms should be available in various languages and written in clear, concise language, avoiding technical jargon. Imagine translators working alongside researchers to ensure diverse populations can understand their choices.

Challenges and Considerations:

- **Balancing clarity with comprehensiveness:** Providing enough information without overwhelming patients with technical details requires careful wording and design.
- **Reaching diverse populations:** Translating consent forms and ensuring accessibility for individuals with disabilities requires additional resources and planning.
- **Evolving regulations:** Data privacy regulations are constantly evolving, so consent forms need to be regularly reviewed and updated to comply with the latest requirements.

4.3. Addressing Algorithmic Bias

Imagine A data mining algorithm as a mirror reflecting the world. But what if the mirror itself is distorted, reflecting an inaccurate and biased image? This is the risk of algorithmic bias, where algorithms trained on skewed data perpetuate existing inequalities in healthcare.

Building a Diverse Foundation: Imagine constructing the algorithm's foundation with data that truly represents the real world. This means incorporating diverse datasets that reflect various demographics, ethnicities, socioeconomic backgrounds, and geographic locations. Think of it as gathering building blocks from various corners of society, ensuring a balanced and representative foundation (Norori et al., 2021).

Explainable Design: Imagine the algorithm not as a black box, but as a transparent window. With explainable functionalities, healthcare professionals can understand how the algorithm arrives at conclusions. This allows them to identify and address potential biases before they lead to unfair outcomes. Think of it as shining a light on the algorithm's inner workings, revealing its logic and decision-making process.

Continuous Vigilance: Like a watchful guardian, regular monitoring is crucial. Fairness metrics and human expert review act as checks and balances, identifying and mitigating potential biases. Imagine a team of experts scrutinizing the algorithm's outputs, ensuring they are fair and unbiased across all populations.

Challenges and Considerations:

- **Data availability:** Acquiring truly diverse datasets can be difficult and time-consuming, requiring collaboration and data sharing initiatives.
- **Explainable AI technology:** While explainable AI techniques are evolving, they are not yet perfect, and interpreting their outputs requires expertise.

- **Bias detection and mitigation:** Identifying and addressing biases can be complex, requiring ongoing monitoring and adjustments to the algorithm.

5. RECENT TECHNIQUES IN HEALTH CARE APPLICATION

5.1. Explainable AI (XAI): Demystifying the Black Box

Imagine a doctor reviewing an X-ray alongside an AI assistant. Instead of a cryptic recommendation, the AI provides a detailed explanation: "I identified a mass in the lung region with 95% confidence based on the following patterns in the X-ray density and texture..." This transparency fostered by XAI builds trust between patients, clinicians, and AI systems, leading to more informed decisions and shared understanding (Dauda et al., 2022).

Challenges and Considerations:

- **Balancing interpretability with accuracy:** Simplifying complex algorithms for human understanding may lead to a loss of accuracy. Striking the right balance requires ongoing research and development.
- **Explainability across different algorithms:** Different AI architectures have varying levels of explainability. Developing universal XAI techniques remains a challenge.
- **Integrating XAI into clinical workflows:** Seamlessly integrating XAI explanations into existing clinical workflows requires careful design and user-friendly interfaces.

5.2. Federated Learning: Privacy-Preserving Collaboration

Imagine individual patient data residing securely on their own devices, like smartphones or wearables. Instead of sharing raw data, anonymized insights generated locally are shared for collective analysis. This decentralized approach, known as federated learning, protects patient privacy while enabling collaborative research on large-scale datasets (Antunes et al., 2022)

Challenges and Considerations:

- **Communication efficiency:** Coordinating data exchange and model updates across numerous devices can be computationally expensive and require efficient communication protocols.
- **Data heterogeneity:** Devices gather data in different formats and with varying quality. Ensuring data quality and consistency across the network poses challenges.
- **Privacy guarantees:** While federated learning protects raw data, ensuring robust privacy measures against potential attacks on the anonymized insights remains crucial.

5.3. Addressing Healthcare Disparities: Data Mining for Equity

Imagine data mining tools analyzing healthcare access and outcomes across different demographics. They identify disparities based on factors like race, ethnicity, socioeconomic status, and geographic location. This valuable insight informs targeted interventions and policy changes, paving the way for equitable healthcare for all (Getzen et al., 2023).

Challenges and Considerations:

- **Data bias:** Data mining algorithms can perpetuate existing biases present in the data. Mitigating these biases requires careful data selection and algorithm design.
- **Community engagement:** Addressing healthcare disparities requires collaborative efforts with affected communities, ensuring their voices and needs are heard and incorporated into solutions.
- **Accountability and transparency:** Monitoring the impact of interventions and ensuring transparency in data use and decision-making is crucial for building trust and ensuring ethical implementation.

The Road Ahead:

Navigating the future of data mining in healthcare demands a multi-faceted approach. By embracing XAI for transparency, leveraging federated learning for privacy-preserving collaboration, and addressing healthcare disparities through data-driven insights, we can harness the power of this technology to build a more equitable and informed healthcare system for all. However, this journey requires addressing ongoing challenges and fostering collaboration among researchers, clinicians, policymakers, and the public. By working together, we can ensure responsible data use and unlock the full potential of data mining to improve human health and well-being.

6. CONCLUSION

The journey into the world of data mining in healthcare reveals a landscape brimming with potential. From the transformative power of drug discovery and optimized clinical trials to the proactive prevention of disease outbreaks, this technology holds the promise to revolutionize healthcare as we know it. Yet, this path is not without its challenges. Ethical considerations and responsible data use are not mere roadblocks, but guiding principles that must be woven into the very fabric of this technological advancement. Guaranteeing patient privacy and data security through robust frameworks, informed consent, and anonymization techniques is paramount. We must strive for transparency in algorithms through explainable AI, fostering trust between patients, clinicians, and the technology itself. Addressing algorithmic bias through diverse data and continuous monitoring ensures fairness and equitable outcomes for all (Cummins.et al., 2023). The future of data mining in healthcare lies in navigating these challenges with a commitment to collaboration. From researchers and clinicians to policymakers and the public, open dialogue and shared responsibility are essential. By working together, we can unlock the full potential of this technology while ensuring ethical and responsible use. Imagine a future where data mining plays a pivotal role in building a healthcare system that is not only efficient and effective but also equitable and accessible for all. This is the future we must strive for, guided by the principles of trust, transparency, and ethical responsibility.

This conclusion emphasizes the ethical imperative of responsible data use, highlights the collaborative effort required, and paints a compelling future vision for healthcare empowered by data mining. Remember to adapt it further to your specific chapter and audience for maximum impact.

REFERENCES

Aiyar, A., & Pingali, P. (2020). Pandemics and food systems-towards a proactive food safety approach to disease prevention & management. *Food Security*, 12(4), 749–756. 10.1007/s12571-020-01074-332837645

Antunes, R. S., André da Costa, C., Küderle, A., Yari, I. A., & Eskofier, B. (2022). Federated learning for healthcare: Systematic review and architecture proposal. [TIST]. *ACM Transactions on Intelligent Systems and Technology*, 13(4), 1–23. 10.1145/3501813

Aye, Y. M., Liew, S., Neo, S. X., Li, W., Ng, H. L., Chua, S. T., Zhou, W.-T., Au, W.-L., Tan, E.-K., Tay, K.-Y., Tan, L. C.-S., & Xu, Z. (2020). Patient-centric care for Parkinson's disease: From hospital to the community. *Frontiers in Neurology*, 11, 502. 10.3389/fneur.2020.0050232582014

Bani Issa, W., Al Akour, I., Ibrahim, A., Almarzouqi, A., Abbas, S., Hisham, F., & Griffiths, J. (2020). Privacy, confidentiality, security and patient safety concerns about electronic health records. *International Nursing Review*, 67(2), 218–230. 10.1111/inr.1258532314398

Bazzano, L. A., Durant, J., & Brantley, P. R. (2021). A modern history of informed consent and the role of key information. *The Ochsner Journal*, 21(1), 81–85. 10.31486/toj.19.010533828429

Chan, C. W., Law, B. M., So, W. K., Chow, K. M., & Waye, M. M. (2017). Novel strategies on personalized medicine for breast cancer treatment: An update. *International Journal of Molecular Sciences*, 18(11), 2423. 10.3390/ijms1811242329140300

Cummins, M. R., Nachimuthu, S. K., Abdelrahman, S. E., Facelli, J. C., & Gouripeddi, R. (2023). Nonhypothesis-driven research: data mining and knowledge discovery. In *Clinical research informatics* (pp. 413–432). Springer International Publishing. 10.1007/978-3-031-27173-1_20

. Dauda, O. I., Awotunde, J. B., AbdulRaheem, M., & Salihu, S. A. (2022). Basic issues and challenges on Explainable Artificial Intelligence (XAI) in healthcare systems. *Principles and methods of explainable artificial intelligence in healthcare*, 248-271.

El-Hagrassy, M. M., Duarte, D., Thibaut, A., Lucena, M. F., & Fregni, F. (2018). Principles of designing a clinical trial: Optimizing chances of trial success. *Current Behavioral Neuroscience Reports*, 5(2), 143–152. 10.1007/s40473-018-0152-y30467533

Fayyad, U., Piatetsky-Shapiro, G., & Smyth, P. (1996). From data mining to knowledge discovery in databases. *AI Magazine*, 17(3), 37–37.

Getzen, E., Ungar, L., Mowery, D., Jiang, X., & Long, Q. (2023). Mining for equitable health: Assessing the impact of missing data in electronic health records. *Journal of Biomedical Informatics*, 139, 104269. 10.1016/j.jbi.2022.10426936621750

Helm, J. E., Alaeddini, A., Stauffer, J. M., Bretthauer, K. M., & Skolarus, T. A. (2016). Reducing hospital readmissions by integrating empirical prediction with resource optimization. *Production and Operations Management*, 25(2), 233–257. 10.1111/poms.12377

Hersh, W. R., Crabtree, M. K., Hickam, D. H., Sacherek, L., Friedman, C. P., Tidmarsh, P., & Kraemer, D. (2002). Factors associated with success in searching MEDLINE and applying evidence to answer clinical questions. *Journal of the American Medical Informatics Association : JAMIA*, 9(3), 283–293. 10.1197/jamia.M099611971889

Hossain, L., Kam, D., Kong, F., Wigand, R. T., & Bossomaier, T. (2016). Social media in Ebola outbreak. *Epidemiology and Infection*, 144(10), 2136–2143. 10.1017/S095026881600039X26939535

Li, R., Niu, Y., Scott, S. R., Zhou, C., Lan, L., Liang, Z., & Li, J. (2021). Using electronic medical record data for research in a Healthcare Information and Management Systems Society (HIMSS) Analytics Electronic Medical Record Adoption Model (EMRAM) stage 7 hospital in Beijing: Cross-sectional study. *JMIR Medical Informatics*, 9(8), e24405. 10.2196/2440534342589

Norori, N., Hu, Q., Aellen, F. M., Faraci, F. D., & Tzovara, A. (2021). Addressing bias in big data and AI for health care: A call for open science. *Patterns (New York, N.Y.)*, 2(10), 100347. 10.1016/j.patter.2021.10034734693373

Nsoesie, E. O., Kraemer, M. U., Golding, N., Pigott, D. M., Brady, O. J., Moyes, C. L., Johansson, M. A., Gething, P. W., Velayudhan, R., Khan, K., Hay, S. I., & Brownstein, J. S. (2016). Global distribution and environmental suitability for chikungunya virus, 1952 to 2015. *Eurosurveillance*, 21(20), 30234. 10.2807/1560-7917.ES.2016.21.20.3023427239817

Park, Y. T., & Atalag, K. (2015). Current national approach to healthcare ICT standardization: Focus on progress in New Zealand. *Healthcare Informatics Research*, 21(3), 144–151. 10.4258/hir.2015.21.3.14426279950

Raghupathi, V. (2019). An empirical investigation of chronic diseases: A visualization approach to medicare in the United States. *International Journal of Healthcare Management*, 12(4), 327–339. 10.1080/20479700.2018.1472849

Raghupathi, W., & Raghupathi, V. (2014). Big data analytics in healthcare: Promise and potential. *Health Information Science and Systems*, 2(1), 1–10. 10.1186/2047-2501-2-325825667

Weth, F. R., Hoggarth, G. B., Weth, A. F., Paterson, E., White, M. P., Tan, S. T., Peng, L., & Gray, C. (2024). Unlocking hidden potential: Advancements, approaches, and obstacles in repurposing drugs for cancer therapy. *British Journal of Cancer*, 130(5), 703–715. 10.1038/s41416-023-02502-938012383

Chapter 3
Design and Development of AI-Powered Healthcare System

A. K. P. Kovendan
https://orcid.org/0000-0002-7232-5571
Vellore Institute of Technology, India

G. N. Balaji
Vellore Institute of Technology, India

Srijita Khatua
Vellore Institute of Technology, India

Harmanpreet Singh
Vellore Institute of Technology, India

Dibyani Chatterjee
Vellore Institute of Technology, India

ABSTRACT

Cancer patient survival is an integral part of the healthcare sector, with researchers offering clinicians snipping information as they consider treatment options that have a big impact on patients' lifestyle decisions. Evidently, no study of predicting survival or death from breast cancer using XGBoost method has been attempted. The goal of this project is to design a prediction system that can forecast both the survival rate and the death rate from breast cancer at an early stage by examining the most limited collection of clinical dataset variables. The potential of the XGBoost method is determined using mainly age at the time of diagnosis along with other

DOI: 10.4018/979-8-3693-3719-6.ch003

Copyright © 2024, IGI Global. Copying or distributing in print or electronic forms without written permission of IGI Global is prohibited.

clinical characteristics, assessed for its relative significance. The project findings show that the XGBoost model fits the testing dataset more effectively, with outcome of accuracy 82.72% approximately.

1. INTRODUCTION

One of the most prevalent malignant tumours in women globally is breast cancer. According to relevant data, every year over than 2.3 million lives are affected worldwide and 685,000 died in 2020 (Benz C. C. (2008)). It continues to be the most common mortality rate for women from breast cancer (Breast Cancer Research Foundation (BCRF)). The project's data came from the METABRIC (Molecular Taxonomy of Breast Cancer) database. Over 1900 breast cancers from throughout the world were examined by the International Consortium) cohort between 1977 and 2005. The METABRIC database includes studies of case types of patients that were compiled using primary pathology reports, investigations that are available for central evaluation with histology slides. The collaboration between researchers of data science and histopathology, in which 10 logistic regression models for multivariables were used, was one of the well-known studies mentioned to each IntClust group, which categorises a sizable number of independent samples for the investigation of gene expression, validates to estimate patient survival periods after hormone therapy (HT) and chemotherapy (CT).

Our effort, however, aims to identify a more comprehensible prognosis indicator using the patient's age, the variables' feature relevance, and their association coefficients. The METABRIC database is utilised to apply the methods Multivariate Linear Regression, Logistic Regression, Random Forest, and XGBoost in order to forecast both the overall patient mortality rate and the survival rate. The project outcomes from such a study and any upcoming research may be very helpful in assisting medical professionals in understanding and making modifications to the optimal course of therapy.

This paper is organized as follows: in section 1, Introduction; in section 2, Relevant work; in section 3, Phases and Method; in section 4, Prognosis Model Construction; in section 5, Our Observations and Results; in section 6, Conclusion.

2. RELEVANT WORK

Numerous studies have been conducted on the use of multivariate regression, logistic regression and random forest to predict breast cancer. Evidently, no study of predicting survival or death from breast cancer using XGBoost method has been attempted.

The authors of (Ferroni et al., 2019)) discuss the value of using a decision support system (DSS) based on machine learning (ML) and random optimization (RO) to extract prognostic data from frequently gathered demographic, clinical, and biochemical data, statistics about people with breast cancer (BC). A DSS model had an accuracy of 86% and a C-index of 0.84 for progression-free survival. With a hazard ratio (HR) of 10.9 (p 0.0001), the model was also able to stratify the testing set into two groups of patients with low- or high-risk of progression.

The study by the authors of (Meifang Li et al., 2020) integrates X-ray analysis with computer-aided diagnostic methods including machine learning and computer vision to examine breast tumour diagnosis strategies. The goal is to increase the detection accuracy of breast cancers. Furthermore, this to estimate various image characteristics, the study integrates breast tumour diagnostic pictures. The best diagnostic pictures are also acquired by experimental research and analysis of the region segmentation technique and pre-processing method of breast detection images, and a practical proposal for the impact of background and other noise on the outcomes of image diagnosis is made.

The authors of (Octaviani, 2019) suggest a random forest for predicting breast cancer. One of the numerous classification methods is random forest, which is an algorithm for huge data categorization. To improve classification performance and accuracy, random forest classification is used to cancer microarray data. This paper is 100 percent accurate.

In the paper (F. Seddik et.al., 2015), the authors' suggested method creates a binary logistic model that divides instances into benign and malignant categories. The Wisconsin Diagnostic Breast Cancer (WDBC) dataset is used to apply the methodology. According to experimental findings, the statistically significant regression model simply takes into account a tumour's size, texture, concavity, and symmetry.

The study by the authors in (S. Kabiraj et al., 2020) uses two well-known ensemble machine learning methods to examine a breast cancer dataset and forecast the development of breast cancer. Breast cancer is predicted using Extreme Gradient Boosting (XGBoost) and Random Forest. For this research, a total of 275 examples with 12 characteristics are used. In this investigation, accuracy rates of 74.73% using the Random Forest method and 73.63% using XGBoost are both achieved.

The authors in (rendhar, S. P. A., & Vasuki, R., 2021). compare the overall results of several categorization algorithms. Utilizing 8 category algorithms, the category algorithms were performed on 8 NCD datasets, a 10-fold cross-validation technique, and algorithms. It has been assessed whether or not to utilize AUC as a sign of accuracy. The authors claim that the NCD datasets contain side-effects and noisy facts. Noise resistance has been demonstrated for KNN, SVM, and NN. They added that the problem with non-essential characteristics may be resolved by using a few pre-processing techniques to raise the accuracy level.

Following our focus on these reviews, we will continue to be committed to using the XGBoost Algorithm to determine the mortality and survival rates from breast cancer and evaluating its accuracy in comparison to other approaches.

2.1 Multivariate Regression

The link between more than one independent variable and a dependent variable is shown using multivariate regression model. This model is intended to evaluate the relative relevance of each variable for forecasting a certain result, however it is most frequently utilised in bigger datasets due to its mathematical complexity. Similar to a linear regression model, this algorithm is based on a number of fundamental presumptions, including that the data are continuous, that the residual error is constant across the entire dataset, that the spread is normally distributed, and that there is some correlation between the input and output variables (Pillai, V., Koohpayegani et al., (2021), Duleba, A. J., & Olive, D. L. (1996), Spanos, A., & Hendry, D. (2011)).

- Multivariate Regression Equation:
$$Y_{ip} = B_{0p} + \sum_{j=1}^{m} B_{jp} X_{ij} + E_{jp} \quad (1)$$
Y_{ip} specifies the anticipated variable for the ith observation, B_{0p} is the intercept for the pth response, and B_{jp} is the jth observation's response, X_{ij} is the jth predictor variable for the ith observation, E_{jp} is the vector, and j^{th} predictor variable slope for the pth answer. The Ordinary Least Squares equation may be used to calculate each model coefficient.

- Ordinary Least Squares Equation:
$$\beta\beta_1 = \frac{\sum_{i=1}^{n}(x_i - \bar{x})(y_i - \bar{y})}{\sum_{i=1}^{n}(x_i - \bar{x})^2} \quad (2)$$
x_i stands for the informative variable, y_i for the expected variable, and β_1 for the model intercept. The equation aids in determining the regression coefficients of the model by computing the smallest sum of squared residuals.

- R-Squared Coefficient Equation:

$$R^2 = 1 - \frac{\sum_{i=1}^{n}(\hat{y}_i - \overline{y})^2}{\sum_{i=1}^{n}(y_i - \overline{y})^2} \quad (3)$$

While it is true that high value of R-Squared coefficients show stronger correlations between the informative and measured variables, it is equally crucial to keep in mind that low value of R-Squared values might provide valuable database insights.

Logistic Regression

A categorical dependent variable's forecasted outcomes are made using the classification approach known as logistic regression (F. Seddik and D. M. Shawky, (2015), Helwig, N. E. (2017). Instead of fitting a regression line into logistic regression, we do it using a "S"-shaped logistic function that predicts two highest values (0 or 1).

- Logistic Regression Equation:
$$\log\frac{Y}{1-Y} = B_0 + B_1 X_1 + B_2 X_2 + B_3 X_3 + \ldots + B_m X_m \quad (4)$$

2.2 Random Forest

An ensemble learning method called Random Forest is widely applied to classification or regression issues. The random forest model is utilised in healthcare sector because it is good at managing complicated datasets by creating several decision trees, and because it can find links between patients having similar features and categorise them respectively (Octaviani, Lidya & Rustam, Zuherman. (2019) Kovendan, A. K. P., et. al., (2018)).

Random Forest models, in contrast to Multivariate Regression models, can tolerate skewed data points and may evaluate a wide range of explanatory factors. However, one disadvantage is that models with a large number of decision trees are frequently computationally inefficient, resulting in longer runtimes and challenges with dataset training.

The Random Forest algorithm's ability to select the best hyperparameters to enhance model performance is one of its important features. Figure 1 illustrates how numerous decision trees are formed using the Random Forest algorithm. There are five parameters needed to be determined: "n estimators," "min samples split," "max samples split," "max features," and "max depth (Kovendan, A. K. P., et. al., (2018)).

Figure 1. Different Branches in Decision Tree Diagram

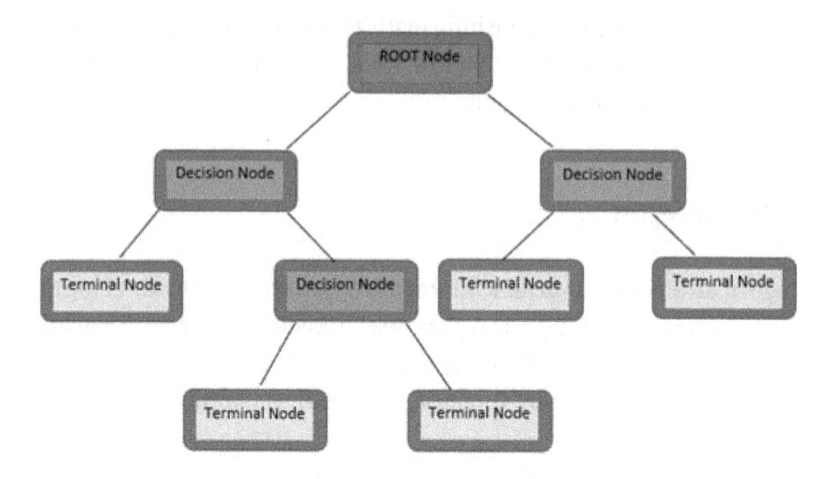

The number of estimators, also known as N estimators, describes how many decision trees are included in the model. The ability of the model to analyse data patterns increases with the quantity of estimators. The training procedures runtime is, however, greatly increased by a large number of estimators.

Maximum and Minimum Sample Splits provide the minimum and maximum number of samples respectively required for a split intermediate node. The ideal value for this parameter, which may be expressed as either a percentage form of samples or as an integer form, would indicate that the model can effectively interpret data correlations without experiencing model underfitting or overfitting problems.

The maximum number of characteristics to consider while determining the best split is represented by the variable max features. Square root, often known as sqrt (n features), is widely employed as a metric in regression situations.

The maximum depth of each tree in the model is indicated by the term max depth. much like n estimators and the ideal value of min/max samples split is required to prevent model under- or overfitting.

3. PHASES AND METHODS

3.1 Hyperparameter Tuning

The implementation of hyperparameter tweaking allowed for the determination of the best split for each parameter. In general, experimental data obtained via trial and error rather than quantitative calculations serve as a superior basis for this strategy's success (Koehrsen, 2018.) In order to get further understanding of the model's performance, the training data were further divided into subsets using K-Fold Cross Validation.

3.2 Performance Metrics

The computation of the mean absolute/mean square error, which compares the precision of the line of the best fit to the original data points, as well as the R2 coefficient, was used to measure model correctness.

3.3 METABRIC Database

Nearly 2000 breast cancer patients' clinical and genetic information is available in the METABRIC database. The scope of our investigation was restricted to just taking into account clinical characteristics (24 from 31 clinical attributes in the database).

These 24 characteristics were the inputs used in our model to calculate patient survival time. Regarding the model's input variables, age_at_diagonosis is the most significant clinical factor.

Table 1. Implemented Features

#	Attributes
1	age_at_diagonosis
2	tumor_size
3	overall_survival
4	type_of_breast_surgery
5	cancer_type_detailed
6	cellularity
7	pam50_+_claudin_low_subtype
8	er_status_measured_by_ihc
9	er_status

continued on following page

Table 1. Continued

#	Attributes
10	her2_status_measured_by_snp6
11	her2_status
12	tumor_other_histologic_subtype
13	hormone_therapy
14	inferred_menopausal_state
15	primary_tumor_laterality
16	nottingham_prognostic_index
17	pr_status
18	oncotree_code
19	chemotherapy
20	cohort
21	neoplasm_histologic_grade
22	lymph_nodes_examined_positive
23	mutation_count
24	radio_therapy

4. PROGNOSIS MODEL CONSTRUCTION

4.1 XGBoost Method

Extreme Gradient Boosting, often known as XGBoost, is a broadly used slope-aided choice tree AI framework. This ensemble additive model is made up of many base learners. The main AI library for backslide, characterisation, and situating challenges, it provides equivalent tree supporting. Figure 2 shows how XGBoost is structured (Mehrotra, R., & Yadav, K. (2022), Liew, X. Y., Hameed, N., & Clos, J. (2021)).

Table 2. Symbols and their Meanings

Symbol	Meaning
p	Number of samples taken
q	Number of features taken
u_i	Features characteristics of the ith sample, $u_i \in R^q$

continued on following page

Table 2. Continued

Symbol	Meaning
v_i	The exact value of the ith sample
$\hat{v}_i$	The expected value of the ith sample
$\hat{v}_i^{(t)}$	The expected value up to the tth tree
$l(\hat{v}_i, \hat{v}_i^{(t)})$	The loss function of the ith sample
$L(v, \hat{v}_i)$	The loss function of total samples taken
$\Omega(f_k)$	Standard expression of objective function to avoid overfitting, where f_k represents the kth DT.

Figure 2. XGBoost

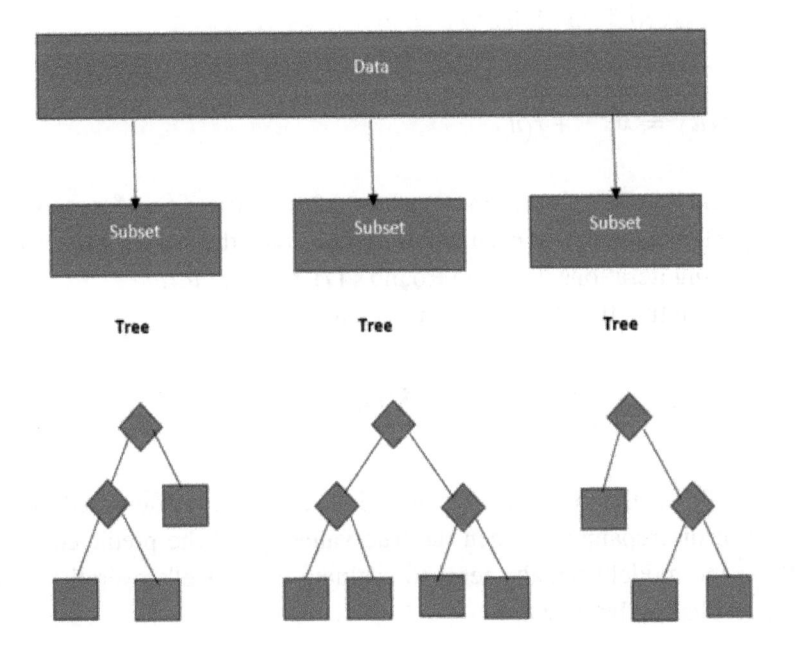

4.2 Model Construction

Table 1 displays the symbols and their meanings.

Given a data collection with q features and p samples, $D = \{(u_i, v_i) | u_i \in R^q, v_i \in R\}$ and $u_i = \{u_{i1}, u_{i2}, \ldots u_{iq} | i = 1,2,\ldots p\}$

This model's main objective is to construct t trees so that the projected value $\hat{v}_i^{(t)}$ up to the tth tree branch meets the following formula.

$$\hat{v}_i^{(0)} = 0$$

$$\hat{v}_i^{(1)} = f_1(u_i) = \hat{v}_i^{(0)} + f_1(u_i)$$

$$\hat{v}_i^{(2)} = f_1(u_i) + f_2(u_i) = \hat{v}_i^{(1)} + f_2(u_i) \ldots \ldots \quad (5)$$

$$\hat{v}_i^{(t)} = \sum_{k=1}^{t} f_k(u_i) = \hat{v}_i^{(t-1)} + f_t(u_i)$$

The gradient boosting algorithm creates a weak classifier $f_k(u_i)$ for each iteration, and the expected value $\hat{v}_i^{(t)}$ for each iteration represents the sum of expected values for the preceding iterations $\hat{v}_i^{(t-1)}$ and Round's DT result $f_t(u_i)$.

The objective function $L^{(t)}$ may be written as

$$\min L^{(t)}(\hat{v}_i, \hat{v}_i^{(t)}) = \min\left(\sum_{i=1}^{p} l(v_i, \hat{v}_i^{(t)}) + \sum_{k=1}^{t} \Omega(f_k)\right) \quad (6)$$

Here $l(\hat{v}_i, \hat{v}_i^{(t)})$ is the loss functions of various types. It is often used to measure the degree of discrepancy between the true value y_i and the predicted value $\hat{v}_i^{(t)}$. $\sum_{k=1}^{t} \Omega(f_k)$ the model's penalty term to evaluate the model's overall complexity and these results can be drawn:

$$\Omega(f_k) = \gamma N_k + \frac{1}{2}\lambda \sum_{j=1}^{N_k} \omega_{kj}^2 \quad (7)$$

where N_k represents the number of leaf nodes in the kth tree, γ represents coefficient the leaf node contraction, ω_{kj} is the score of the jth leaf node in the kth tree, and λ is the penalty coefficient the leaf node ω's score. Cross validation can be used to maximize the value of $\Omega(f_k)$.

In formula (5), replace with the predicted value $\hat{v}_i^{(t)}$ of the kth sample in the t round. The following equation may be derived by iteration of objective function of formula (6) and then applying approximation upto second-order of the Taylor expansion at $\hat{v}_i^{(t-1)}$ (using Chen's derivation (H. Li, Y. Cao, (2020))):

$$min\, L^{(t)} = min\left(\sum_{i=1}^{p}\left[g_i f_t(u_i) + \frac{1}{2}h_i f_t^2(u_i)\right] + \Omega(f_t)\right) \tag{8}$$

Here g_i is the first derivative and h_i second derivative of the loss function $l(u_i, \hat{u}_i^{(t)})$.
Total sample points on the jth leaf node in the DT is defined as $I_j = \{i | q(u_i) = j\}$, where ω denotes the leaf node's score and $r(u)$ denotes the structural function that projects the sample point x to location j of the leaf node. This allows us to describe the DT result as $\omega_{r(u)}$. Think of each DT $f(u)$ as containing an independent outcomes $\omega_{r(u)}$ of this tree and its tree structure $r(x)$, which are indicated as follows:

$$f(u) = \omega_{r(u)},\ \omega \in R^T,\ r:R \xrightarrow{d} \{1,2,3,.....,T\} \tag{9}$$

When formula (9) is substituted in formula (8), the next equation may be created.

$$min\, L^{(t)} = min\left(\sum_{j=1}^{T}\left[G_i \omega_{t,j} + \frac{1}{2}(H_j + \lambda)\omega_{i,j}^2\right] + \gamma N_t\right) \tag{10}$$

where $G_j = \sum_{i \in I_j} g_i$ and $H_j = \sum_{i \in I_j} h_i$
the actual label for the samples is either 1 or 0, this study uses the widely-used log loss function as lack of function.

$$l(v_i, \hat{v}_i^{(t)}) = -(v_i log(c_i) + (1 - v_i) log(1 - c_i))$$

where

$$c_i = \frac{1}{1 + e^{-\hat{v}_i^{(t)}}} \tag{11}$$

The probability of p samples $V_i = v(i = 1,2,....,p)$ can be obtained according to binomial distribution formula in probability.

$$P\{V_1 = v_1, V_2 = v_2, ...V_p = v_p\} = \prod_{i=1}^{p} c_i^{v_i}(1 - c_i)^{(1-v_i)} \tag{12}$$

We take the logarithm of formula to get the highest chance that C meets this requirement (12)

$$\ln C = \sum_{i=1}^{p} v_i \ln c_i + \sum_{i=1}^{p} (1 - v_i) \ln(1 - c_i) \qquad (13)$$

In this situation, we must meet the lnC maximal maximum probability function. The minimal value of the loss function may be comparable if the loss function is configured to be lnC. Then the values of g_i and h_i may be calculated using formula (11) to represent the loss function.

$$g_i = c_i - v_i \qquad (14)$$

$$h_i = c_i(1 - c_i) \qquad (15)$$

Similar to how we may select the softargmax function as the loss function for multiclassification issues.

$$l(v, c) = -\sum_{q=1}^{Q} y_q \log c_q, \text{ where } c_q = \frac{e^{p_i^{q_0}}}{\sum_{q=1}^{Q} e^{p_i^{q_0}}} \qquad (16)$$

where Q denotes a total of Q categories and q is the category of labels. Formula (16) degenerates into formula (11) when $Q = 2$.

5. OUR OBSERVATIONS AND RESULTS

With regard to the 24 clinically important characteristics that may be employed in future research to demonstrate a strong association to patient mortality rate and treatment alternatives, our study's findings were both valuable and consistent with the initial premise. We are able to accurately find the death rate XGBoost algorithm with an accuracy of 82.7272% approximately.

Figure 3. Death Rate According to Age Prediction through XGB Method

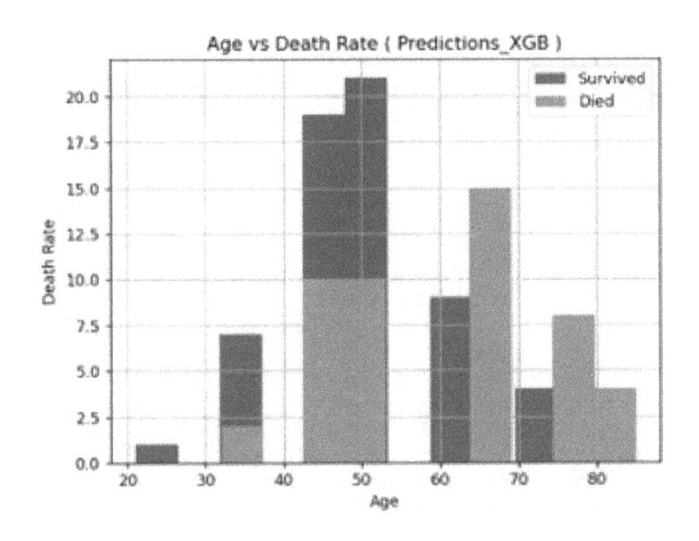

Figures 4, 5, and 6 below show the findings for three distinct algorithms along with the degree of accuracy that was achieved.

Table 3. Accuracy Obtained

ML Algorithm	Accuracy
Multivariate Regression	81.81818181818183%
Logistic Regression	78.18181818181819%
Random Forest	77.27272727272727%
XGBoost	82.72727272727273%

Figure 4. Death Rate According to Age Prediction through MVLR Method

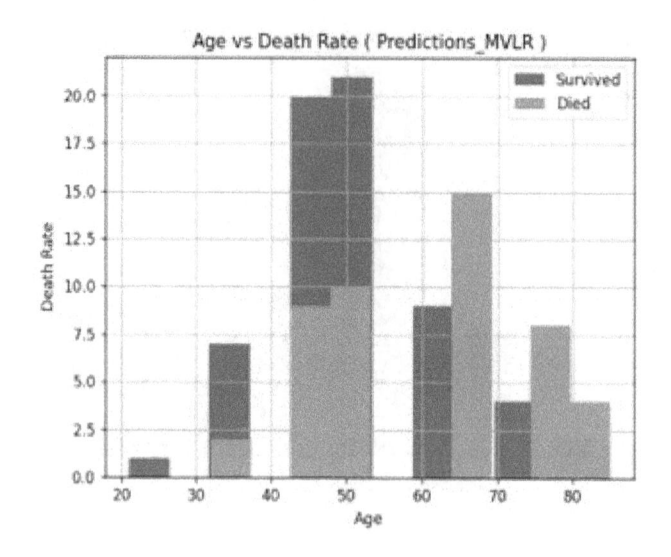

Figure 5. Death Rate According to Age Prediction through LR Method

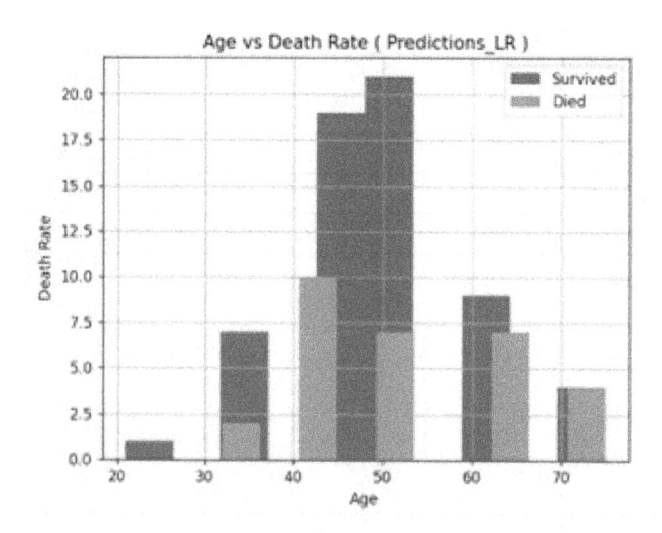

Figure 6. Death Rate According to Age Prediction through RF Method

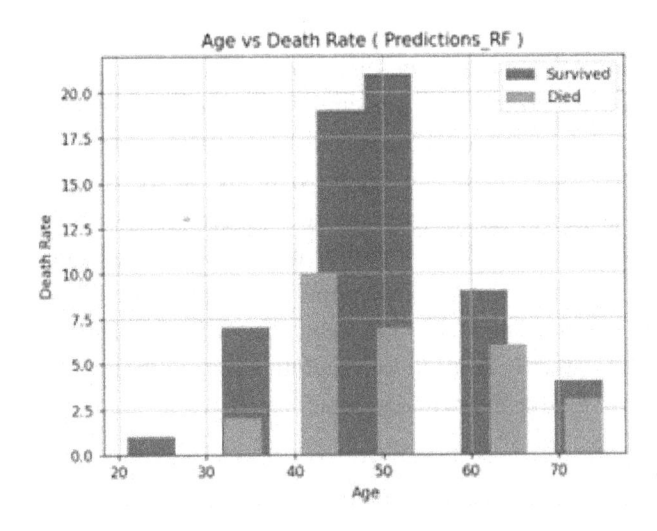

The comparison of the different methods at the different age of diagnosis is shown in Figure 7.

Figure 7. Comparison of the Methods at Different Age of Diagnosis

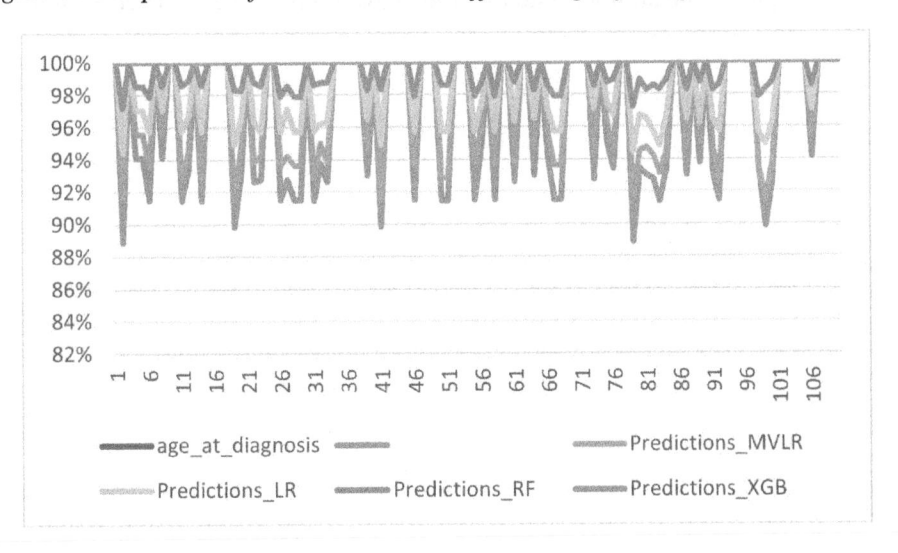

6. CONCLUSION

In the field of oncology, machine learning (ML) has just reached an advanced stage in the creation of prognostic classification models of cancer survival and progression. Our discovery represents a substantial advance in knowledge of clinical and genetic characteristics, which will help scientists and medical professionals enhance the treatment choices and quality of life for patients. In addition to the foregoing signs, the study may broaden its scope to include genetic disorders and subtypes defined by gene expression, which would be useful to provide more accurate forecasts. One of the difficulties in this discipline is to improve prediction accuracy by employing more sophisticated Machine Learning (ML) and Deep Learning (DL) models. This approach may be used to integrate a histopathological evaluation on bigger and more diverse real-world datasets.

Data Availability

Dataset is collected from METABRIC (Molecular Taxonomy of Breast Cancer International Consortium) database (El-Bendary, N., & Belal, N. A. (2020)) .

Conflict of interest statement

For this paper, the authors state that they have no possible conflicts of interest.

REFERENCES

Benz, C. C. (2008). Impact of aging on the biology of breast cancer. *Critical Reviews in Oncology/Hematology*, 66(1), 65–74. 10.1016/j.critrevonc.2007.09.00117949989

Breast cancer statistics and resources: Breast Cancer Research Foundation: BCRF. Breast Cancer Research Foundation. Retrieved July 21, 2022,

Burt, J. R., Torosdagli, N., Khosravan, N., RaviPrakash, H., Mortazi, A., Tissavirasingham, F., Hussein, S., & Bagci, U. (2018). Deep learning beyond cats and dogs: Recent advances in diagnosing breast cancer with deep neural networks. *The British Journal of Radiology*, 91(1089), 20170545. 10.1259/bjr.2017054529565644

Bustan, M. N., & Poerwanto, B. (2021). Logistic Regression Model of Relationship between Breast Cancer Pathology Diagnosis with Metastasis. *Journal of Physics: Conference Series*, 1752(1), 1752. 10.1088/1742-6596/1752/1/012026

Chi, B. W., & Hsu, C. C. (2012). A hybrid approach to integrate genetic algorithm into dual scoring model in enhancing the performance of credit scoring model. *Expert Systems with Applications*, 39(3), 2650–2661. 10.1016/j.eswa.2011.08.120

Duleba, A. J., & Olive, D. L. (1996). Regression analysis and multivariate analysis. *Seminars in Reproductive Endocrinology*, 14(2), 139–153. 10.1055/s-2007-10163228796937

El-Bendary, N., & Belal, N. A. (2020). A feature-fusion framework of clinical, genomics, and histopathological data for METABRIC breast cancer subtype classification. *Applied Soft Computing*, 91, 106238. 10.1016/j.asoc.2020.106238

Ferroni, P., Zanzotto, F. M., Riondino, S., Scarpato, N., Guadagni, F., & Roselli, M. (2019). Breast Cancer Prognosis Using a Machine Learning Approach. *Cancers (Basel)*, 11(3), 328. 10.3390/cancers1103032830866535

Gensheimer, M. F., Henry, A. S., Wood, D. J., Hastie, T. J., Aggarwal, S., Dudley, S. A., Pradhan, P., Banerjee, I., Cho, E., Ramchandran, K., Pollom, E., Koong, A. C., Rubin, D. L., & Chang, D. T. (2019). Automated Survival Prediction in Metastatic Cancer Patients Using High-Dimensional Electronic Medical Record Data. *Journal of the National Cancer Institute*, 111(6), 568–574. 10.1093/jnci/djy17830346554

Helwig, N. E. (2017). *Multivariate Linear Regression*. University of Minnesota.

Howlader, N., Cronin, K. A., Kurian, A. W., & Andridge, R. (2018). Differences in Breast Cancer Survival by Molecular Subtypes in the United States. *Cancer Epidemiology, Biomarkers & Prevention*, 27(6), 619–626. 10.1158/1055-9965. EPI-17-062729593010

Hueman, M. T., Wang, H., Yang, C. Q., Sheng, L., Henson, D. E., Schwartz, A. M., & Chen, D. (2018). Creating prognostic systems for cancer patients: A demonstration using breast cancer. *Cancer Medicine*, 7(8), 3611–3621. 10.1002/cam4.162929968970

Kabiraj, S., ….. "Breast Cancer Risk Prediction using XGBoost and Random Forest Algorithm," 2020 11th International Conference on Computing, Communication and Networking Technologies (ICCCNT), Kharagpur, India, 2020,1-4 10.1109/ICCCNT49239.2020.9225451

Kourou, K., Exarchos, T. P., Exarchos, K. P., Karamouzis, M. V., & Fotiadis, D. I. (2014). Machine learning applications in cancer prognosis and prediction. *Computational and Structural Biotechnology Journal*, 13, 8–17. 10.1016/j.csbj.2014.11.00525750696

H. Li, Y. Cao, S. Li, J. Zhao and Y. Sun, "XGBoost Model and Its Application to Personal Credit Evaluation," in IEEE Intelligent Systems, vol. 35, no. 3, 52-61, 1 May-June 2020, .10.1109/MIS.2020.2972533

Li, J., Zhou, Z., Dong, J., Fu, Y., Li, Y., Luan, Z., & Peng, X. (2021). Predicting breast cancer 5-year survival using machine learning: A systematic review. *PLoS One*, 16(4), e0250370. 10.1371/journal.pone.025037033861809

Li, M., Ruan, B., Yuan, C., Song, Z., Dai, C., Fu, B., Qiu, J., Maseleno, A., Yuan, X., & Balas, V. E. (2020). Intelligent system for predicting breast tumors using machine learning. *Journal of Intelligent & Fuzzy Systems*, 39(4), 4813–4822. 10.3233/JIFS-179967

Liew, X. Y., Hameed, N., & Clos, J. (2021). An investigation of XGBoost-based algorithm for breast cancer classification. *Machine Learning with Applications*, 6, 100154. 10.1016/j.mlwa.2021.100154

Mehrotra, R., & Yadav, K. (2022). Breast cancer in India: Present scenario and the challenges ahead. *World Journal of Clinical Oncology*, 13(3), 209–218. 10.5306/wjco.v13.i3.20935433294

Octaviani, L., & Rustam, Z. (2019). Random forest for breast cancer prediction. *AIP Conference Proceedings*, 2168, 020050. 10.1063/1.5132477

Pillai, V., Koohpayegani, S. A., Ouligian, A., Fong, D., & Pirsiavash, H. (2021). Consistent Explanations by Contrastive Learning. *2022 IEEE/CVF Conference on Computer Vision and Pattern Recognition (CVPR)*, 10203-10212.

Seddik, F., & Shawky, D. M. "Logistic regression model for breast cancer automatic diagnosis," *2015 SAI Intelligent Systems Conference (IntelliSys)*, London, UK, 2015, 150-154 10.1109/IntelliSys.2015.7361138

Spanos, A., & Hendry, D. (2011). The multivariate linear regression model. *Statistical Foundations of Econometric Modeling*, 571–607.

Torre, L. A., Bray, F., Siegel, R. L., Ferlay, J., Lortet-Tieulent, J., & Jemal, A. (2015). Global cancer statistics, 2012. *CA: a Cancer Journal for Clinicians*, 65(2), 87–108. 10.3322/caac.2126225651787

Chapter 4
Applications of AI Techniques in Healthcare and Wellbeing

S. C. Vetrivel
https://orcid.org/0000-0003-3050-8211
Kongu Engineering College, India

V. P. Arun
JKKN College of Engineering and Technology, India

R Maheswari
Kongu Engineering College, India

T. P. Saravanan
Kongu Engineering College, India

ABSTRACT

The integration of Artificial Intelligence (AI) techniques in healthcare and wellbeing systems has witnessed significant advancements, offering transformative solutions to traditional healthcare paradigms. This chapter provides a comprehensive overview of the diverse applications of AI in the healthcare sector, highlighting its potential to enhance diagnostics, treatment planning, personalized medicine, and overall patient outcomes. AI techniques, including machine learning and deep learning algorithms, have demonstrated remarkable capabilities in analyzing large datasets such as medical images, genetic information, and electronic health records. These technologies enable more accurate and timely disease detection, improving diagnostic accuracy and aiding healthcare professionals in making informed decisions. In treatment planning, AI-driven systems contribute to the development of personalized

DOI: 10.4018/979-8-3693-3719-6.ch004

Copyright © 2024, IGI Global. Copying or distributing in print or electronic forms without written permission of IGI Global is prohibited.

therapeutic strategies. By leveraging patient-specific data, AI models can predict treatment responses, optimize drug regimens, and minimize adverse effects.

1. INTRODUCTION TO AI IN HEALTHCARE

1.1. Overview of Artificial Intelligence

Artificial Intelligence (AI) is a multidisciplinary field of computer science that focuses on the development of intelligent machines capable of performing tasks that typically require human intelligence. The overarching goal of AI is to create systems that can learn, reason, problem-solve, and adapt to changing environments (Alexandrova, 2012). The field encompasses various subfields, including machine learning, natural language processing, computer vision, robotics, and expert systems. Machine learning, a subset of AI, involves the use of algorithms and statistical models to enable systems to improve their performance on a specific task through experience. Natural language processing focuses on enabling computers to understand, interpret, and generate human language. Computer vision allows machines to interpret and make decisions based on visual data. Robotics integrates AI to develop intelligent machines capable of interacting with the physical world. AI applications are diverse, ranging from virtual assistants and recommendation systems to autonomous vehicles and healthcare diagnostics. As AI technologies advance, ethical considerations, transparency, and responsible development practices become increasingly important to ensure the responsible and beneficial deployment of AI systems in various domains.

1.2. Evolution of AI in Healthcare

The evolution of artificial intelligence (AI) in healthcare has been a transformative journey, revolutionizing the way medical professionals deliver care and manage patient data. In the early stages, AI applications in healthcare primarily focused on automating administrative tasks and streamlining workflow processes. As technology advanced, machine learning algorithms became more sophisticated, enabling AI systems to analyze vast amounts of medical data with unprecedented speed and accuracy. Diagnostic tools powered by AI, such as image recognition algorithms for medical imaging, have significantly improved the speed and accuracy of disease detection. Natural language processing (NLP) has been instrumental in extracting valuable insights from unstructured clinical notes, making it easier for healthcare providers to access and utilize patient information effectively (Ahmed et al., 2020; Al-Zewairi et al., 2017). Furthermore, AI has played a pivotal role in personalized medicine, tailoring treatment plans based on individual patient characteristics, genetics, and historical health data. The integration of AI in healthcare has not only enhanced diagnostic capabilities but has also facilitated predictive analytics for disease prevention and early intervention. As the field continues to evolve, ethical considerations, data privacy, and regulatory frameworks become critical components to address, ensuring the responsible and ethical deployment of AI technologies in healthcare settings. Overall, the evolution of AI in healthcare holds immense promise for improving patient outcomes, reducing costs, and advancing medical research and innovation.

1.3. Importance and Impact of AI in Healthcare

Artificial Intelligence (AI) has emerged as a transformative force in healthcare, revolutionizing the industry by enhancing efficiency, accuracy, and patient outcomes. One of the primary advantages of AI in healthcare is its ability to analyze vast amounts of data quickly and identify patterns that may be beyond the scope of human capability. This enables healthcare professionals to make more informed decisions, leading to improved diagnosis and treatment planning. AI applications, such as machine learning algorithms, can process and interpret medical images, such as X-rays and MRIs, with remarkable accuracy, aiding in early detection of diseases like cancer and facilitating timely interventions. In addition to diagnostic capabilities, AI plays a crucial role in personalized medicine (Ahmed & Liang, 2019). By analyzing an individual's genetic makeup, lifestyle factors, and health history, AI algorithms can tailor treatment plans to match the specific needs of each patient. This not only maximizes the efficacy of treatments but also minimizes adverse effects, showcasing the potential for more targeted and efficient healthcare delivery. Another significant impact of AI in healthcare is its contribution to predictive analytics. By analyzing patient data over time, AI algorithms can predict disease progression and identify high-risk individuals. This proactive approach allows healthcare providers to intervene early, preventing or mitigating the severity of certain conditions. This not only improves patient outcomes but also helps in resource allocation, reducing the burden on healthcare systems. Furthermore, AI-powered virtual health assistants and chatbots have proven valuable in enhancing patient engagement and providing real-time support. These tools can offer personalized health advice, medication reminders, and monitor patients' vital signs remotely, enabling continuous care beyond traditional clinical settings. This can be particularly beneficial for individuals with chronic conditions, fostering a more patient-centric and accessible healthcare model (Arnold & Wade, 2015). Despite these remarkable advancements, the integration of AI in healthcare also presents challenges, including concerns about data privacy, ethical considerations, and the need for regulatory frameworks. Striking a balance between harnessing the potential of AI and addressing these challenges is crucial to realizing the full benefits of AI in healthcare. As technology continues to evolve, ongoing research, collaboration, and ethical guidelines will be essential to maximize the positive impact of AI on the health and well-being of individuals worldwide.

2. FUNDAMENTALS OF HEALTHCARE AND WELLBEING

2.1. Basics of Healthcare Systems

The fundamentals of healthcare and wellbeing encompass a broad spectrum of elements, with the healthcare system playing a pivotal role in promoting and maintaining individual and community health. At its core, a healthcare system is a complex network of institutions, professionals, and resources dedicated to delivering medical services and ensuring the overall well-being of a population (Aucejo et al., 2020). This system is designed to provide preventive, curative, rehabilitative, and palliative care, addressing a wide range of health issues. One key aspect of healthcare fundamentals is accessibility. An effective healthcare system strives to ensure that healthcare services are accessible to all members of society without discrimination. This involves not only the physical availability of healthcare facilities but also financial accessibility, considering the affordability of services. Achieving universal health coverage, where everyone has access to essential healthcare services without facing financial hardship, is a fundamental goal for many healthcare systems worldwide. Quality and safety are critical components of healthcare fundamentals. Quality healthcare ensures that services are evidence-based, effective, and provided by qualified professionals. Patient safety measures are in place to minimize the risk of harm during the course of medical interventions. Standardization of medical practices, accreditation of healthcare facilities, and ongoing quality improvement initiatives contribute to maintaining high standards of care within the healthcare system. Healthcare systems also emphasize the importance of preventive care. Fundamentals of healthcare include promoting healthy behaviors, preventing diseases, and identifying risk factors early on. Public health campaigns, immunization programs, and screenings are examples of initiatives aimed at reducing the burden of illness on both individuals and society as a whole. In terms of organization, healthcare systems are often structured into primary, secondary, and tertiary levels of care. Primary care serves as the first point of contact for individuals seeking healthcare, focusing on preventive care and managing common health issues. Secondary and tertiary care involve specialized medical services and interventions, such as surgery or intensive care, for more complex health conditions (Badawi et al., 2014). The fundamentals of healthcare systems are also closely tied to healthcare policy and governance. Governments, regulatory bodies, and healthcare organizations work together to establish policies, regulations, and guidelines that guide the delivery of healthcare services. Effective governance ensures the equitable distribution of resources, ethical practices, and accountability within the healthcare system.

2.2. Challenges in Healthcare

The challenges in healthcare under the fundamentals of healthcare and wellbeing are multifaceted and can vary across different regions and healthcare systems. However, several common challenges persist globally (Baumgartner et al., 2021). Addressing these challenges requires collaboration among governments, healthcare providers, researchers, and communities. Solutions often involve a combination of policy changes, technological advancements, and community engagement to create a more inclusive and effective healthcare system. Here are some key challenges:

- **Access to Healthcare:** Disparities in access to healthcare services exist, both within and between countries. Economic, geographical, and social factors can limit individuals' ability to access necessary healthcare, leading to unequal health outcomes.
- **Cost of Healthcare:** The rising cost of healthcare is a significant challenge, affecting individuals, families, and governments. High healthcare costs can lead to financial barriers, limiting access to necessary treatments and preventive care.
- **Quality of Care:** Ensuring consistent and high-quality healthcare is challenging. Disparities in healthcare quality can result from variations in healthcare provider practices, resources, and infrastructure.
- **Health Information Technology:** The integration of health information technology, including electronic health records (EHRs) and telemedicine, presents challenges related to interoperability, data security, and ensuring that technology enhances rather than hinders patient care.
- **Preventive Care and Health Promotion:** Encouraging preventive measures and health-promoting behaviors is a fundamental aspect of healthcare. However, challenges include promoting healthy lifestyles, preventing chronic diseases, and ensuring individuals have access to regular screenings and vaccinations.
- **Workforce Shortages:** Many regions face shortages of healthcare professionals, including doctors, nurses, and other allied health workers. This shortage can strain healthcare systems and lead to increased workloads for existing staff.

- **Global Health Threats:** Emerging infectious diseases, pandemics, and global health threats, such as the COVID-19 pandemic, highlight the need for coordinated international responses and robust public health infrastructure.
- **Mental Health:** Mental health challenges, including stigma, access to mental health services, and the integration of mental health into primary care, continue to be significant issues in healthcare.
- **Aging Population:** The aging population in many countries poses challenges in terms of increased demand for healthcare services, long-term care, and managing chronic conditions associated with aging.
- **Healthcare Policy and Governance:** Developing effective healthcare policies, governance structures, and regulatory frameworks is crucial for ensuring equitable access to quality healthcare and addressing the evolving needs of populations.
- **Health Disparities:** Disparities in health outcomes based on factors such as race, ethnicity, socioeconomic status, and gender persist. Addressing these disparities requires a comprehensive and holistic approach.
- **Bioethical and Legal Issues:** Healthcare faces complex bioethical and legal challenges, including issues related to patient autonomy, informed consent, medical privacy, and the ethical use of emerging technologies.

2.3. Importance of Wellbeing

The importance of wellbeing is a fundamental aspect of healthcare, encompassing both physical and mental dimensions. At the core of healthcare principles lies the recognition that individuals thrive when their overall wellbeing is nurtured and maintained. Physical health is a cornerstone, as it directly influences one's ability to lead a fulfilling life. Regular exercise, balanced nutrition, and preventive healthcare measures contribute to the maintenance of physical wellbeing, reducing the burden of illness on individuals and society. Equally crucial is the emphasis on mental health within the framework of wellbeing. Mental and emotional stability are integral components of overall health, impacting cognitive function, interpersonal relationships, and daily functioning (Beam & Kohane, 2018; Bono et al., 2020). Recognizing the significance of mental health has led to a shift in healthcare paradigms, with a growing emphasis on holistic approaches that address both the body and the mind. Interventions such as counseling, psychotherapy, and stress management techniques are integral components of healthcare strategies aimed at promoting mental wellbeing. Moreover, the interconnectedness of physical and mental health underscores the need for a comprehensive healthcare system that addresses the multifaceted nature of wellbeing. Lifestyle factors, including diet, exercise, sleep, and stress management, play pivotal roles in preventing diseases and promoting overall health. Healthcare practitioners increasingly recognize the importance of patient education, empowering individuals to make informed choices that positively impact their wellbeing. Beyond individual health, the concept of wellbeing extends to community and societal levels (Brodeur et al., 2021). Healthy individuals contribute to the productivity and resilience of communities, fostering social cohesion and economic stability. Therefore, public health initiatives and policies that prioritize wellbeing can have far-reaching implications, promoting a society where individuals are not merely free from illness but actively engaged in activities that enhance their quality of life.

3. DATA IN HEALTHCARE

3.1. Importance of Data in Healthcare

Data plays a crucial role in the healthcare sector, contributing significantly to the improvement of patient outcomes, operational efficiency, and overall quality of care. One of the key aspects of the importance of data in healthcare is its role in supporting evidence-based decision-making. Healthcare professionals rely on accurate and timely data to make informed choices about patient treatment plans, medication prescriptions, and diagnostic interventions. This data-driven approach ensures that healthcare providers can offer the most effective and personalized care to patients, leading to better health outcomes. Furthermore, data in healthcare is instrumental in facilitating medical research and innovation. Researchers can leverage large datasets to identify patterns, trends, and correlations that may lead to breakthroughs in disease understanding, prevention, and treatment. This continuous cycle of data collection and analysis fosters a dynamic environment for scientific advancements, ultimately benefiting both healthcare professionals and patients alike. In healthcare management, data serves as a powerful tool for improving operational efficiency and resource allocation. Hospitals and healthcare organizations can use data to optimize workflows, reduce wait times, and enhance resource utilization, leading to cost savings and improved patient satisfaction. Data analytics also aids in predicting and preventing potential issues, such as identifying high-risk patients and implementing proactive interventions to prevent complications. Patient engagement and empowerment are also enhanced through the effective use of data in healthcare. Electronic health records (EHRs) enable patients to access their medical information, track their health metrics, and actively participate in shared decision-making with healthcare providers. This transparency and involvement empower patients to take a more proactive role in managing their health, leading to better compliance with treatment plans and improved overall well-being.

3.2. Types of Healthcare Data

Healthcare data can be categorized into various types, each serving different purposes and contributing to the overall management and improvement of healthcare services. Understanding and effectively utilizing these different types of healthcare data are crucial for improving patient care, enhancing healthcare outcomes, and optimizing healthcare systems (Burns et al., 2020). However, it's essential to prioritize patient privacy and adhere to ethical and legal standards when handling healthcare data. Following are some key types of healthcare data:

Electronic Health Records (EHRs) and Electronic Medical Records (EMRs):
o **EHRs:** These are comprehensive digital records of a patient's health information. EHRs are designed to be shared across different healthcare settings, providing a holistic view of a patient's medical history, medications, allergies, test results, and more.
o **EMRs:** Similar to EHRs, EMRs are digital versions of paper charts in a clinician's office. They contain patient information, such as medical history, diagnoses, medications, immunization dates, allergies, and treatment plans.

Medical Imaging Data:
o This includes data from various imaging techniques like X-rays, CT scans, MRI scans, ultrasounds, and more. These images aid in diagnosing and monitoring conditions.

Clinical Data:
o Clinical data encompasses a wide range of information collected during patient care, such as vital signs (heart rate, blood pressure, temperature), laboratory results, pathology reports, and other clinical observations.

Administrative and Billing Data:
o This type of data includes information related to healthcare administration and billing processes. It involves patient demographics, insurance details, billing codes, and other financial aspects of healthcare services.

Genomic and Molecular Data:
o With advancements in genomics, healthcare now involves the collection and analysis of genetic information. Genomic data provides insights into an individual's genetic makeup, allowing for personalized medicine and targeted therapies.

Public Health Data:
o This type of data is collected at a population level and is used to monitor and improve public health. It includes information about disease out-

breaks, vaccination rates, environmental factors, and epidemiological studies.

Patient-Generated Health Data (PGHD):
o   PGHD is data collected directly from patients, often through wearable devices or mobile apps. It includes information about daily activities, exercise, sleep patterns, and other lifestyle factors.

Research and Clinical Trial Data:
o   Data generated from clinical trials and medical research contribute to the advancement of medical knowledge. This includes data on drug efficacy, treatment outcomes, and patient responses.

Healthcare Surveys and Patient Feedback:
o   Surveys and patient feedback provide valuable information about patient satisfaction, healthcare experiences, and areas for improvement in healthcare services.

Healthcare Analytics Data:
o   This involves the use of data analytics tools to derive insights from various healthcare data sources, enabling better decision-making, resource allocation, and predictive modeling.

Telehealth and Remote Monitoring Data:
o   With the rise of telehealth, data collected from virtual consultations and remote monitoring devices contribute to the management of chronic conditions and preventive healthcare.

3.3. Data Collection and Storage

Data collection and storage in healthcare play a pivotal role in modern healthcare systems, facilitating improved patient care, research, and overall operational efficiency. The process of collecting healthcare data involves gathering information from various sources, including electronic health records (EHRs), medical devices, wearable technologies, and patient-reported data (Butler & Kern, 2016). EHRs, in particular, have become a cornerstone in healthcare data collection, as they centralize comprehensive patient information such as medical history, medications, diagnoses, and treatment plans. Healthcare organizations must adhere to strict regulations and ethical standards when collecting and storing patient data. Compliance with regulations like the Health Insurance Portability and Accountability Act (HIPAA) in the United States ensures the confidentiality, integrity, and availability of patient information. Secure and standardized data collection methods help protect sensitive patient data from unauthorized access, ensuring patient privacy and maintaining trust in healthcare systems. Data storage in healthcare involves the secure retention of vast amounts of patient information (Carter et al., 2013). Cloud-based storage solutions have gained popularity due to their scalability, accessibility, and cost-effectiveness. However, concerns regarding data security and privacy necessitate robust encryption protocols and stringent access controls. Many healthcare institutions also implement on-premises storage solutions with advanced security measures to maintain control over sensitive data. Interoperability is a critical aspect of data storage in healthcare, ensuring that different systems and applications can seamlessly exchange and use information. Standardized formats, such as Health Level Seven (HL7) and Fast Healthcare Interoperability Resources (FHIR), enable the integration of diverse healthcare data sources. This interoperability enhances care coordination, facilitates research collaborations, and supports the development of innovative healthcare solutions. Data analytics and artificial intelligence (AI) are increasingly utilized in healthcare data storage, helping extract valuable insights from large datasets. Predictive analytics, machine learning algorithms, and data mining enable healthcare professionals to identify trends, predict disease outbreaks, and personalize treatment plans. These technologies also contribute to ongoing medical research, ultimately advancing the understanding and treatment of various health conditions.

4. MACHINE LEARNING IN HEALTHCARE

4.1. Introduction to Machine Learning

Machine Learning (ML) is a transformative field that leverages algorithms and statistical models to enable computers to learn patterns and make predictions or decisions without explicit programming. In the context of healthcare, ML holds immense potential to revolutionize various aspects of the industry, from diagnostics and treatment planning to personalized medicine and healthcare management (Chan et al., 2018). The integration of ML in healthcare aims to enhance efficiency, accuracy, and overall patient outcomes. Healthcare generates vast amounts of data, including patient records, medical images, genomic information, and clinical notes. Machine Learning algorithms can analyze this data to uncover valuable insights, identify patterns, and predict outcomes. This data-driven approach facilitates more precise diagnostics, early detection of diseases, and tailored treatment plans. Additionally, ML algorithms can assist healthcare professionals in making informed decisions by providing evidence-based recommendations and predictions. One significant application of Machine Learning in healthcare is in medical imaging. ML algorithms can be trained on large datasets of medical images to detect abnormalities, tumors, or other anomalies with high accuracy. This not only expedites the diagnostic process but also reduces the risk of human error (Clifton et al., 2012;

Cloutier et al., 2019). Furthermore, predictive modeling using ML can help forecast disease progression, allowing for proactive intervention and personalized treatment strategies. In the realm of personalized medicine, Machine Learning plays a crucial role in analyzing genetic and molecular data to understand individual variations in response to treatment. By identifying biomarkers and genetic patterns, ML enables the development of targeted therapies, minimizing adverse effects and optimizing treatment outcomes. This shift towards personalized medicine is indicative of the potential for ML to revolutionize healthcare practices, moving from a one-size-fits-all approach to more tailored and effective interventions.

However, the integration of Machine Learning in healthcare also poses challenges, including data privacy concerns, ethical considerations, and the need for regulatory frameworks. As ML applications become more prevalent in healthcare, addressing these challenges will be essential to ensure the responsible and ethical use of technology for the benefit of patients and healthcare providers alike..

4.2. Applications of Machine Learning in Healthcare

Machine Learning (ML) has shown significant promise in various applications within the healthcare sector, transforming the way medical data is analyzed, diagnosed, and treated. These applications of machine learning in healthcare have the potential to improve patient outcomes, enhance efficiency, and contribute to the overall advancement of the healthcare industry. However, it is crucial to address challenges related to data privacy, ethics, and regulatory compliance in the deployment of these technologies. Below given are some key applications of machine learning in healthcare:

- **Disease Prediction and Diagnosis:** ML algorithms can analyze large datasets, including patient records, medical images, and genomic data, to identify patterns and predict the likelihood of certain diseases. This is particularly valuable for early detection and diagnosis.
- **Medical Imaging:** ML is extensively used in medical imaging for tasks such as image segmentation, object detection, and classification. It helps in improving the accuracy and efficiency of diagnostic processes, especially in fields like radiology and pathology.
- **Drug Discovery and Development:** ML accelerates the drug discovery process by analyzing biological data, identifying potential drug candidates, and predicting their efficacy. This can lead to more efficient and cost-effective drug development.
- **Personalized Medicine:** ML algorithms analyze patient data, including genetic information, to tailor treatments to individual patients. This enables

healthcare providers to develop personalized treatment plans that are more effective and have fewer side effects.
- **Health Monitoring and Wearables:** ML algorithms can analyze data from wearable devices and other health monitoring tools to provide real-time insights into a person's health. This is valuable for continuous monitoring of chronic conditions and early detection of health issues.
- **Clinical Decision Support Systems:** ML-powered decision support systems assist healthcare professionals by providing relevant information and suggestions based on patient data. This aids in making more informed and timely clinical decisions.
- **Fraud Detection and Healthcare Management:** ML helps in identifying fraudulent activities, such as insurance claims fraud, by analyzing patterns in data. It also aids in optimizing hospital operations, resource allocation, and patient flow management.
- **Natural Language Processing (NLP) in Healthcare:** NLP, a subset of ML, is used to extract valuable information from unstructured medical data, such as clinical notes and research papers. This facilitates better data utilization for research, diagnosis, and treatment planning.
- **Remote Patient Monitoring:** ML enables the development of systems that continuously monitor and analyze patient data remotely. This is particularly useful for managing chronic conditions, allowing for early intervention and reducing the need for frequent hospital visits.
- **Epidemiology and Public Health:** ML can analyze large-scale healthcare data to predict disease outbreaks, track the spread of infectious diseases, and assist in public health planning and resource allocation.

4.3. Case Studies of ML in Diagnosis and Treatment

These case studies demonstrate the versatility and potential impact of machine learning in improving the diagnosis and treatment of various medical conditions. As technology continues to advance, the integration of machine learning in healthcare is likely to play an increasingly significant role in enhancing patient care.

Cancer Diagnosis with Deep Learning:

- **Problem:** Detecting cancerous tumors in medical images is a challenging task that requires accuracy.
- **Solution:** Researchers have developed deep learning models, such as convolutional neural networks (CNNs), to analyze medical images

like mammograms and identify patterns indicative of cancer. Google's DeepMind, for instance, has worked on breast cancer detection using AI.

Diabetes Management with Predictive Analytics:

- **Problem:** Predicting and managing blood glucose levels in diabetes patients is crucial for effective treatment.
- **Solution:** Machine learning algorithms have been applied to analyze patient data, including glucose levels, diet, and activity, to predict future blood sugar levels. This enables personalized treatment plans and proactive management to prevent complications.

Alzheimer's Disease Prediction:

- **Problem:** Early detection of Alzheimer's disease is challenging but crucial for better patient outcomes.
- **Solution:** Machine learning models have been trained on various data types, including brain imaging, genetic information, and cognitive assessments, to predict the likelihood of developing Alzheimer's disease. These models assist in early diagnosis and intervention.

Drug Discovery and Development:

- **Problem:** Traditional drug discovery is a time-consuming and expensive process.
- **Solution:** Machine learning accelerates drug discovery by predicting potential drug candidates, optimizing molecular structures, and identifying drug interactions. Atomwise, for example, uses deep learning for virtual screening of potential drug compounds.

Personalized Cancer Treatment with Genomic Data:

- **Problem:** Traditional cancer treatments may not be effective for every patient due to genetic variations.
- **Solution:** Machine learning analyzes genomic data to identify specific genetic markers and predict which treatments are most likely to be effective for an individual patient. This approach leads to more personalized and targeted cancer therapies.

Sepsis Detection in Intensive Care Units (ICUs):

- **Problem:** Early detection of sepsis in ICU patients is critical for timely intervention and improved outcomes.
- **Solution:** Machine learning models have been developed to analyze real-time patient data, including vital signs and laboratory results, to predict the onset of sepsis. These models help clinicians identify at-risk patients early, leading to prompt treatment.

5. NATURAL LANGUAGE PROCESSING (NLP) IN HEALTHCARE

5.1. Overview of NLP

Natural Language Processing (NLP) in healthcare refers to the application of artificial intelligence (AI) and computational linguistics to enable computers to understand, interpret, and generate human-like text. In the healthcare sector, NLP plays a crucial role in extracting valuable insights from unstructured data present in clinical notes, medical records, and other textual sources (Coburn & Gormally, 2020; Cooke et al., 2016). The primary goal is to enhance the efficiency of healthcare processes, improve patient outcomes, and facilitate evidence-based decision-making. One of the key aspects of NLP in healthcare is the ability to process and analyze large volumes of text data rapidly. With the proliferation of electronic health records (EHRs), NLP algorithms can extract pertinent information from these records, such as patient demographics, medical history, and treatment plans. This not only streamlines administrative tasks but also assists healthcare professionals in making informed decisions by providing a comprehensive view of a patient's health journey. Moreover, NLP in healthcare extends beyond data extraction to sentiment analysis and contextual understanding. By analyzing the sentiment in patient narratives, healthcare providers can gain insights into the emotional well-being of patients, helping in personalized care and patient engagement. Contextual understanding enables NLP systems to interpret medical jargon, abbreviations, and contextual nuances present in clinical documentation, contributing to more accurate and meaningful analyses. NLP applications in healthcare also include clinical decision support systems, where these technologies assist healthcare providers in diagnosing diseases, recommending treatment plans, and predicting patient outcomes. By leveraging the wealth of information embedded in medical literature and research articles, NLP contributes to evidence-based medicine, allowing practitioners to stay updated on the latest advancements and integrate them into their clinical practice (Costanza-Chock, 2020). Despite the potential benefits, challenges exist in implementing NLP in healthcare, including the need for robust data privacy and security measures, ensuring compliance with healthcare regulations, and addressing the inherent variability and complexity of medical language. However, as technology continues to advance and more healthcare organizations adopt NLP solutions, the field holds immense promise for transforming the way healthcare data is utilized, ultimately improving patient care and outcomes.

5.2. NLP Applications in Healthcare

Natural Language Processing (NLP) has emerged as a powerful tool in the healthcare sector, revolutionizing various aspects of patient care, administrative tasks, and medical research. One significant application of NLP in healthcare is in clinical documentation. By automating the extraction of information from unstructured clinical notes, NLP helps healthcare professionals save time and improve accuracy in medical records. This not only enhances the efficiency of healthcare providers but also contributes to better patient outcomes by ensuring comprehensive and up-to-date medical histories (Crawford, 2020). Another crucial area where NLP is making substantial contributions is in disease surveillance and epidemiology. NLP algorithms can analyze vast amounts of textual data from sources such as electronic health records, social media, and news articles to detect and monitor disease outbreaks. This real-time analysis enables healthcare authorities to respond promptly to emerging health threats, implement preventive measures, and allocate resources effectively, ultimately enhancing public health strategies. Furthermore, NLP facilitates the development of clinical decision support systems. These systems leverage natural language understanding to interpret medical literature, guidelines, and patient data, assisting healthcare professionals in making well-informed and evidence-based decisions. This application of NLP not only improves the quality of patient care but also helps in reducing medical errors and optimizing treatment plans. In addition to clinical applications, NLP is instrumental in patient engagement and support (Daher et al., 2017). Chatbots and virtual assistants equipped with NLP capabilities enable patients to interact with healthcare systems more effectively. These tools can provide information about medications, appointment scheduling, and general health inquiries, enhancing patient experience and fostering a sense of empowerment and involvement in their own healthcare. Lastly, NLP plays a pivotal role in biomedical research and literature mining. By analyzing vast amounts of scientific literature, NLP systems can extract valuable insights, identify trends, and accelerate the discovery of new medical knowledge. This application not only aids researchers in staying abreast of the latest developments but also supports the advancement of medical science and the discovery of novel treatments and therapies. Overall, the integration of NLP in healthcare applications holds great promise in transforming the industry, improving patient outcomes, and advancing medical research.

6. COMPUTER VISION IN HEALTHCARE

6.1. Imaging and Diagnostics

Imaging and diagnostics play a pivotal role in revolutionizing healthcare through the integration of computer vision technologies. Computer vision in healthcare refers to the application of artificial intelligence (AI) algorithms and image processing techniques to analyze medical images, thus aiding in the early detection, diagnosis, and treatment of various conditions. Advanced imaging modalities, such as magnetic resonance imaging (MRI), computed tomography (CT), X-rays, and ultrasound, generate vast amounts of medical data that can be overwhelming for human interpretation (D'Alfonso, 2020; De Pue et al., 2021). Computer vision algorithms excel in extracting meaningful insights from these images by identifying patterns, anomalies, and relevant features. These technologies enhance the accuracy and efficiency of diagnostic processes, leading to quicker and more precise medical assessments. Additionally, computer vision contributes to the automation of tasks such as tumor detection, organ segmentation, and disease classification, allowing healthcare professionals to focus on interpretation and decision-making. The continuous evolution of computer vision in healthcare promises to improve patient outcomes, streamline workflows, and foster a more proactive approach to disease management.

6.2. Robotics and Surgery

Robotics and surgery have undergone a transformative evolution in the healthcare sector, thanks to the integration of computer vision technologies. Computer vision, a subset of artificial intelligence, empowers machines to interpret and make decisions based on visual data. In the context of robotics and surgery, computer vision plays a pivotal role in enhancing precision, efficiency, and safety. In robotic surgery, computer vision enables robotic systems to perceive the surgical environment with a level of detail and accuracy that surpasses human capabilities. Advanced imaging technologies, such as three-dimensional (3D) reconstruction and augmented reality, allow robots to visualize the patient's anatomy in real-time. This heightened visual acuity aids surgeons in navigating complex anatomical structures with unparalleled precision during minimally invasive procedures (Labovitz et al., 2017). Computer vision algorithms also assist in tracking and compensating for patient movements, contributing to improved surgical outcomes.

Moreover, computer vision in robotics facilitates the development of autonomous or semi-autonomous surgical robots. These robots can utilize visual information to adapt to dynamic changes in the operating field, making decisions in real-time based on the surgeon's input and predefined parameters. The integration of machine learning algorithms further refines the robot's ability to recognize and respond to diverse surgical scenarios, contributing to a more personalized and adaptive approach to patient care. In the field of computer vision-assisted surgery, the technology extends beyond the operating room. Pre-operative planning benefits from the analysis of medical imaging data, such as CT scans and MRIs, to create detailed maps of the patient's anatomy (Moreb et al., 2020). During surgery, computer vision aids in instrument tracking, enabling surgeons to precisely control robotic tools and ensure accurate incisions. Postoperative monitoring and analysis benefit from computer vision algorithms that can assess patient recovery, identify potential complications, and contribute to data-driven decision-making for optimal postoperative care.

7. PREDICTIVE ANALYTICS AND MODELING

7.1. Predictive Analytics in Healthcare

Predictive analytics in healthcare, situated under the broader category of Predictive Analytics and Modeling, has emerged as a pivotal tool revolutionizing the healthcare industry. This specialized field leverages advanced statistical algorithms and machine learning techniques to analyze historical data and identify patterns, trends, and potential future outcomes. The primary goal is to anticipate health-related events, streamline decision-making processes, and ultimately improve patient outcomes. In the realm of healthcare, predictive analytics is employed for a myriad of purposes. One significant application involves predicting disease occurrences and patient outcomes (Naylor, 2018; Rajkomar et al., 2019). By analyzing extensive datasets that include patient demographics, medical history, and diagnostic test results, healthcare professionals can forecast the likelihood of diseases such as diabetes, cardiovascular conditions, or even infectious diseases. This enables early intervention and personalized treatment plans tailored to individual patient needs, thereby enhancing the effectiveness of healthcare delivery. Moreover, predictive analytics plays a crucial role in resource optimization within healthcare systems. Hospitals and healthcare organizations utilize predictive models to forecast patient admission rates, allocate resources efficiently, and manage staff levels effectively. This proactive approach aids in reducing overcrowding, improving resource utilization, and ultimately enhancing the overall quality of care provided to patients.

7.2. Disease Prediction and Prevention Models

Predictive analytics and modeling play a pivotal role in the realm of disease prediction and prevention, offering innovative approaches to foresee and mitigate potential health threats. These models harness advanced statistical techniques and machine learning algorithms to analyze vast datasets containing information about individuals' health, lifestyle, genetic factors, and environmental influences. By leveraging these data, predictive models can identify patterns and correlations that may serve as early indicators of diseases. One key aspect of disease prediction models involves the use of electronic health records (EHRs) and patient data to build predictive algorithms (Salvador-Meneses et al., 2019; Upadhyay & Khandelwal, 2019). These algorithms can predict the likelihood of an individual developing a particular disease based on their medical history, genetic predispositions, and lifestyle choices. This personalized approach enables healthcare professionals to intervene proactively, providing targeted interventions and preventive measures tailored to an individual's unique risk profile. Furthermore, the integration of genetic information into predictive models has led to significant advancements in disease prediction. Genomic data analysis allows for the identification of genetic markers associated with various diseases, enabling the development of models that can assess an individual's genetic susceptibility to certain conditions (Zhou et al., 2019). This information empowers individuals and healthcare providers to implement preventive measures, such as lifestyle modifications or early screening, to reduce the risk of disease onset. In addition to individual-level predictions, predictive analytics is also employed at the population level to anticipate disease outbreaks and epidemics. By analyzing patterns in large-scale data, such as social media trends, environmental factors, and geographical information, these models can identify potential hotspots for disease emergence. Public health authorities can then allocate resources strategically and implement targeted interventions to curb the spread of infectious diseases. The continuous refinement of predictive models is driven by advancements in technology, including the incorporation of artificial intelligence and deep learning techniques.

These sophisticated models can discern complex relationships within datasets and adapt to changing patterns over time. This adaptability enhances their ability to accurately predict disease trends and recommend effective prevention strategies (Ura et al., 2012). While predictive analytics and modeling offer promising avenues for disease prediction and prevention, ethical considerations, such as privacy concerns and data security, must be carefully addressed. Striking a balance between the potential benefits of these models and protecting individual privacy is crucial to ensure the responsible and effective use of predictive analytics in healthcare. As these models evolve, they have the potential to revolutionize disease prevention by enabling timely interventions, improving healthcare outcomes, and ultimately reducing the burden of diseases on individuals and healthcare systems.

7.3. Personalized Medicine

Personalized medicine, within the realm of predictive analytics and modeling, represents a transformative approach to healthcare that tailors medical treatment and interventions to the individual characteristics of each patient. Predictive analytics plays a crucial role in this paradigm by leveraging advanced algorithms and statistical models to analyze vast amounts of patient data, including genetic information, lifestyle factors, environmental influences, and clinical histories. Through the integration of these diverse datasets, predictive models can identify patterns, correlations, and potential risk factors, enabling healthcare professionals to make more informed decisions about personalized treatment plans.

In the context of personalized medicine, genetic information is a key component that predictive analytics leverages for modeling. Genetic data, obtained through techniques such as genomic sequencing, allows for the identification of specific genetic variations associated with diseases, drug responses, and susceptibility to certain conditions. Predictive models can analyze this genetic information to predict an individual's likelihood of developing a particular disease, their response to specific medications, and the potential risks and benefits of different treatment options (VanderWeele, 2019). Furthermore, predictive analytics in personalized medicine goes beyond genetics to incorporate other factors influencing health. Lifestyle data, including diet, physical activity, and environmental exposures, is considered to provide a more comprehensive understanding of an individual's health profile. Predictive models can assess how these lifestyle factors interact with genetic information, enabling healthcare providers to recommend personalized interventions that consider both genetic predispositions and environmental influences. In the realm of treatment optimization, predictive analytics aids in predicting individual responses to medications. By analyzing a patient's genetic makeup and other relevant data, models can anticipate how an individual is likely to respond to a specific drug, including potential side effects and efficacy. This information empowers healthcare providers to prescribe medications that are more tailored to an individual's unique characteristics, improving the overall effectiveness of treatments while minimizing adverse reactions.

8. AI IN DRUG DISCOVERY AND DEVELOPMENT

8.1. Drug Discovery Process

The integration of Artificial Intelligence (AI) in the drug discovery process has revolutionized the traditional methodologies, accelerating and enhancing the efficiency of drug development. The AI-driven drug discovery process typically begins with target identification, where machine learning algorithms analyze biological data to identify potential drug targets, such as specific proteins or genes associated with a disease (Wang et al., 2020). Subsequently, AI algorithms aid in virtual screening, predicting and assessing the interactions between potential drug candidates and target molecules. This expedites the identification of lead compounds for further development. Machine learning models also play a crucial role in optimizing drug design by predicting the pharmacokinetic and toxicity profiles of candidate compounds (Dodge et al., 2012). Furthermore, AI facilitates data integration from diverse sources, including genomics, proteomics, and clinical data, enabling a more comprehensive understanding of disease mechanisms. Additionally, AI-driven algorithms contribute to patient stratification, predicting responders to specific treatments based on individual patient characteristics.

8.2. Role of AI in Drug Development

The role of artificial intelligence (AI) in drug development has revolutionized the field of drug discovery and development, offering unprecedented advancements in efficiency, speed, and accuracy. AI plays a crucial role in various stages of the drug development process, from target identification and validation to lead optimization and clinical trial design. Machine learning algorithms analyze vast datasets, including genomics, proteomics, and chemical structures, to identify potential drug targets and predict the therapeutic efficacy of compounds (Diener et al., 1985; Diener et al., 1999). This enables researchers to prioritize and focus on the most promising candidates, significantly reducing the time and resources required for drug discovery. Additionally, AI enhances the optimization of drug candidates by predicting their pharmacokinetics and toxicity profiles, leading to more informed decisions in the preclinical phase. In clinical trials, AI aids in patient stratification, identifying suitable biomarkers, and optimizing trial designs to increase the likelihood of success (Dooris et al., 2018). The integration of AI technologies in drug development not only accelerates the pace of innovation but also holds the potential to deliver more precise and personalized therapies, ultimately improving patient outcomes.

8.3. Drug Repurposing and Accelerated Research

Drug repurposing, also known as drug repositioning, is a strategy in drug discovery and development that involves identifying new uses for existing drugs. This approach has gained significant traction in recent years, thanks to the integration of Artificial Intelligence (AI) into drug discovery processes. AI in drug discovery expedites the identification of potential candidates for repurposing by analyzing vast datasets, including biological and chemical information (Dubberly & Pangaro, 2007; Dubberly & Pangaro, 2019). Machine learning algorithms can sift through these datasets to uncover hidden relationships between drugs and diseases, providing valuable insights for researchers. Accelerated research under AI in drug discovery and development involves the use of advanced technologies to streamline and expedite the traditionally time-consuming phases of drug development. AI algorithms can analyze large-scale genomic and proteomic data, predict drug-target interactions, and optimize compound structures, significantly reducing the time and cost associated with bringing a new drug to market. By leveraging AI, researchers can identify promising drug candidates more efficiently, prioritize compounds with higher success probabilities, and design clinical trials with greater precision. This transformative approach not only enhances the speed of drug development but also increases the likelihood of discovering novel therapeutic applications for existing drugs through the repurposing strategy.

9. VIRTUAL HEALTH ASSISTANTS AND CHATBOTS IN HEALTHCARE

Virtual Health Assistants (VHAs) and chatbots have emerged as transformative technologies in the healthcare industry, playing pivotal roles in enhancing patient engagement, improving efficiency, and delivering personalized care (European Commission, 2019; Fawaz & Samaha, 2021; Fioramonti et al., 2022). These intelligent systems leverage artificial intelligence (AI) and natural language processing (NLP) to interact with users, providing a wide range of healthcare-related services. One significant application of VHAs and chatbots in healthcare is patient communication and education. These tools facilitate seamless communication between healthcare providers and patients, offering information on medications, treatment plans, and lifestyle recommendations. VHAs can address patient queries, provide medication reminders, and offer real-time support, thereby enhancing patient compliance and overall health outcomes. Furthermore, these technologies contribute to the optimization of administrative processes within healthcare organizations. Chatbots integrated into electronic health record (EHR) systems can streamline appointment scheduling, prescription refills, and billing inquiries (Fokkinga et al., 2020). By automating routine administrative tasks, VHAs enable healthcare professionals to focus more on direct patient care, reducing administrative burdens and improving operational efficiency. In the realm of mental health, virtual health assistants and chatbots have proven to be valuable tools. They provide a confidential and easily accessible platform for individuals to express their feelings, receive emotional support, and access mental health resources (Frisch et al., 1992). These technologies can offer mental health assessments, coping strategies, and even crisis intervention, bridging gaps in mental health services and reaching a wider audience.

10. ETHICAL AND REGULATORY CONSIDERATIONS

10.1. Ethical Issues in AI in Healthcare

Ethical issues in AI within the healthcare domain have become increasingly prominent, raising concerns and necessitating careful consideration of both ethical and regulatory aspects. One major concern revolves around patient privacy and the security of sensitive health data (Genç & Arslan, 2021). As AI systems process vast amounts of personal information to make predictions or recommendations, ensuring robust safeguards against unauthorized access and data breaches is imperative. Moreover, there is a growing ethical dilemma regarding transparency and accountability in AI algorithms (Gillespie et al., 2014). The complex nature of these algorithms often makes it challenging to understand their decision-making processes, leading to the "black box" problem. Stakeholders, including healthcare professionals and patients, need transparency to trust AI systems and hold them accountable for their actions. Additionally, biases in AI models pose a significant ethical challenge, as they can perpetuate existing disparities in healthcare outcomes. Addressing these biases requires constant vigilance and rigorous testing to ensure fair and equitable AI applications (Glanville, 2009; Graham et al., 2019). Striking a balance between innovation and ethical considerations is crucial, necessitating comprehensive regulatory frameworks that evolve alongside technological advancements to uphold the ethical principles of beneficence, autonomy, justice, and privacy in healthcare AI systems.

10.2. Privacy and Security Concerns

Privacy and security concerns occupy a central position within the realm of ethical and regulatory considerations, especially in the rapidly evolving landscape of technology and data-driven environments. With the proliferation of digital platforms, the collection, storage, and utilization of personal information have become ubiquitous, giving rise to heightened apprehensions about individual privacy. Ethically, the responsible handling of sensitive data is imperative to ensure that individuals retain control over their personal information, fostering a sense of trust between users and technology providers (Gregory et al., 2019). On the regulatory front, governments and international bodies are grappling with the task of creating and enforcing laws that strike a delicate balance between enabling innovation and safeguarding privacy. The General Data Protection Regulation (GDPR) in Europe and similar initiatives globally underscore the need for transparency, consent, and robust security measures to protect against unauthorized access and data breaches. Striking an ethical equilibrium requires ongoing collaboration between stakeholders, including technology developers, policymakers, and the public, to establish norms that protect privacy while enabling the benefits of technological advancements (Hagey & Horwitz, 2021). In this complex landscape, addressing privacy and security concerns is not merely a legal obligation but a fundamental ethical imperative that underpins the responsible development and deployment of technology.

11. FUTURE TRENDS AND INNOVATIONS

The future of healthcare and wellbeing is poised for transformative advancements through the integration of cutting-edge Artificial Intelligence (AI) techniques. One prominent trend is the increasing use of machine learning algorithms for personalized medicine. AI can analyze vast amounts of patient data, including genetic information, lifestyle factors, and historical health records, to tailor treatment plans that are uniquely suited to individual needs. This not only enhances the efficacy of medical interventions but also minimizes adverse effects, ultimately leading to more efficient and patient-centric healthcare. Another significant innovation in AI for healthcare involves the application of natural language processing (NLP) and sentiment analysis to improve patient communication and support. Chatbots equipped with advanced language models can engage in empathetic and context-aware conversations with individuals, providing real-time support, answering queries, and even detecting emotional cues. Such AI-driven interactions have the potential to enhance mental health support, facilitate preventive care, and contribute to overall patient satisfaction. Furthermore, the development of AI-powered diagnostic tools is set to revolutionize disease detection and monitoring. Computer vision algorithms, when applied to medical imaging data such as X-rays, MRIs, and CT scans, can assist healthcare professionals in identifying abnormalities and diagnosing conditions with greater accuracy and speed (Hekkert & van Dijk, 2011; Hu et al., 2021). This not only expedites the diagnostic process but also enables early intervention, significantly improving patient outcomes. The integration of blockchain technology with AI is also a promising trend in healthcare. Blockchain can enhance the security and integrity of health data, ensuring that sensitive patient information remains confidential while still being accessible to authorized parties. Combining blockchain with AI allows for the creation of decentralized, interoperable health records that streamline data sharing among different healthcare providers, leading to more comprehensive and collaborative patient care. In the realm of wellbeing, AI-driven applications are increasingly focused on preventive measures. Wearable devices equipped with AI algorithms can monitor vital signs, detect irregularities, and provide proactive health insights. These devices empower individuals to take charge of their wellbeing by adopting healthier lifestyles, adhering to fitness routines, and managing stress levels effectively. As the field of AI in healthcare and wellbeing continues to evolve, ethical considerations, data privacy, and regulatory frameworks will play crucial roles in shaping the responsible and effective implementation of these technologies. Nevertheless, the ongoing convergence of AI techniques with healthcare promises a future where personalized, efficient, and accessible healthcare and wellbeing solutions become integral components of our daily lives.

12. CHALLENGES AND LIMITATIONS

Artificial Intelligence (AI) holds immense promise in transforming healthcare and wellbeing, but it also faces several challenges and limitations that need careful consideration. One significant challenge is the integration of AI into existing healthcare systems. Many healthcare facilities operate with outdated or incompatible IT infrastructure, making it difficult to seamlessly incorporate AI technologies. The interoperability issues between different software and hardware platforms can hinder the effective deployment of AI solutions, limiting their potential impact on patient care. Another major concern is the ethical and privacy implications of AI in healthcare. The use of AI often involves handling large volumes of sensitive patient data. Maintaining the privacy and security of this information is crucial, and there is a constant need for robust regulations and safeguards to prevent unauthorized access or misuse of personal health data. Striking the right balance between utilizing AI for improved diagnostics and treatments while respecting patient confidentiality is an ongoing challenge (Khan et al., 2021). Furthermore, the lack of standardized protocols and guidelines for AI applications in healthcare poses a significant limitation. The diversity of healthcare settings, patient populations, and medical conditions makes it challenging to create universally applicable algorithms and models. Developing standardized frameworks and protocols that can be adapted across different healthcare contexts is essential for the widespread adoption and effectiveness of AI in healthcare. The interpretability and explainability of AI models in healthcare represent another hurdle. In critical medical decision-making, it is essential for healthcare professionals to understand how AI algorithms arrive at their conclusions (Kjell & Diener, 2020). Black-box algorithms that lack transparency may lead to skepticism and hinder the acceptance of AI technologies among healthcare practitioners. Striving for more interpretable AI models is crucial to gaining trust and fostering collaboration between AI systems and healthcare professionals. Moreover, the potential for bias in AI algorithms is a pressing concern. If the training data used to develop AI models is not representative or if biases exist in the data, the algorithms may produce results that disproportionately impact certain demographic groups. This raises ethical issues and could contribute to healthcare disparities. Addressing biases in AI algorithms requires careful consideration during the development and training phases, as well as ongoing monitoring and refinement to ensure fair and equitable outcomes.

13. CONCLUSION

AI techniques have emerged as transformative tools in the realm of healthcare and wellbeing, offering unprecedented opportunities for improving patient outcomes, enhancing diagnostic accuracy, and optimizing treatment strategies. The integration of machine learning, natural language processing, and predictive analytics has paved the way for more personalized and efficient healthcare solutions. While challenges such as data privacy and ethical considerations remain, the potential benefits of AI in healthcare are vast. As technology continues to advance, the synergy between artificial intelligence and healthcare promises to revolutionize the industry, ultimately contributing to a more accessible, cost-effective, and patient-centric approach to wellbeing. The ongoing collaboration between healthcare professionals and AI systems holds the promise of ushering in a new era of precision medicine and comprehensive healthcare management.

REFERENCES

Ahmed, Z., & Liang, B. T. (2019, March). Systematically dealing practical issues associated to healthcare data analytics. In *Future of Information and Communication Conference* (pp. 599-613). Springer.

Ahmed, Z., Mohamed, K., Zeeshan, S., & Dong, X. (2020). Artificial intelligence with multi-functional machine learning platform development for better healthcare and precision medicine. *Database (Oxford)*, 2020, baaa010. Advance online publication. 10.1093/database/baaa01032185396

Al-Zewairi, M., Biltawi, M., Etaiwi, W., & Shaout, A. (2017). Agile software development methodologies: Survey of surveys. *Journal of Computer and Communications*, 5(05), 74–97. 10.4236/jcc.2017.55007

Alexandrova, A. (2012). Well-being as an object of science. *Philosophy of Science*, 79(5), 678–689. 10.1086/667870

Arnold, R. D., & Wade, J. P. (2015). A definition of systems thinking: A systems approach. *Procedia Computer Science*, 44, 669–678. 10.1016/j.procs.2015.03.050

Aucejo, E. M., French, J., Ugalde Araya, M. P., & Zafar, B. (2020). The impact of COVID-19 on student experiences and expectations: evidence from a survey. J. Public Econ. 191, 104271–104271. doi: .2020.10427110.1016/j.jpubeco

Badawi, O., Brennan, T., Celi, L. A., Feng, M., Ghassemi, M., Ippolito, A., Johnson, A., Mark, R. G., Mayaud, L., Moody, G., Moses, C., Naumann, T., Nikore, V., Pimentel, M., Pollard, T. J., Santos, M., Stone, D. J., & Zimolzak, A. (2014). Making big data useful for health care: A summary of the inaugural mit critical data conference. *JMIR Medical Informatics*, 2(2), e3447. 10.2196/medinform.344725600172

Baumgartner, J., Ruettgers, N., Hasler, A., Sonderegger, A., & Sauer, J. (2021). Questionnaire experience and the hybrid system usability scale: Using a novel concept to evaluate a new instrument. *International Journal of Human-Computer Studies*, 147, 102575–102575. 10.1016/j.ijhcs.2020.102575

Beam, A. L., & Kohane, I. S. (2018). Big data and machine learning in health care. *Journal of the American Medical Association*, 319(13), 1317–1318. 10.1001/jama.2017.1839129532063

Bono, G., Reil, K., & Hescox, J. (2020). Stress and wellbeing in urban college students in the U.S. during the COVID-19 pandemic: Can grit and gratitude help? *International Journal of Wellbeing*, 10(3), 39–57. 10.5502/ijw.v10i3.1331

Brodeur, A., Clark, A. E., Fleche, S., & Powdthavee, N. (2021). COVID-19, lockdowns and well-being: Evidence from Google trends. *Journal of Public Economics*, 193, 104346–104346. 10.1016/j.jpubeco.2020.10434633281237

Burns, D., Dagnall, N., & Holt, M. (2020). Assessing the impact of the COVID-19 pandemic on student wellbeing at universities in the United Kingdom: A conceptual analysis. *Frontiers in Education*, 5, 5. 10.3389/feduc.2020.582882

Butler, J., & Kern, M. L. (2016). The PERMA-profiler: A brief multidimensional measure of flourishing. *International Journal of Wellbeing*, 6(3), 1–48. 10.5502/ijw.v6i3.526

Carter, K., Banks, S., Armstrong, A., Kindon, S., & Burkett, I. (2013). Issues of disclosure and intrusion: Ethical challenges for a community researcher. *Ethics & Social Welfare*, 7(1), 92–100. 10.1080/17496535.2013.769344

Chan, L., Swain, V. D., Kelley, C., de Barbaro, K., Abowd, G. D., & Wilcox, L. (2018). Students' experiences with ecological momentary assessment tools to report on emotional well-being. *Proceedings of the ACM on Interactive, Mobile, Wearable and Ubiquitous Technologies*, 2(1), 1–20. 10.1145/3191735

Clifton, D. A., Gibbons, J., Davies, J., & Tarassenko, L. (2012, June). Machine learning and software engineering in health informatics. In 2012 first international workshop on realizing ai synergies in software engineering (raise) (pp. 37-41). IEEE. 10.1109/RAISE.2012.6227968

Cloutier, S., Ehlenz, M., & Afinowich, R. (2019). Cultivating community wellbeing: Guiding principles for research and practice. *International Journal of Community Well-being*, 2(3-4), 277–299. 10.1007/s42413-019-00033-x

Coburn, A., & Gormally, S. (2020). Defining well-being in community development from the ground up: A case study of participant and practitioner perspectives. *Community Development Journal: An International Forum*, 55(2), 237–257. 10.1093/cdj/bsy048

Cooke, P. J., Melchert, T. P., & Connor, K. (2016). Measuring well-being: A review of instruments. *The Counseling Psychologist*, 44(5), 730–757. 10.1177/0011000016633507

Costanza-Chock, S. (2020). *Design justice: Community-led practices to build the worlds we need*. The MIT Press. 10.7551/mitpress/12255.001.0001

Crawford, D. N. (2020). Supporting student wellbeing during COVID-19. Tips from regional and remote Australia.

D'Alfonso, S. (2020). AI in mental health. *Current Opinion in Psychology*, 36, 112–117. 10.1016/j.copsyc.2020.04.00532604065

Daher, M., Carré, P. D., Jaramillo, A., Olivares, H., & Tomicic, A. (2017). Experience and meaning in qualitative research: a conceptual review and a methodological device proposal. Forum Qual. Sozialforschung 18. 10.17169/fqs-18.3.2696

De Pue, S., Gillebert, C., Dierckx, E., Vanderhasselt, M.-A., De Raedt, R., & Van den Bussche, E. (2021). The impact of the COVID-19 pandemic on wellbeing and cognitive functioning of older adults. *Scientific Reports*, 11(1), 4636. 10.1038/s41598-021-84127-733633303

Diener, E., Emmons, R. A., Larsen, R., & Griffin, S. (1985). The satisfaction with life scale. *Journal of Personality Assessment*, 49(1), 71–75. 10.1207/s15327752jpa4901_1316367493

Diener, E., Suh, E. M., Lucas, R. E., & Smith, H. L. (1999). Subjective well-being: Three decades of progress. *Psychological Bulletin*, 125(2), 276–302. 10.1037/0033-2909.125.2.276

Dodge, R., Daly, A., Huyton, J., & Sanders, L. (2012). The challenge of defining wellbeing. *International Journal of Wellbeing*, 2(3), 222–235. 10.5502/ijw.v2i3.4

Dooris, M., Farrier, A., & Froggett, L. (2018). Wellbeing: The challenge of 'operationalising' an holistic concept within a reductionist public health programme. *Perspectives in Public Health*, 138(2), 93–99. 10.1177/1757913917711204 28574301

Dubberly, H., & Pangaro, P. (2007). Cybernetics and service-craft: Language for behavior-focused design. *Kybernetes*, 36(9/10), 1301–1317. 10.1108/03684920710827319

Dubberly, H., & Pangaro, P. (2019). Cybernetics and design: Conversations for action. *Design Research Foundations*, 85–99. 10.1007/978-3-030-18557-2_4

European Commission. (2019). A definition of artificial intelligence: Main capabilities and scientific disciplines. Shaping Europe's digital future. Retrieved from https://digital-strategy.ec.europa.eu/en/library/definition-artificial-intelligence-main-capabilities-and-scientific-disciplines

Fawaz, M., & Samaha, A. (2021). E-learning: Depression, anxiety, and stress symptomatology among Lebanese university students during COVID-19 quarantine. *Nursing Forum*, 56(1), 52–57. 10.1111/nuf.1252133125744

Fioramonti, L., Coscieme, L., Costanza, R., Kubiszewski, I., Trebeck, K., Wallis, S., Roberts, D., Mortensen, L. F., Pickett, K. E., Wilkinson, R., Ragnarsdottír, K. V., McGlade, J., Lovins, H., & De Vogli, R. (2022). Wellbeing economy: An effective paradigm to mainstream post-growth policies? *Ecological Economics*, 192, 107261. 10.1016/j.ecolecon.2021.107261

Fokkinga, S. F., Desmet, P. M. A., & Hekkert, P. (2020). Impact-centered design: Introducing an integrated framework of the psychological and behavioral effects of design. *International Journal of Design*, 14(2), 97–116.

Frisch, M. B., Cornell, J., Villanueva, M., & Retzlaff, P. J. (1992). Clinical validation of the quality of life inventory: A measure of life satisfaction for use in treatment planning and outcome assessment. *Psychological Assessment*, 4(1), 92–101. 10.1037/1040-3590.4.1.92

Genç, E., & Arslan, G. (2021). Optimism and dispositional hope to promote college students' subjective well-being in the context of the COVID-19 pandemic. *Journal of Positive School Psychology*, 5(2), 87–96. 10.47602/jpsp.v5i2.255

Gillespie, T. (2014). The relevance of algorithms. In Gillespie, T., Boczkowski, P. J., & Foot, K. A. (Eds.), *Media Technologies* (pp. 167–194). The MIT Press. 10.7551/mitpress/9042.003.0013

Glanville, R. (2009). Article. *System Science and Cybernetics*, 3, 59–86.

Graham, S., Depp, C., Lee, E. E., Nebeker, C., Tu, X., Kim, H.-C., & Jeste, D. V. (2019). Artificial intelligence for mental health and mental illnesses: An overview. *Current Psychiatry Reports*, 21(11), 116. 10.1007/s11920-019-1094-031701320

Gregory, T., Engelhardt, D., Lewkowicz, A., Luddy, S., Guhn, M., Gadermann, A., Schonert-Reichl, K., & Brinkman, S. (2019). Validity of the middle years development instrument for population monitoring of student wellbeing in Australian school children. *Child Indicators Research*, 12(3), 873–899. 10.1007/s12187-018-9562-3

Hagey, K., & Horwitz, J. (2021). Facebook tried to make its platform a healthier place. It got angrier instead. *Wall Street Journal*, 1–16.

Hekkert, P., & van Dijk, M. (2011). *Vision in design - a guidebook for innovators*. BIS Publishers.

Hu, C., Chen, C., & Dong, X.-P. (2021). Impact of COVID-19 pandemic on patients with neurodegenerative diseases. *Frontiers in Aging Neuroscience*, 13, 664965. 10.3389/fnagi.2021.66496533897410

Khan, I., Shah, D., & Shah, S. S. (2021). COVID-19 pandemic and its positive impacts on environment: An updated review. *International Journal of Environmental Science and Technology*, 18(2), 521–530. 10.1007/s13762-020-03021-333224247

Kjell, O. N. E., & Diener, , E. (2020). Abbreviated Three-Item Versions of the Satisfaction with Life Scale and the Harmony in Life Scale Yield as Strong Psychometric Properties as the Original Scales. *Journal of Personality Assessment*, 0, 1–2. 10.1080/00223891.2020.173709332167788

Labovitz, D. L., Shafner, L., Reyes Gil, M., Virmani, D., & Hanina, A. (2017). Using artificial intelligence to reduce the risk of nonadherence in patients on anticoagulation therapy. *Stroke*, 48(5), 1416–1419. 10.1161/STROKEAHA.116.01628128386037

Moreb, M., Mohammed, T. A., & Bayat, O. (2020). A novel software engineering approach toward using machine learning for improving the efficiency of health systems. *IEEE Access : Practical Innovations, Open Solutions*, 8, 23169–23178. 10.1109/ACCESS.2020.2970178

Naylor, C. D. (2018). On the prospects for a (deep) learning health care system. *Journal of the American Medical Association*, 320(11), 1099–1100. 10.1001/jama.2018.1110330178068

Rajkomar, A., Dean, J., & Kohane, I. (2019). Machine learning in medicine. *The New England Journal of Medicine*, 380(14), 1347–1358. 10.1056/NEJMra181425930943338

Salvador-Meneses, J., Ruiz-Chavez, Z., & Garcia-Rodriguez, J. (2019). Compressed kNN: K-Nearest Neighbors with Data Compression. *Entropy (Basel, Switzerland)*, 21(3), 234. 10.3390/e2103023433266949

Upadhyay, A. K., & Khandelwal, K. (2019). Artificial intelligence-based training learning from application. *Development and Learning in Organizations*, 33(2), 20–23. Advance online publication. 10.1108/DLO-05-2018-0058

Ura, K., Alkire, S., & Zangmo, T. (2012). *GNH and GNH Index*. Centre for Bhutan Studies.

VanderWeele, T. J. (2019). Measures of community well-being: A template. *International Journal of Community Well-being*, 2(3-4), 253–275. 10.1007/s42413-019-00036-8

Wang, F., Kaushal, R., & Khullar, D. (2020). Should health care demand interpretable artificial intelligence or accept "black box" medicine? *Annals of Internal Medicine*, 172(1), 59–60. 10.7326/M19-254831842204

Zhou, Y., Zhao, L., Zhou, N., Zhao, Y., Marino, S., Wang, T., Sun, H., Toga, A. W., & Dinov, I. D. (2019). Predictive big data analytics using the UK Biobank data. *Scientific Reports*, 9(1), 1–10. 10.1038/s41598-019-41634-y30979917

Chapter 5
Artificial Intelligence in Records Structures Research:
A Systematic Literature Review and Research Agenda

P. Immaculate Rexi Jenifer
SASTRA University (Deemed), India

M. Rajakumaran
SASTRA University (Deemed), India

A. Dennis Ananth
SASTRA University (Deemed), India

S. Markkandeyan
https://orcid.org/0000-0002-7408-1523
SASTRA University (Deemed), India

R. G. Gokila
SASTRA University (Deemed), India

ABSTRACT

AI has received expanded interest from the data systems (IS) studies network in recent years. There is, however, a developing difficulty that studies on AI should enjoy a loss of cumulative building of information, which has overshadowed IS research formerly. This look at addresses this subject, by way of engaging in a scientific literature overview of AI studies in IS between 2005 and 2020. The seek

DOI: 10.4018/979-8-3693-3719-6.ch005

approach ended in 1877 research, of which 98 had been diagnosed as primary research and a synthesise of key issues which might be pertinent to this take a look at is presented. In doing so, this has a look at makes important contributions, namely (i) an identification of the modern mentioned enterprise price and contributions of AI, (ii) research and sensible implications on the use of AI and (iii) opportunities for destiny AI studies inside the shape of the AI research.

1. INTRODUCTION

It has been asserted that AI has the ability to revolutionize a wide range of sectors and businesses, including delivery chains, pharmaceuticals, and autos. According to studies, artificial intelligence (AI) offers opportunities to reimagine business models, change the nature of work in the future, boost productivity, and even enhance human talents. The International Data Corporation (IDC) projects that global spending on AI will reach about $98 billion in 2023, more than twice the $37.5 billion that was spent in 2019. This indicates the increased interest in using AI to transform economies. However, there is disagreement over what AI is and how it differs from other virtual technologies. The increase in interest in AI in recent years can be traced to a few factors.

This systematic review's objectives are to:

1. Determine AI's claimed business value and contributions; and
2. Look at the practical effects on AI use.
3. Determine the prospects for upcoming AI studies in IS research.

The chapter is organized as follows. First, a summary of relevant AI research in the topic of IS is given. After that, the systematic literature review technique is described and the study's limitations are noted. The state-of-the-art in AI research is then discussed, along with the technology's purported contributions and business value as well as a definitional examination. A discussion, some consequences, and a future study agenda follow. A conclusion and suggestions for more research round out the work.

2. BACKGROUND AND RELATED WORK

This section commences with an overview of extant information systems literature on AI. The lack of clarity concerning the concept and classification of AI are discussed.

AI has a history a good deal longer than is commonly understood, in fields from technological know-how and philosophy ranging all the way lower back to historical Greece (Dennehy, 2020), however its contemporary new release owes much to Alan Turing (Turing, 1950) and conventionin Dartmouth College in 1956 (McCorduck, 2004), wherein the term "Artificial Intelligence" turned into formally coined and described throughJohn McCarthy on the time as "the technology and engineering of making clever machines". Russel and Norvig (2020) referred to it because the "the beginning of synthetic intelligence." One of the initial paradigms of AI changed into that it revolved round high-degree cognition. Not the capacity to comprehend concepts, understand items, or execute complicated motor abilties shared with the aid of maximum animals, however the potential to engage in multi-step reasoning, to recognize the meaning of natural language, to layout innovative artefacts, to generate novel plans that attain dreams, and even to purpose about their very own reasoning (Langley, 2011).This standard human like intelligence changed into called strong AI (Kurzweil, 2005). For sturdy AI, the number one method has targeted on symbolic reasoning, that computer systems aren't honestly numeric calculators but instead fashionable symbol manipulators. As stated by Newell and Simon (1976) in their physical image machine hypothesis, shrewd behaviour seems to require the capacity to interpret and control symbolic systems. While this technique showed promise to start with (Newell & Simon, 1963), many branches of AI have retreated from this approach due its difficulty and the lack of progress coming in to the twenty first century. It remains yet unsure on while and if sturdy AI could be made a reality.

The distinction between susceptible AI and robust AI is likewise worried with rule adherence, i.e., the way machines interact with regulations. Abubakar, A. M, distinguishes rule-based selection making wherein machines strictly appreciate the regulations set via builders from rule following decision making which machines follow guidelines which have not been strictly precise to them. Rule-based choice-making suits weak AI, whilst rule-following selection making is an try that tends towards robust AI. An instance of rule-following decision making is neural networks (NN), which allow algorithms to examine from themselves. Strong AI could be machines making their very own regulations after which comply with them, which isn't always possible at the degree of right now (Abubakar, A. M).

AI has long gone thru many peaks and troughs in view that its early inception in the Fifties, normally called AI "summers and winters" Goel, U. (2019). Since 2010, but, AI can be stated to have yet again entered a summer season period, specially because of sizeable improvements within the computing power of computer systems and the get right of entry to to huge amounts of information Goel, U. (2019).This resurgence in AI research is the result of 3 breakthroughs: (1) the creation of a far extra sophisticated elegance of algorithms; (2) the appearance available on the market of low-cost pixy processors capable of appearing massive quantities of calculations in some milliseconds; and (three) the supply of very massive, correctly annotated databases taking into consideration more state-of-the-art learning of wise systems (Wamba, S. F. (2018).

Despite the duration of time the field has existed, there is still no usually regular definition (Allen, 1998, Bhatnagar et al., 2018, Brachman, 2006, Hearst and Hirsh, 2000, Nilsson, 2009). This is not considered a problem but, as many clinical ideas simplest get proper definitions after they have matured enough, rather than at their conception, and given the complexity and breadth of AI, it could now not be viable to expect AI to have a set definition yet. Still, this doesn't mean that the subject must be omitted, in particular with therecent advancements and advancements referring to the sphere (Austin, P., Tu, J., Ho, J., Levy, D., & Lee, D. (2013). However, without a clear definition of the time period, "it is difficult for policymakers to assess what AI structures might be capable of do within the close to destiny, and how the sphere may get there. There is no common framework to determine which varieties of AI systems are even applicable" (Austin, P., Tu, J., Ho, J., Levy, D., & Lee, D. (2013). A similar subject has been echoed with the aid of Monett and Lewis (2018), that "theories of intelligence and the purpose of Artificial Intelligence (A.I.) have been the source of a whole lot confusion both within the discipline and amongst the majority".

In the years right now preceding and after the 1956 Dartmouth conference wherein the time period turned into coined, whilst the concept for AI become first brewing in educational cognizance, many researchers (might later end up well-known for his or her contributions to AI) formulated many theories and recommendations that focused on the commonplace features of mind and (Badjatiya, P., Gupta, S., Gupta, M.,&Varma, V. (2017).While these idea leaders were influential, the sphere of AI as we know it owes greater to Kolbjørnsrud, V., Amico, R., & Thomas, R. J. (2017). While this is in part due to their very own attendance of the famous 1951 Dartmouth conference, it is in all likelihood extra on the grounds that they went on to set up 3 leading research centres which fashioned the move of though concerning AI for years. Their own opinion on AI become as follows;

"By 'popular wise action' we wish to suggest the identical scope of intelligence as we see in human motion: that during any actual scenario behaviour appropriate to the ends of the device and adaptive to the demands of the environment can arise, within some limits of speed and complexity" (Ballew, B. (2009).Intelligence usually way "the capability to remedy tough problems" (Minsky, 1958).

"AI is involved with techniques of accomplishing dreams in situations in which the data available has a certain complicated character. The strategies that should be used are related to the trouble supplied with the aid of the state of affairs and are similar whether the trouble solver is human, a Martian, or a computer program" (Trappl, R. (1986)).

With the variety of separate critiques on what AI is, lacking agreement on a general evaluation (i.E., criteria, benchmark tests, milestones) makes it extremely challenging for the field to maintain healthy boom (DeCanio, S. J. (2016)).

Table 1. Primary Studies by Journal and Conference

Channel	Title	Number of studies	Primary studies
Journal(n=9)	European Journal of Information Systems	3	P3, P4, P12
	Journal of Strategic Information Systems	4	P15, P20, P23, P24, P25
	Journal of Information Technology	4	P10, P13, P17
	Journal of The Association of Information Systems	3	P7, P11
	Information systems journal	4	P10, P13, P17
	International Journal of Information Management	4	P6, P8, P15
	International Journal of Information Management	3	P5, P9, P16
Conference(n=2)	European Journal of Information Systems	24	P15, P20, P25

3. COMPARING AI MODELS FOR RECORD-KEEPING APPLICATIONS

Deep Learning for Tabular Data:

Deep learning models have gained interest for tabular data due to their success in other domains (e.g., images, text). Tabular data consists of heterogeneous features represented as vectors. Using deep learning allows constructing multi-modal pipelines where tabular data can be combined with other types of data (e.g., images, audio).

Baseline Models:

Establishing effective baselines is crucial. Recent work identifies two powerful architectures: **ResNet-like architecture**: A strong baseline often missing in prior studies.
Transformer adaptation for tabular data: Outperforms other solutions on most tasks.

Comparison with Gradient Boosted Decision Trees (GBDT):

Despite advances in deep learning, GBDT remains a strong competitor for tabular data. No universally superior solution exists; performance depends on the specific problem.

4. ARTIFICIAL INTELLIGENCE IN DOCUMENT ADMINISTRATION

Numerous industries, including records management, have seen a considerable increase in the use of artificial intelligence. Businesses are realizing more and more how artificial intelligence may enhance records management procedures including retention, retrieval, and classification (Rjab&Mellouli, 2019).

Artificial intelligence has several advantages for records administration, including better accuracy, less manual labor, and enhanced efficiency. Organizations may automate records management processes and free up employee time for more strategic and value-added work by utilizing AI technologies like machine learning and natural language processing. AI may also assist firms with record identification and classification, assuring regulatory compliance and lowering the possibility of sensitive data handling errors or exposure. 2019's Rjab& Mellouli3.Systematic

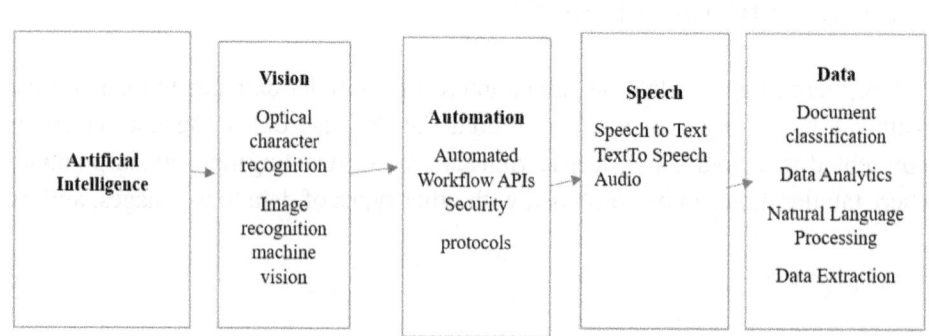

Figure 1. AI Process Diagram

Artificial Intelligence	Vision	Automation	Speech	Data
	Optical character recognition	Automated Workflow APIs	Speech to Text	Document classification
	Image recognition machine vision	Security protocols	TextTo Speech Audio	Data Analytics
				Natural Language Processing
				Data Extraction

5. LITERATURE REVIEW METHODOLOGY

A thorough literature research was done to look into artificial intelligence's potential in records management. The methodology comprised a methodical search and analysis of pertinent research publications from a variety of sources, including Scopus and Web of Science. The selection of articles was based on inclusion criteria that included publications in reputable journals or conference proceedings, as well as an emphasis on artificial intelligence in records administration. A total of thirty papers were included in the systematic literature review after the articles were screened for quality and relevancy. The application of AI technologies for record classification, retrieval, and retention, as well as the difficulties and consequences of using AI in this setting, were all explored in these articles on the subject of artificial intelligence in records management.

6. THE AIM OF THE RESEARCH

The goal of this research query is to become aware of and categorise the contributions of the number one studies. These contributions (see Table 10), adapted from Shaw (2003) and Paternoster, Giardino, Unterkalmsteiner, Gorschek, and Abrahamsson (2014) consist of six forms of contributions, namely (i) framework, approach, technique, (ii) hints, (iii) training found out, (iv) version, (v) tool, and (vi) advice/implication.

Table 2. Contribution Type

Title	Description
Framework/Method/ Technique	The contribution of the study is a particular framework, method, or technique used to facilitate the construction and management of software and systems.
Guidelines	A list of advice or recommendations based on synthesis of the obtained research results.
Lessons Learned	The set of outcomes directly based on the research results obtained from the data analysis.
Model	The representation of an observed reality in concepts or related concepts after a conceptualisation process.
Tool	A technology, program, or application that is developed in order to support different aspects of information
Advice/Implication	A discursive and generic recommendation based on opinion.

7. EMERGING TRENDS IN AI FOR RECORDS STRUCTURES

AI is transforming how records are organized and managed across different sectors. Some new developments in AI for record structures include:

1. Utilizing Natural Language Processing (NLP) for Record Categorization: NLP methods are increasingly utilized to automatically classify records based on their content, enabling more efficient organization and retrieval of data from unstructured sources.

Implementing Semantic Understanding for Context-Based Organization: AI is now capable of understanding the semantic context of records, allowing systems to organize them based on meaning rather than just keywords. This enhances navigation and improves the relevance of retrieved information. Leveraging Graph Databases for Mapping Relationships: AI-powered graph databases help in representing intricate relationships among records, enabling users to uncover insights that may not be obvious through traditional databases. Automated Generation of Metadata: AI algorithms can now generate metadata like tags and descriptions for records automatically, reducing manual effort and enhancing the accuracy and consistency of metadata across records. utilizing Predictive Analytics for Record Management: AI-driven predictive analytics models predict future record management needs, aiding organizations in optimizing their strategies and resource allocation effectively. Integrating Blockchain for Secure Record Keeping: Combining blockchain technology with AI ensures that records are tamper-proof and immutable, safeguarding their integrity and authenticity from unauthorized alterations. Personalized Record Arrangement: AI systems can analyze user behaviour to personalize record organization, delivering relevant information tailored to individual needs, thus enhancing user experience and productivity. Employing Robotic Process Automation (RPA) for Efficient Record Handling: RPA technologies automate repetitive record management tasks, streamlining processes, reducing errors, and freeing up human resources for more valuable activities. Implementing Federated Search for Distributed Records: AI algorithms enable federated search capabilities, allowing users to access information stored across different systems and locations, promoting collaboration and knowledge sharing. Continuous Learning for Enhanced Record Organization: AI systems are designed to continuously learn and improve their record organization capabilities by adapting to evolving data patterns and user preferences, ensuring optimized and relevant record structures.

These emerging AI trends in record structures are reshaping organizational practices, leading to more efficient, intelligent, and adaptive record management approaches.

Figure 2. AI and Machine Learning Trends

2023 Emerging AI and Machine Learning Trends

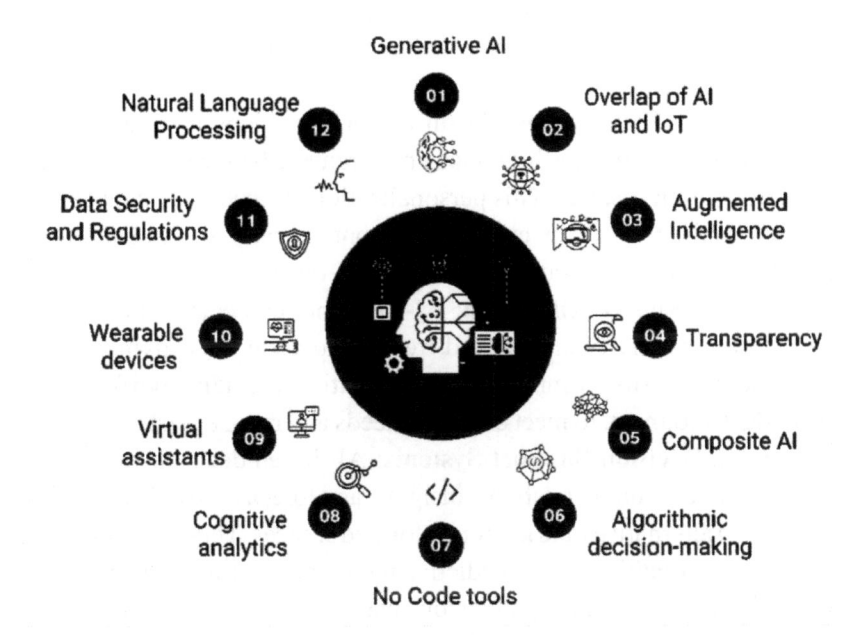

- 01 Generative AI
- 02 Overlap of AI and IoT
- 03 Augmented Intelligence
- 04 Transparency
- 05 Composite AI
- 06 Algorithmic decision-making
- 07 No Code tools
- 08 Cognitive analytics
- 09 Virtual assistants
- 10 Wearable devices
- 11 Data Security and Regulations
- 12 Natural Language Processing

8. ANALYZING THE INFLUENCE OF ARTIFICIAL INTELLIGENCE ON INFORMATION MANAGEMENT

The impact of AI on information management is significant and diverse, transforming how organizations manage, analyze, and extract insights from extensive data sets. Here is a detailed examination of its effects:

1. **Enhanced Data Processing Efficiency**: AI algorithms, especially machine learning and deep learning models, facilitate quicker and more effective processing of large data quantities. Tasks like data cleaning, standardization, and conversion can be automated, reducing the time and manual effort needed for data preparation.

2. **Improved Data Quality and Precision**: AI-driven data validation and cleansing methods enhance data quality by recognizing and rectifying errors, disparities, and duplicates in datasets. This ensures that organizations operate with precise and dependable information, leading to better decision-making results.
3. **Advanced Data Analysis and Insight Generation**: AI supports advanced data analysis techniques such as predictive analytics, pattern recognition, and anomaly detection. By unveiling hidden patterns, trends, and correlations within data, AI empowers organizations to derive actionable insights and make data-informed decisions with increased certainty.
4. **Tailored User Experiences**: AI allows organizations to offer tailored user experiences by analyzing individual preferences, behaviors, and interactions with information systems. This personalization enriches user engagement, satisfaction, and efficiency by customizing content, suggestions, and interactions to each user's specific requirements and preferences.
5. **Optimized Resource Allocation**: AI-based predictive analytics models help organizations predict future demand, trends, and resource needs more accurately. This enables them to optimize resource allocation, including staffing, inventory, and budget allotment, to meet expected needs and reduce waste or deficiencies.
6. **Automated Decision Support Systems**: AI-driven decision support systems offer real-time recommendations, insights, and forecasts to aid decision-makers in assessing alternatives and making informed choices. These systems utilize past data, current conditions, and predictive modeling to propose the most efficient courses of action, enhancing decision-making speed and accuracy.
7. **Enhanced Security and Risk Management**: AI technologies like machine learning-based anomaly detection and behavior analysis reinforce cybersecurity measures by identifying and mitigating security threats instantly. Moreover, AI helps organizations evaluate and manage risks more competently by studying historical data, recognizing potential vulnerabilities, and implementing proactive risk mitigation strategies.
8. **Streamlined Business Processes**: AI-powered automation tools, such as robotic process automation (RPA) and intelligent document processing (IDP), simplify routine and repetitive tasks in different business procedures. By automating data entry, document processing, and workflow management, organizations can enhance operational efficiency, decrease errors, and free up human resources for more strategic endeavors.
9. **Enhanced Compliance and Regulatory Adherence**: AI supports organizations in upholding compliance with regulatory standards and industry norms by automating compliance monitoring, reporting, and auditing procedures. AI-based systems can analyze vast data volumes to pinpoint compliance risks, detect

potential violations, and ensure conformity to relevant regulations, reducing the likelihood of penalties or legal problems.
10. **Fostering Innovation and Competitive Edge**: AI enables organizations to innovate and distinguish themselves by using data-driven insights to create new products, services, and business models. By leveraging AI technologies for information management, organizations can gain a competitive advantage by anticipating market trends, recognizing emerging opportunities, and providing innovative solutions that meet evolving customer demands.

In conclusion, AI's impact on information management is transformative, enhancing efficiency, accuracy, personalization, and innovation throughout various data processing and decision-making aspects. By embracing AI technologies, organizations can fully leverage their data assets and secure a strategic advantage in today's data-centric business environment.AI technologies are reshaping the landscape of records systems across various sectors, enriching efficiency, accuracy, and accessibility. Below are numerous AI technologies actively changing records systems:NLP empowers machines to comprehend and interpret human language. In records systems, NLP aids in text extraction, sentiment analysis, and document summarization, streamlining the organization and search of extensive textual data. ML algorithms can sift through vast datasets to recognize patterns, trends, and anomalies. Within records systems, ML is utilized for classification, categorization, and prediction tasks, automating processes like document sorting, archival, and retrieval. AI-driven image recognition technologies can analyze and interpret visual data embedded in records. This is especially beneficial for systems handling scanned documents, images, or photographs, enabling automated tagging, indexing, and content extraction.

Speech recognition tech transforms spoken language into text, enabling hands-free data input and transcription of audio files. For records systems, speech recognition simplifies the automatic transcription of meetings, interviews, and other dialogues, making them searchable and accessible. RPA automates repetitive tasks by replicating human actions in digital systems. Within records management, RPA streamlines data entry, validation, and routine administrative tasks, increasing efficiency and reducing errors. Blockchain technology establishes a secure and unalterable ledger for tracking transactions. In records systems, blockchain can create secure audit trails, guaranteeing the integrity and authenticity of records, often required in trust-based contexts.

1. **Predictive Analytics:** Predictive analytics algorithms forecast future outcomes and trends by examining historical data. In records systems, predictive analytics aids in anticipating document access patterns, storage needs, and compliance risks, allowing for proactive decisions and resource allocation.
2. **Federated Learning:** Federated learning allows AI models to be trained across multiple decentralized data sources without sharing raw data. In records systems, federated learning enhances privacy and robustness of AI models for personalized content recommendations and predictive maintenance tasks.
3. **Semantic Web Technologies:** Semantic web technologies enable machines to grasp the meaning and context of information online. In records systems, these technologies improve data sharing and interoperability across diverse systems and platforms.
4. **Cognitive Search:** Cognitive search systems use AI techniques to offer more contextually relevant search results. In records systems, cognitive search boosts the retrieval and discovery of records by understanding user intent and context, leading to efficient information discovery and decision-making.

Organizations leveraging these AI technologies can elevate their records systems to become more intelligent, automated, and adaptive, ultimately enhancing productivity, compliance, and decision-making capabilities.

9.AI RESEARCH AGENDA FOR RECORDS STRUCTURES

Creating a roadmap for AI research in records structures involves identifying crucial areas where AI advancements can enhance the organization, management, and utilization of records.

The proposed research agenda highlights key areas for exploration:

1. AI-Driven Record Classification and Categorization:

Enhance AI algorithms to automatically classify and categorize records based on their content, context, and metadata. Investigate methods to improve the precision and complexity of record classification, particularly for diverse datasets.

Semantic Understanding and Contextual Organization: Utilize AI techniques to comprehend the semantic significance of records and organize them based on contextual relations and domain-specific knowledge. Explore integrating external knowledge sources like ontologies to enhance record organization I-Enabled Record Linkage and Relationship Mapping: Develop AI approaches to identify and link related records across various datasets, including entity resolution techniques. Explore constructing graph-based representations of record connections for exploration and data discovery. Automated Metadata Generation and Enrichment: Research auto-generation of metadata for records and enriching them by extracting key entities and relationships from unstructured data. Investigate leveraging AI to enhance metadata consistency and accuracy across record collections.AI-Powered Record Retention and Disposition: Develop AI models to determine record retention based on legal requirements, organizational policies, and business value. Investigate optimizing record retention strategies using AI technology.AI-Enhanced Record Access and Retrieval: Explore AI-driven methods to enhance record access and retrieval efficiency, including personalized search and recommendation systems. Investigate AI methods to improve record discoverability based on user preferences.AI-Assisted Record Preservation and Long-Term Accessibility Develop AI techniques to assess digital record integrity, authenticity, and preservation over time. Explore AI automation for record migration to ensure long-term accessibility. Ethical and Fair AI in Records Management: Study ethical considerations and biases related to AI use in records management. Develop guidelines for the responsible and fair use of AI in records management. Interdisciplinary Collaboration and Knowledge Sharing: Foster collaboration between AI researchers, records management professionals, and other stakeholders to tackle challenges. Promote sharing research findings to advance AI in records structures. Evaluation and Benchmarking of AI Solutions: Establish evaluation metrics for AI-driven solutions in records management. Conduct empirical evaluations to assess the effectiveness of AI techniques in record management scenarios. By focusing on these areas, researchers can advance AI in records structures, addressing key challenges and improving record organization and management across various domains.

10. CHALLENGES AND OPPORTUNITIES IN AI-ENABLED RECORDS MANAGEMENT

Developing a research agenda for AI in records structures involves identifying key areas where advancements in AI can contribute to improving the organization, management, and utilization of records. Here's a proposed research agenda outlining several important areas for investigation:

1. **AI-Driven Record Classification and Categorization**:
    o   Develop more robust and scalable AI algorithms for automatically classifying and categorizing records based on their content, context, and metadata.

- o Investigate techniques for improving the accuracy and granularity of record classification, especially for complex and heterogeneous datasets.
2. **Semantic Understanding and Contextual Organization**:
    - o Explore AI-driven approaches for understanding the semantic meaning of records and organizing them based on contextual relationships and domain-specific knowledge.
    - o Investigate methods for integrating external knowledge sources, such as ontologies and domain-specific taxonomies, to enhance the contextual organization of records.
3. **AI-Enabled Record Linkage and Relationship Mapping**:
    - o Develop AI techniques for automatically identifying and linking related records across disparate datasets, including techniques for entity resolution and relationship inference.
    - o Investigate approaches for constructing and analyzing graph-based representations of record relationships to facilitate exploration and discovery of interconnected data.
4. **Automated Metadata Generation and Enrichment**:
    - o Explore AI-driven methods for automatically generating and enriching metadata for records, including techniques for extracting key entities, attributes, and relationships from unstructured data.Investigate approaches for leveraging AI to improve the consistency, accuracy, and completeness of metadata across diverse record collections.
5. **AI-Powered Record Retention and Disposition**:
    - o Develop AI-driven models for determining record retention and disposition schedules based on factors such as legal requirements, organizational policies, and business value.
    - o Investigate techniques for leveraging AI to optimize record retention strategies, balancing compliance obligations with storage costs and information retrieval needs.
6. **AI-Enhanced Record Access and Retrieval**:
    - o Explore AI-driven approaches for improving the efficiency and effectiveness of record access and retrieval, including techniques for personalized search, recommendation, and navigation
    - o Investigate methods for leveraging AI to enhance the discoverability of records by automatically identifying and surfacing relevant information based on user context and preferences.
7. **AI-Assisted Record Preservation and Long-Term Accessibility**:
    Develop AI techniques for assessing the integrity, authenticity, and preservation risk of digital records over time, including methods for detecting and mitigating degradation, obsolescence, and loss.Investigate approaches

for leveraging AI to automate the migration, emulation, or transformation of records to ensure their long-term accessibility and usability across evolving technological environments.

8. **Ethical and Fair AI in Records Management**:
   o Investigate ethical considerations and potential biases associated with the use of AI in records management, including issues related to privacy, transparency, accountability, and fairness.
   o Develop guidelines and best practices for ensuring the responsible and equitable use of AI in records structures, taking into account diverse stakeholder perspectives and societal impacts.
9. **Interdisciplinary Collaboration and Knowledge Sharing**:
   o Foster interdisciplinary collaboration between AI researchers, records management professionals, archivists, librarians, and other stakeholders to address the complex challenges at the intersection of AI and records structures.Promote knowledge sharing and dissemination of research findings through conferences, workshops, publications, and collaborative projects to advance the field and inform practice.Develop standardized evaluation metrics and benchmarking frameworks for assessing the performance, reliability, and scalability of AI-driven solutions for records management.Conduct comparative studies and empirical evaluations to validate the effectiveness and efficiency of AI techniques in real-world record management scenarios, using diverse datasets and use cases.

By focusing research efforts on these key areas, researchers can advance the state-of-the-art in AI for records structures, addressing critical challenges and opportunities to enhance the organization, management, and utilization of records in diverse domains.

11. CHALLENGES AND OPPORTUNITIES IN AI-ENHANCED RECORDS MANAGEMENT

When it comes to AI-enhanced records management, organizations are faced with both challenges and opportunities that demand careful consideration. Let's delve into some key aspects:

Challenges:

1. **Data Quality and Integration:** The effectiveness of AI algorithms in records management can be hindered by poor data quality and a lack of integration across different sources. Inaccurate metadata, incomplete records, and data silos pose obstacles for precise analysis and decision-making.
2. **Privacy and Security Concerns:** Managing records with AI power can raise privacy and security issues, especially when dealing with sensitive or identifiable data. Ensuring compliance with data protection laws and guarding against unauthorized access are imperative.
3. **Bias and Fairness:** AI algorithms may unintentionally perpetuate biases present in historical data, resulting in unjust outcomes. Rectifying bias and promoting fairness in AI-powered records management necessitates meticulous attention to data selection, algorithm design, and model assessment.
4. **Interpretability and Transparency:** The intricate nature of AI algorithms can make it challenging to interpret their decisions and rationale. Lack of transparency may erode trust in AI systems, particularly in scenarios where accountability and explainability are crucial.
5. **Resource Constraints:** Implementation of AI-enabled records management systems may demand substantial investments in technology, infrastructure, and expertise. Smaller organizations might encounter limitations and difficulties in adopting and sustaining AI solutions.
6. **Ethical Considerations:** Ethical dilemmas may surface in AI-enhanced records management, concerning consent, transparency, and responsible technology use. Balancing the advantages of AI-driven automation with ethical standards and societal values requires thoughtful deliberation and ethical frameworks.

12.OPPORTUNITIES:

AI technologies can automate routine tasks, streamline processes, and augment records management efficiency. Automated data entry, classification, and retrieval functionalities can save time and resources, enabling organizations to focus on higher-value tasks. AI-driven analytics can unveil valuable insights from vast data sets, empowering informed decision-making and strategic planning. Predictive analytics, anomaly detection, and trend analysis can aid in identifying patterns, risks, and opportunities in records management processes. AI algorithms can tailor user experiences by delivering personalized content, recommendations, and insights according to individual preferences. Personalized search results, content suggestions, and user interfaces can enhance user satisfaction and engagement.

AI technologies can help organizations maintain regulatory compliance and mitigate risks related to records management. Automated compliance monitoring, audit trails, and risk assessment tools can identify and address compliance gaps and vulnerabilities.AI-powered innovation in records management can grant organizations a competitive edge by unlocking new pathways for efficiency, insight, and value creation. Embracing cutting-edge AI technologies can position organizations as frontrunners in their field.AI-enabled records management systems can scale to handle large data volumes and adapt to evolving organizational needs. Scalable AI algorithms, cloud-based solutions, and flexible architectures can support growth and evolution over time.AI-fueled analytics can facilitate knowledge discovery and collaboration, unveiling hidden insights and promoting information exchange. Advanced search capabilities, semantic analysis, and collaborative filtering can nurture innovation and knowledge sharing within organizations.AI-driven records management systems can continuously learn and enhance, refining algorithms, optimizing processes, and adapting to changing environments. Feedback mechanisms, model retraining, and performance monitoring can propel ongoing improvement and innovation.By addressing challenges effectively and leveraging the opportunities brought by AI-enhanced records management, organizations can fully unleash the potential of their data assets, boost operational efficiency, and foster innovation in the digital era.

13. FUTURE DIRECTIONS OF AI IN ARCHIVAL SCIENCE

The future of AI in archival science holds immense potential for transforming how archival materials are preserved, accessed, and utilized. Here are several future directions in which AI is likely to impact archival science:

AI technologies will play a significant role in automating and improving the digitization and preservation of archival materials. Advanced image recognition algorithms can assist in digitizing handwritten or damaged documents, while machine learning models can aid in the detection and restoration of deteriorating or fragile materials.

The semantic context of archival records, enabling more accurate categorization, description, and contextualization of materials. Natural language processing (NLP) techniques will facilitate the extraction of meaningful information from textual documents, enhancing access and discoverability for researchers.

AI algorithms will automate the generation and enrichment of metadata for archival materials, reducing the manual effort required for cataloging and indexing. By analyzing the content and context of records, AI systems can assign descriptive metadata tags, identify related items, and enrich existing metadata with additional contextual information. AI-powered retrieval systems will provide more intelligent and personalized access to archival collections. These systems will leverage machine learning models to understand user preferences and behavior, delivering tailored search results, recommendations, and contextual insights based on individual research interests and objectives.

As born-digital records become increasingly prevalent, AI technologies will be essential for preserving and managing these materials effectively. AI-driven tools for file format identification, emulation, and migration will ensure the long-term accessibility and usability of digital archival materials across evolving technological platforms.

AI-powered transcription and translation tools will streamline the processing of multilingual and handwritten archival materials. These tools will leverage speech recognition and optical character recognition (OCR) technologies to automatically transcribe audio recordings and digitize handwritten documents, making them more accessible to a global audience. Predictive analytics models will assist archivists in making informed decisions about collection management and resource allocation. By analyzing usage patterns, preservation risks, and collection gaps, AI systems can recommend priorities for digitization, conservation, and acquisition efforts, ensuring the long-term sustainability of archival repositories.

AI-enabled collaborative platforms will facilitate knowledge sharing and collaboration among archival institutions and researchers. These platforms will leverage AI technologies to aggregate and analyze metadata from diverse archival collections, enabling cross-institutional research projects, data integration, and interdisciplinary collaborations. Future developments in AI for archival science will prioritize ethical considerations, transparency, and accountability. Archivists and AI researchers will collaborate to develop ethical guidelines, best practices, and governance frameworks for the responsible use of AI in archival contexts, ensuring that AI technologies align with professional standards and ethical principles. As AI becomes increasingly integral to archival practice, education and training programs will incorporate AI skills and competencies into archival curricula. Archivists will acquire proficiency in AI tools and techniques, enabling them to harness the full potential of AI technologies for advancing archival science and preserving cultural heritage.

Overall, the future of AI in archival science holds promise for revolutionizing how archival materials are managed, accessed, and interpreted. By embracing AI technologies and practices, archival institutions can enhance the discoverability, accessibility, and relevance of their collections, ensuring that they continue to serve as valuable resources for researchers, educators, and communities around the world.

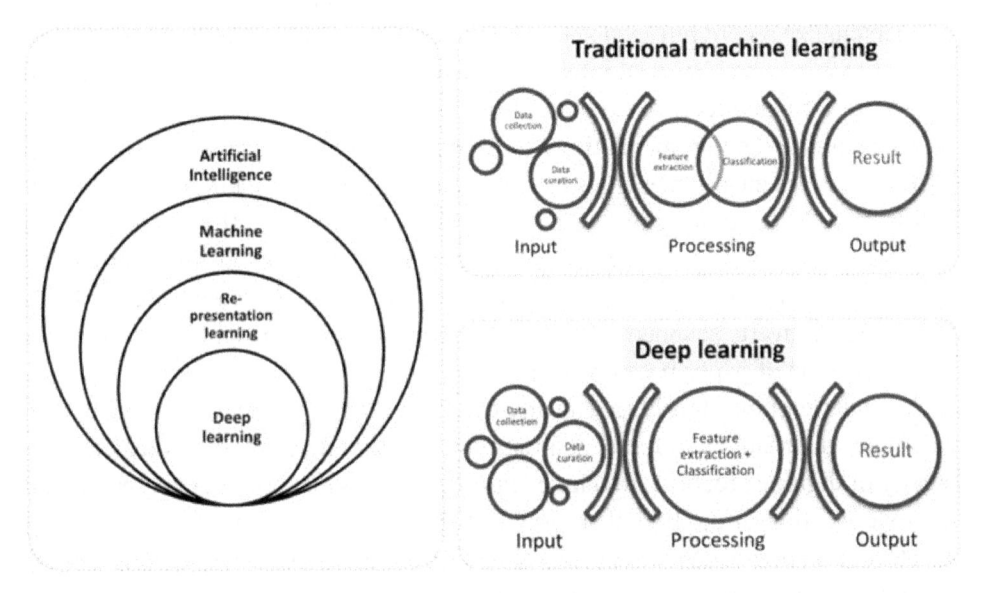

Figure 3. Operational Diagram

14. THE ROLE OF MACHINE LEARNING IN RECORDKEEPING

Machine learning (ML) plays a pivotal role in recordkeeping by automating tasks, improving efficiency, and enhancing decision-making processes. Here's how machine learning contributes to recordkeeping:

Machine learning algorithms can automate data entry tasks by extracting relevant information from various sources such as documents, forms, emails, and databases. This reduces manual data entry errors and accelerates the process of capturing information into recordkeeping systems.

Machine learning models can classify and categorize records based on their content, structure, or metadata attributes. This enables automated organization and indexing of records, making it easier to retrieve and manage large volumes of information efficiently. Machine learning algorithms can analyze historical data to predict future trends, patterns, and events related to record management. For example, predictive analytics can forecast storage needs, identify potential compliance risks, and optimize resource allocation for recordkeeping activities.

Machine learning techniques can identify anomalies or deviations from expected patterns within records, indicating potential compliance issues or irregularities. By monitoring data streams in real-time, machine learning models can detect unauthorized access, data breaches, or fraudulent activities, helping organizations maintain regulatory compliance and data integrity. Machine learning algorithms can personalize record retrieval and recommendation systems based on user preferences, behavior, and historical interactions with records. By analyzing user queries, access patterns, and feedback, machine learning models can deliver more relevant search results and recommendations, enhancing user satisfaction and productivity. NLP techniques enable machines to understand and process natural language text within records, facilitating tasks such as sentiment analysis, entity extraction, and summarization. NLP-powered analytics can extract insights from unstructured textual data, enabling more comprehensive analysis and decision-making. OCR technology converts scanned images of text into machine-readable text, enabling the digitization of paper-based records.

Machine learning algorithms can improve OCR accuracy by learning to recognize patterns and variations in fonts, handwriting, and layout structures, enhancing the quality of digitized records. Machine learning systems can continuously learn and improve over time through feedback loops and iterative refinement. By incorporating user feedback, performance metrics, and new data sources, machine learning models can adapt to changing requirements and environments, ensuring that recordkeeping processes remain effective and efficient.

Overall, machine learning empowers organizations to streamline recordkeeping processes, extract valuable insights from data, and optimize decision-making in record management. By leveraging machine learning technologies, organizations can enhance the accuracy, efficiency, and accessibility of their recordkeeping systems, ultimately improving organizational performance and compliance outcomes.

15. EVALUATING AI EFFECTIVENESS IN RECORDS STRUCTURES RESEARCH

Evaluating the effectiveness of AI in records structures research involves assessing various aspects, including accuracy, efficiency, scalability, usability, and impact on organizational objectives. Here are several key factors to consider when evaluating AI effectiveness in records structures research: Measure the accuracy of AI algorithms in tasks such as record classification, categorization, extraction, and retrieval. Evaluate the precision, recall, and F1-score of AI models compared to manual or baseline methods.

Assess the efficiency and speed of AI-enabled processes compared to traditional manual approaches. Measure the time taken to complete tasks such as data entry, classification, or retrieval using AI algorithms. Evaluate the scalability of AI solutions to handle large volumes of records and diverse data types. Measure the performance of AI systems under varying workloads and data volumes to ensure scalability and responsiveness. Assess the usability and user experience of AI-enabled recordkeeping systems. Conduct user studies and surveys to evaluate user satisfaction, ease of use, and perceived usefulness of AI features and functionalities. Evaluate the robustness and resilience of AI algorithms against noise, errors, and adversarial attacks. Test AI models under different conditions and scenarios to assess their reliability and performance in real-world environments. Measure the generalization and adaptability of AI models across different datasets, domains, and use cases. Evaluate the transferability of AI solutions to new contexts and scenarios to assess their versatility and applicability. Assess the impact of AI-enabled recordkeeping on organizational objectives such as productivity, cost savings, compliance, and decision-making. Quantify the benefits and value generated by AI solutions in terms of tangible outcomes and business metrics. Consider the ethical and societal implications of AI in records structures research. Evaluate the fairness, transparency, and accountability of AI algorithms to ensure responsible and ethical use of AI technologies. Compare the performance of AI-enabled recordkeeping systems with baseline methods or alternative approaches. Conduct controlled experiments or A/B testing to validate the effectiveness of AI solutions against existing practices. Assess the long-term impact and sustainability of AI in records structures research. Evaluate the scalability, maintainability, and future-proofing of AI solutions to ensure continued effectiveness and relevance over time.By considering these factors and conducting rigorous evaluations, researchers can assess the effectiveness of AI in records structures research, identify areas for improvement, and inform the development of more advanced and impactful AI solutions for recordkeeping.

16. CONCLUSION

In conclusion, our systematic literature review of artificial intelligence (AI) in records structures research reveals a growing body of literature exploring the application of AI techniques in various aspects of recordkeeping. Through this review, we have identified key trends, challenges, and opportunities in the intersection of AI and records management, as well as outlined a comprehensive research agenda for future investigations. Our review highlights the following key findings: AI technologies such as natural language processing (NLP), machine learning (ML), and semantic understanding are increasingly being leveraged to automate record classification, improve metadata generation, enhance search and retrieval capabilities, and support decision-making processes in recordkeeping.

While AI holds promise for revolutionizing records management, it also presents challenges such as data quality issues, privacy concerns, bias, and interpretability. However, there are significant opportunities for improving efficiency, accuracy, and decision-making through AI-enabled recordkeeping solutions. We propose a research agenda encompassing key areas for future investigations, including AI-driven record classification, semantic understanding, automated metadata generation, predictive analytics, and ethical considerations. These areas represent critical avenues for advancing the field of AI in records structures research and addressing the complex challenges and opportunities therein. In summary, our systematic literature review provides valuable insights into the current state of AI in records structures research and outlines a roadmap for future research endeavours. By addressing the identified research agenda, scholars, practitioners, and policymakers can contribute to the development of innovative AI solutions that enhance the organization, management, and utilization of records in diverse contexts, ultimately advancing the field of recordkeeping and contributing to the broader goals of information management and knowledge preservation.

REFERENCES:

Abubakar, A. M., Behravesh, E., Rezapouraghda, H., & Yildiz, S. B. (2019). Applying artificial intelligence technique to predict knowledge hiding behavior. *International Journal of Information Management*, 49, 45–57. 10.1016/j.ijinfomgt.2019.02.006

Agarwal, S., Kumar, S., & Goel, U. (2019). Stock market response to information diffusion through internet sources: A literature review. *International Journal of Information Management*, 45, 118–131. 10.1016/j.ijinfomgt.2018.11.002

Ali, O., Shrestha, A., Soar, J., & Wamba, S. F. (2018). Cloud computing-enabled healthcare opportunities, issues, and applications: A systematic review. *International Journal of Information Management*, 43, 146–158. 10.1016/j.ijinfomgt.2018.07.009

Allen, J. F. (1998). AI growing up: The changes and opportunities. *AI Magazine*, 19(4), 13–23.

Austin, P., Tu, J., Ho, J., Levy, D., & Lee, D. (2013). Using methods from the data-mining and machine-learning literature for disease classiffcation for heart failure subtypes. *Journal of Clinical Epidemiology*, •••, 398–407. 10.1016/j.jclinepi.2012.11.00823384592

Badjatiya, P., Gupta, S., Gupta, M., & Varma, V. (2017). Deep learning for hate speech detection in tweets. *26th International World Wide Web Conference*. 10.1145/3041021.3054223

Dejoux, C., & L'eon, E. (2018). *M´etamorphose des managers* (1st ed.). Pearson.

Dennehy, D. (2020). Ireland post-pandemic: Utilizing AI to kick-start economic recovery. *Cutter Business Technology Journal*, 33(11), 22–27.

Kolbjørnsrud, V., Amico, R., & Thomas, R. J. (2017). Partnering with AI: How organizations can win over skeptical managers. *Strategy and Leadership*, 45(1), 37–43. 10.1108/SL-12-2016-0085

Kurzweil, R. (2005). *The singularity is near*. Viking.

Lacity, M., Willcocks, L., & Andrew, C. (2015). *Robotic process automation: Mature capabilities in the energy sector*. LSE Research Online Documents on Economics.

Langley, P. (2011). Artificial Intelligence. *AISB Quarterly*.

LeCun, Y., Bengio, Y., & Hinton, G. (2015). Deep Learning.Nature, 521, 436–444.
Leidner, D., & Kayworth, T. (2006). A review of culture in information systems research: Toward a theory of information technology culture conflict. *Management Information Systems Quarterly*, 30(2), 357–399.

McCarthy, J. (1988). Mathematical logic in arti

cial intelligence. *Daedalus*, 117(1), 297–311.

McCorduck, P. (2004). *Machines who think: A personal inquiry into the history and prospects artificial intelligence* (2nd ed.). A. K. Peters. 10.1201/9780429258985

.McCulloch, W. S., & Pitts, W. H. (1943). A logical calculus o

ideas immanent in neural activity.Bulletin o Mathematical Biophysics, 5, 115–133 .

Turing, A. M. (1950). *I.—Computing machinery and intelligence.Mind, LIX, 433–460.*
U.S. National Science and Technology Council. (2016).*Preparing for the future artificial intelligence*. Government Printing Office.

Chapter 6
The Use of Artificial Intelligence in Health Communication:
A Research on ChatGPT

Nural Imik Tanyildizi
https://orcid.org/0000-0002-9177-759X
Fırat University, Turkey

Ilkay Yıldız
https://orcid.org/0000-0002-6260-9730
Bingöl Üniversitesi, Turkey

ABSTRACT

Communication is of great importance in health services. Nowadays, new media, especially the internet, are frequently used in health communication. Artificial intelligence has also begun to be used in healthcare. Artificial intelligence studies generally aim to develop artificial methods that imitate human ways of thinking. In addition, it is predicted that some programs produced based on artificial intelligence will affect health communication processes in daily use. The most important of these programs is the ChatGPT (Chatbot Generative Pre-trained Transformer) program. The purpose of this study is to reveal the benefits and drawbacks of using the ChatGPT program in health communication by providing a qualitative framework. For this purpose, a semi-structured interview was conducted with 30 people over the age of 18, determined by a purposeful sampling method. In line with the data obtained, the use of Chat GPT in health communication was tried to be explained.

DOI: 10.4018/979-8-3693-3719-6.ch006

INTRODUCTION

This article provides an analysis of the uses of ChatGPT and artificial intelligence in healthcare communication. ChatGPT is an advanced language model that uses deep learning techniques to generate human-like responses to natural language input. It is part of the family of generative pre-training transformer (GPT) models developed by OpenAI in November 2022 and is currently one of the largest publicly available language models (Dave, Athaluri, Singh, 2023:1). ChatGPT is an advanced language model that uses deep learning techniques to produce human-like responses to natural language input (Radford et al., 2018:2). Artificial intelligence (AI), which is seen as a multidisciplinary approach of both computer and linguistic science (Yağar, 2023:1228), has achieved success in tasks such as understanding, answering, coding, summarizing and inferring (Zhang and Li, 2021:832). ChatGBT produces answers to questions the way people do and uses combinations that give answers as if they are experts on this subject. It also uses existing language models in web pages, books, articles, and conversations on social media (Uc-Cetina et al., 2022:2).

ChatGPT is on its way to be adopted all over the world as the latest developing technology. This situation arises from the very wide use of technology and especially the development of software (Metz, 2022; Reed, 2022). However, these developments also bring about various debates. There is concern that artificial intelligence may change the roles that humans traditionally have to undertake by doing the work done by humans. (Else, 2023:614; Stokel-Walker, 2023:621). Artificial intelligence, which causes such difficulties to arise, provides both positive and negative opinions by responding to many problems in actions such as text creation, writing and speaking. As a result, ChatGPT is among the most transformative artificial intelligence tools and is increasingly being developed. It also presents challenges and opportunities for institutions and organizations, societies and individuals (Dwivedi, et al. 2023: 57).

When we look at the studies on the use of ChatGPT within the scope of health communication, it is seen that the number of academic studies is low. In their study, Devivedi, et.al., (2023) discusses ChatGPT from a multidisciplinary perspective and also touches upon its use in health and health communication. Devivedi, et.al., states that ChatGPT has witnessed transformations in the field of health and aims to provide quality service by providing easier access from remote areas within the scope of health communication (2023: 45). Yağar (2023) also provided information regarding health communication in her study on the use of ChayGPT in the field of health. From the patient's perspective, when ChatGPT is used as a virtual assistant, it allows patients to access health-related issues, get information, reach the necessary results related to themselves, and use it as a consultancy service (2023:1234). Dave, et.al. (2023:2) examined ChatGPT in the field of medicine. The study believes that ChatGPT will facilitate the development of virtual assistants within the scope of health communication. Menichettia, et.al. (2023:3) stated in his study that the widespread use of ChatGPT in health communication is possible through greater knowledge on issues related to its use in an accountable, honest and reliable manner. Marchetti, et.al. (2001:1), states in his study that the creative intelligence that emerged with the development of information and communication technologies supports the communication between health institutions and them. Marchetti, et.al., however, stated that such computer-based applications are difficult because communication is more fluent and faster in speech. In their study on message production in health communication, Lim and Schmälzle (2023) produced messages both through artificial intelligence and humans to raise awareness about folic acid. As a result of the study, it was revealed that the messages produced by artificial intelligence ranked higher in terms of quality and clarity. The use of artificial intelligence is becoming important in terms of the understandability of messages in health communication (2023:2). In their study, Kreps and Neuhauser (2013) emphasized the importance of urgency in health communication. The study was carried out with a 2-year pilot application, with participants consisting of 30 patients and 4 employees. It has been difficult to gather the necessary information from patients to enable decisions to be made about an intestinal disease, such as determining treatment courses and performing surgery when necessary. Artificial intelligence has been used to prevent this and ensure fast, urgent health communication. As a result of the study, it was observed that by using artificial intelligence in health communication, the quality of communication increased, more harmonious and sensitive messages were produced, and a smart, interesting and interactive health communication was achieved (2013:209). In another study by Neuhauser, Kreps, et.al (2013), in the same project, it was investigated whether visualization and design elements made with artificial intelligence were effective in health communication. Visual and design-supported contents regarding patients' conditions and treatment methods were created with artificial intelligence. As a result of the study, it was revealed that design and visualizations further strengthen health communication. Nadarzynski, et.al. (2019) used a semi-structured interview technique via social media for the use of artificial intelligence in healthcare services. As a result of the study, it was revealed that the use of chatbots in health communication was approached positively, but hesitations towards artificial intelligence continued. Nadarzynski, et.al., stated that as a solution to this, those who design artificial intelligence should take a user-centered approach that addresses users' concerns and offers other experiences (2019:1). Nancy, et.al. (2013)'s study is important in that it shows the usefulness of knowledge-based and symbolic artificial intelligence approaches in the use of artificial intelligence in health communication. It is emphasized that knowledge-based artificial intelligence will make it easier to use modeling in other multidisciplinary fields in health communication (2013: 140). Hu (2015) examined empirical articles published in English between 2008 and 2012 on the use of new media in health communication. As a result of the study, it was concluded that the most discussed topics within the scope of health communication are websites, web and computer-based intervention programs, online forums and support groups, e-mails, and web 2.0-based social media applications. Another important result is that technologies such as the virtual world, virtual reality and artificial intelligence are not given sufficient importance (2015:260). Golan, et.al. (2024) used the interview method with graduate students in their study to reveal students' ideas about the use of artificial intelligence in health communication. As a result of the study, opinions emerged that the accuracy of information regarding health communication is high, comprehensive and clear due to the ease in which artificial intelligence produces and presents information (2024:357). Qian, Yuan (2024) administered a survey to 364 people in study. Participants were asked what their expectations were for communicating with chatbots and human doctors about their mental health. The study concluded that participants had higher expectations from human doctors, even though chatbots produced faster solutions. Additionally, it has been observed that when chatbots make participants feel emotionally closer, participants change their behavior (2024:5). An important result obtained from the study is that adding affectionate words and sentences to the texts designed for artificial intelligence, for example, using sentences expressing affection such as 'I understand you', 'I am sorry to hear this', 'You are stressed right now', provided emotional support to the participants (2024: 3). Amanawa Imomoemi, Amanawa (2024:178) discussed areas where artificial intelligence contributes to public health communication. It has been concluded that with training on artificial intelligence, especially in public health communication, this field will be transformed, service will be provided at better standards and the ability to act faster in emergency situations will be developed. Antel, et.al. (2022:3046) examined articles addressing artificial intelligence and virtual reality issues in health communication. Chow, et al. (2023) pointed out that ChatCPT's health condition did not develop more negatively during the process. Anand, D, et al. (2022) found that the use of computer-aided artificial intelligence will be beneficial in the field of health, especially in the detection of cancerous diseases. Accordingly, the conclusion obtained from the articles in the literature is that these developing technologies provide better information in order to better guide patients' decision-making processes, and that communication-oriented applications and trainings can be used to improve health communication.

ChatGPT, which has become important for institutions and organizations, has begun to be used effectively in the field of health. Although there are many studies in the literature in the field of health, the number of studies specifically addressing the subject of health communication is quite low. The main purpose of this study is to reveal the acceptability of ChatGPT by individuals within the scope of health communication. Another aim of the study is to reveal whether individuals have knowledge about what ChatGPT, a newly developing technology, is and what its usage areas include. The importance of the study lies in the fact that studies on artificial intelligence within the scope of health communication are not sufficient. In addition, the use of the interview method in the study and the collection of data through one-on-one interviews with individuals make the study important. In this context, first of all, the interview questions were created by taking the opinions of experts. Later, interviews were held with 30 people within the framework of questions. As a result of the interview, it was concluded that individuals did not have knowledge of how to use ChatGPT within the scope of health communication. Some of the participants are not familiar with ChatGPT.

USE OF ARTIFICIAL INTELLIGENCE IN HEALTH COMMUNICATION

Artificial intelligence was invented in 1956 in a Dartmouth workshop. Artificial intelligence, which has been constantly developing since then, has become controversial all over the world and in every line of business. Activities that were unimaginable a few years ago can be completed by artificial intelligence without any human intervention. Artificial intelligence refers to comprehensive systems that analyze the environment, use intelligence to operate, and use the freedom given to achieve specified goals (Kumar, et.al. 2024:2). Artificial intelligence and communication should not be considered separately from each other. Software and various applications that play an important role in the development of artificial intelligence are communication-based. In addition to being communication-based, artificial intelligence develops better communication skills and eliminates communication barriers that may arise. In this way, communication between individuals gains speed, communication becomes easier and information exchange becomes higher quality. Koçyiğit and Darı exemplified this situation as follows: Artificial intelligence can instantly translate many different languages into their native languages with various translation software. It can also use symbols developed for the hearing impaired (2023:432). Developments in artificial intelligence are frequently used in daily life. People can chat with digital chat robots throughout the day through different applications they use on their smart devices. This increases the speed of communication, the development of positive communication skills, the use of empathic language, and allows people to evaluate each other more closely (Hohenstein, et.al., 2023:1).

ChatGPT (Generative Pre-trained Transformer) is presented as an open tool that is easily accessible to everyone, developed by OpenAI on November 30, 2022 (https://chat.openai.com). ChatGPT is defined as a game changer in every field, as it creates a model change in academic terms in health communication (Sallam, et.al. 2023:2;

Dis, et.al. 2023: 224). ChatGPT works through various algorithms to understand natural language structures and provide answers created with artificial intelligence (Koçyiğit, Darı, 2023:433). Salvagno, et al. (2023:1) listed the features of ChatGPT as follows: *"(a) write a small text on a given topic; (b) get information on a topic of interest; (c) compose an email or message with a certain tone, specific content, and intended for a particular person; (d) correct the shape of a text or change its wording; (e) solve problems."* With these features, ChatGPT has the capacity to minimize communication problems and produce understandable, accurate and contextual answers. ChatGPT's reliability, wide scope, multilingualism and largely free nature make it different (Yıldız, Alper, 2024:523). Due to these features, ChatGPT has begun to be used more in health communication. By sorting, classifying and combining health issues, it can give quicker advice to people. It can also produce faster solutions to problems.

Health communication is a fundamental clinical skill required for effective clinical diagnosis, treatment decision making, and achieving optimal patient outcomes (Butow, Hoque, 2020:49). Research shows that if healthcare professionals have high communication skills within the scope of health communication, there is a positive increase in patients' capacity to understand, remember and follow medical conversations and recommendations, and to self-manage their diseases (Duffy, et.al.2004; Heisler, et.al. 2002; Renzi, et.al. 2001; Safran, et.al. 1998; Sullivan, et.al. 2000; Zachariae, et.al. 2003). There is still a need for time for artificial intelligence to replace these communication skills and to be used effectively in health communication. Because human communication does not only consist of a few features such as the ability to use language, good speaking and pronunciation, and high listening ability. Transferring the body language, clothing, tone of voice and emphasis that support non-verbal communication in humans to artificial intelligence is an extremely complex process. However, despite all the negative situations experienced, progress has been made in developing frameworks that increase behavioral interaction in artificial intelligence, model and calculate it (Butow, Hoque, 2020:51). These advances are also extremely important in health communication. Because in health communication, the answers to questions such as whether people are in pain, whether they are stressed, whether they are anxious or not can be understood more easily through emotional coding. With artificial intelligence, it can read many such behavioral codes and detect the posture of the face and the movements of the eyes. It is inevitable for health communication to further develop such codes of behavior in the future.

Although there are many positive aspects of artificial intelligence in health communication, it should be acknowledged that there are also concerns and fears. The use of artificial intelligence may not be welcomed in cases such as difficulty in learning new developing technology, lack of widespread training, lack of familiarity and facing uncertainty (Bulut, et.al. 2024:56). For all these reasons, there may be difficulties in adopting, applying and transferring artificial intelligence technologies to people. One of the obstacles to the development of artificial intelligence in health communication is the infrastructure problem. As the technological infrastructure remains inadequate, the usage rate of artificial intelligence is also decreasing. In order to prevent this, strategic plans should be implemented, financial resources should be provided to develop the infrastructure, and familiarity should be ensured by organizing training and various programs (Sebetci, 2024:3). As a result, when using artificial intelligence and ChatGPT in health communication, it should be known how this technology should be handled, the purposes for which it will be used should be specified, and whether the results obtained are accurate and reflect reality should be carefully examined. In addition, it should not be forgotten that it is obligatory to protect the privacy and confidentiality of any information entered into ChatGPT.

Generally speaking, Dave, et.al. (2023:02) listed the advantages, limitations and ethical aspects of ChatGPT in the field of health and medicine as follows:

"Advantages and Applications

1. Produces formally structured text.
2. Has eloquent vocabulary
3. Can be used as a rapid search engine
4. Produced text skips conventional plagiarism cheks
5. Searches and analyzes available literatüre
6. Can be used for medical education
7. Can act as a conversational agent
8. Can be used for patient monitoring and prompt
9. Follow up in case of exacerbation of risk factors

Limitations and Ethical Concerns

1. May infringe copyright laws
2. Medico-legal complications may arise
3. Sometimes gives inaccurate results
4. Sometimes gives biased and harmful results
5. Unable to differentiate between reliable and unreliable sources
6. Sometimes produces irrelevant references."

ChatGPT can significantly reduce the time it takes to perform various tasks by providing various conveniences in the field of health communication. If ChatGPT is used, the remaining time can be spent with better quality, can be included in production processes, effective communication, and can be used to do other necessary work.

As a result, as artificial intelligence applications such as ChatGPT begin to play larger roles in our lives, their benefits in the field of health communication cannot be ignored. In this context, as the communication that people expect from artificial intelligence approaches normal human intelligence, the use cases of ChatCPT will increase further.

METHODOLOGY OF THE STUDY

The aim of this study is to reveal the benefits and drawbacks of using the ChatGPT program in health communication for people. Additionally, within the scope of ChatGPT applications in health communication, an evaluation has been made about the future of artificial intelligence.

The research was designed and conducted as a qualitative research. Qualitative research is a method that is inquisitive, interpretive and strives to understand the problem in its natural environment (Guba ve Lincoln, 1994; Klenke, 2016, Baltacı 2019). Qualitative research, which uses qualitative data collection methods such as observation, interview and document analysis regarding the solution of a problem, refers to a subjective-interpretive process aimed at perceiving previously known or unrecognized problems and dealing with natural phenomena related to the problem in a realistic manner (Seale, 1999).

The study group determined to obtain data in the research was determined by the snowball sampling method. In the snowball sampling method, a reference person is selected regarding the subject of the study and other people are reached through this person (Biernacki, and Waldorf, 1981). In qualitative research, data is collected through interviews, observations and documents (Creswell, 2021). For this reason, a semi-structured interview form was created in the research. The interview form was developed by the researchers. While creating the form, the opinions of experts on health communication and artificial intelligence were taken. The form contains 13 questions. 3 of these questions are about age, gender and education level. The remaining 10 questions are given below:

- Do you use digital applications in the field of health?
- Should digital applications be used in the field of health?
- -What do you think about the use of artificial intelligence in health communication?

- Do you know what ChatGPT is?
- Have you used the ChatGPT application for health-related issues?
- Do you think ChatGPT should be used in the healthcare field?
- What might be the advantages of using ChatGPT in health communication?
- What might be the disadvantages of using ChatGPT in the field of healthcare?
- What do you think about the future of artificial intelligence applications in the field of healthcare?
- Are traditional methods or artificial intelligence applications more effective in health communication?

Semi-structured interview forms were applied by researchers online. The answers were transferred to Microsoft Word. After this stage, the data obtained was read and categorized. In line with the data obtained, the categories created for content analysis were collected under 7 headings. These are: The status of using digital applications in the field of health, the opinion about the use of artificial intelligence in health communication, the usage status of the ChatGPT application in health communication, the advantages of using ChatGPT in health communication, the disadvantages of using ChatGPT in health communication, the future of the use of artificial intelligence in health communication, traditional methods and artificial intelligence in health communication. Comparison of the use of intelligence applications. The data obtained according to the determined categories were analyzed with the content analysis method.

DATA ANALYSIS AND FINDINGS

The population of the research consists of university graduates over the age of 18. The researcher first reached two people in his close circle. Later, other people were reached through them. The age range of the people participating in the research is between 18 and 60. 16 of the people participating in the research were women and 14 were men. In the research, a semi-structured interview form was applied to 30 people reached by snowball sampling method. The interviews were recorded with the permission of the participants. The answers given to the questions in this form were analyzed with content analysis. The data obtained as a result of the qualitative analysis were shown in tables. Since the answers given to some open-ended questions were multiple choices, the table was not used. The findings obtained as a result of the analysis were given below:

Table 1. Participants' Usage of Digital Applications in the Field of Health.

Yes I'm using	25
No I do not use	3
I use it sometimes	2
Total	30

When the research participants' usage of digital applications in the field of health was examined, it was seen that 27 people used these applications. 3 people do not use it. Based on these data, it is possible to say that digital applications in the field of health are used by the majority of participants.

Table 2. Participants' Opinions about the use of Digital Applications in the Field of Health

Yes Should Be Used	27
No It Should Not Be Used	3
Total	30

When the participants' opinions about the use of digital applications in health communication are examined, it is seen that 27 people have a positive view on the use of digital applications in health communication, while 3 people have a negative view on the use of digital applications in health communication. People with negative views prefer face-to-face communication.

Table 3. Participants' Opinions about the use of Artificial Intelligence in Health Communication

I find artificial intelligence applications unnecessary in health communication.	3
Artificial intelligence applications in health communication benefit people.	12
Artificial intelligence applications in health communication provide convenience in the field of health.	6
Artificial intelligence applications in health communication save time.	7
Artificial intelligence applications in health communication are promising but insufficient.	2
Total	30

Looking at the participants' answers to the interview questions, it can be said that the participants are generally positive about the use of artificial intelligence applications in health communication. 12 people stated that artificial intelligence would be beneficial in health communication, 6 people stated that it would provide convenience, and 7 people stated that it would save time. The remaining 5 people stated that artificial intelligence applications in health communication are unnecessary and insufficient.

Table 4. Participants' Awareness of ChatGPT

Yes I know	3
No, I do not know	27
Total	30

In the research, before asking questions about ChatGPT to the participants, it was wanted to find out whether they knew ChatGPT. All but 3 of the participants stated that they were aware of this practice.

Table 5. Participants' use of ChatGPT on Health-Related Issues

Yes I Used	6
No I didn't use it	24
Total	30

When the answers given to the question about the participants' usage of ChatGPT were evaluated, it was seen that 24 people did not use the application and only 6 people used this application in health communication. In line with these data, although almost all of the participants knew the ChatGPT application, they did not use this application in health communication.

Table 6. Participants' Opinions about the use of ChatGPT in Health Communication

Yes it should be used	3
No it should not be used	27
Total	30

In the study, participants were asked about their thoughts on the use of ChatGPT in health communication. 27 of the participants said that "it should be used". The remaining 3 people stated that "it is unnecessary to use it". It is possible to say that the participants largely support the ChatGPT application. Moreover, the answers in the tables above also support this situation (Table 2, Table 3).

Table 7. Advantages of using ChatGPT in Health Communication According to Participants

Using ChatGPT application in health communication saves time.	14
Using ChatGPT application in health communication informs people about the disease	9
Using ChatGPT application in health communication reduces the workload of doctors.	4
It is unnecessary to use ChatGPT application in health communication	1

continued on following page

Table 7. Continued

Using ChatGPT application in health communication saves time.	14
There is no benefit in using the ChatGPT application in health communication.	2
Total	30

When the participants were asked about the advantages of using ChatGPT in health communication, 14 of the participants stated that it saved time, 9 stated that it informed people about the disease, and 4 stated that it reduced the workload of doctors. 2 participants argued that there was no advantage, and 1 participant argued that the use of ChatGPT in health communication was unnecessary. Some of the answers given by the participants to this question are given below:

> "With this application, patients can find answers to some minor health problems without going to the doctor. Thus, they save time."
> "With this application, there is no need to go to the doctor unnecessarily. We especially save time and money."
> "With this application, we may not have to waste time in the hospital."
> "ChatGPT can ease the workload of doctors and healthcare professionals. We do not keep doctors busy unnecessarily."
> "ChatGPT has no advantage. Because virtual communication in the field of health can lead to misinformation. It can cause people to experience greater health problems."

Table 8. Disadvantages of using ChatGPT in Health Communication According to Participants

ChatGPT application in health communication may provide incorrect information to patients.	18
The application of ChatGPT in health communication may cause patients to worry unnecessarily.	4
Using ChatGPT application in health communication may cause healthcare workers to become unemployed.	5
In health communication, ChatGPT application cannot explain as much as a doctor.	3
Total	30

When we look at the answers to the disadvantages of ChatGPT in health communication, more than half of the participants emphasized that "patients may be misinformed". 5 participants stated that "health workers will face the problem of becoming unemployed". 4 participants stated that "sometimes people will worry unnecessarily as a result of the information they receive from here." 3 people stated that this application cannot provide the necessary explanation to patients as much as the doctor does. Some of the answers given by the participants to this question are given below:

"This application is after all an artificial intelligence, it is not real, so it may give false information to patients."

"Since the patient does not explain his/her problem face to face, the wrong diagnosis may be made. In this case, the patient will be misinformed."

"Since the doctor does not examine the patient, the patient may be given incorrect information. In other words, the diagnosis of the disease may be incorrect."

"The patient may express himself incorrectly. Since he is not in the examination, sometimes patients may feel upset for no reason."

"Sometimes patients can worry even about a simple illness."

"If ChatGPT becomes widespread, the rate of going to hospitals may decrease in the future. Everyone first gets information on ChatGPT. They do not go to the doctor immediately. This may cause healthcare workers to become unemployed."

"A machine cannot be as good as a human. It is not possible to be as descriptive as a doctor, especially in the field of health."

Table 9. Participants' Opinions about the Future of Artificial Intelligence Applications in the Field of Healthcare

It will become common in the healthcare field	14
It will create problems in the field of health	5
It will make things easier in the field of healthcare.	8
It can be used in limited places	3
Total	30

When asked about their thoughts on the future of ChatGPT, nearly half of the participants said that it would "become widespread in the future." 8 participants stated that "it will provide convenience in the field of healthcare". Based on these data, it is possible to say that more than half of the participants think that the future of ChatGPT is promising. 5 participants believe that it will "cause problems" due to providing incorrect information in the field of health. 3 participants stated that "its use will be limited". Some of the answers given by the participants to this question are given below:

"ChatGPT will become very widespread in the future, even doctors will not feel the need to examine except for some cases. Artificial intelligence will do everything."

"Health communication can only be done through artificial intelligence programs in the coming years. This saves both time and money. In short, ChatGPT will be widely used in the future."

> "With this application, people will be able to find solutions to their diseases immediately. Many people will use this application. Even country governments will support these applications in health communication. These applications will become widespread."
>
> "Even if this application is used in the future, it cannot become widespread. Because artificial intelligence cannot treat or solve everything on its own. It will definitely be limited to certain health issues. For example, it cannot perform surgery."
>
> "It will cause problems in health communication because it misinforms people and will not be used."
>
> "With this application, there may be different interpretations of the diagnosis between the doctor and artificial intelligence. This will reduce trust and cause chaos."

Table 10. Participants' Preferences Regarding Artificial Intelligence Applications and Traditional Applications in Health Communication

I prefer traditional methods in health communication.	6
I prefer artificial intelligence applications in health communication	5
Both applications should be used when necessary in health communication.	19
Total	30

Finally, the participants were asked whether they preferred artificial intelligence applications or traditional applications in health communication. To this question, 2/3 of the participants said that both applications can be used together. In other words, they argued that artificial intelligence applications can be used when necessary, but this should not eliminate traditional health communication. While 6 participants stated that they would prefer traditional methods, 5 participants stated that they preferred artificial intelligence applications in health communication. Some of the answers given by the participants to this question are given below:

> "Artificial intelligence applications should be used, but not alone. There should definitely be traditional health communication along with them. I think the two applications should be used together."
>
> "The two applications should be used together, and the deficiency in one should be filled by the other."
>
> "I always prefer face-to-face communication techniques in health communication. I think that communication established in virtual environments will not be beneficial."

"I think artificial intelligence applications alone may be sufficient in health communication. I may prefer it. It can save time and money. Also, technology is advancing a lot. I think artificial intelligence will be an inevitable end in the future."

DISCUSSION AND CONCLUSION

Today, health communication has gone beyond just the patient-doctor-nurse relationship and has covered a broader area. So much so that it seems that medical science can no longer keep up with health-related issues on its own (Yıldız, Tanyıldızı, 2015:126).

In this context, it is inevitable to start using various applications and integrate the necessary technologies into health communication. One of these technologies and applications is ChatGPT, which is a state-of-the-art product. ChatGPT is one of the latest technology products that uses an effective language model and has both advantages and various applications in terms of health and health communication. The most important goal of ChatGPT is to imitate human behavior and intelligence in the most perfect way. Although ChatGPT offers important opportunities in terms of health communication, it also brings with it various challenges. For this reason, ChatGPT should be evaluated meticulously in terms of health communication. These evaluation criteria for artificial intelligence, which is thought to be particularly beneficial, should also be developed.

Before ChatGPT is used in the field of health communication, as in every field, reliability, ethical approaches, prejudices in society, fears, threats, and limitations to be applied by institutions should be comprehensively addressed. For example, ChatGPT can easily perform many tasks in health communication. However, in ChatGPT, more thought also needs to be given to how data should be protected. The pieces of Dwivedi (2023) and Yağar (2023) were achieved in this process. In addition, it should not be forgotten that ChatGPT cannot always provide the correct information, and just like humans, users cannot find answers to everything they want. While benefiting from the benefits of ChatGPT and the innovations it brings, the application phase of the methods should also be improved. In this regard, Chow et al. (2023) stated that problems may arise in the use of ChatCPT as a new model in the field of health. He also emphasized that information should be confirmed on issues such as accuracy and security.

In the study conducted on the use of ChatGPT in health communication, the most general results are as follows: It was stated that most people who participated in the research were of the opinion that both traditional methods and artificial intelligence applications such as ChatGPT were necessary in health communication, and that the use of both methods together was growth-oriented. It is possible to say that various digital applications in the field of health are used by the participants. Opinions towards ChatGPT are generally positive. Participants who expressed negative opinions attach more importance to face-to-face communication. Participants who were positive about ChatGPT stated that ChatGPT would be useful, provide convenience to people, save time in work, ease the workload of employees, and inform people about diseases more quickly and easily. The majority of participants are aware of the studies on ChatGPT. Although participants are aware of ChatGPT, a new digital application, the number of people using it is low. Although the number of people using ChatGPT is low, most of the participants support this application. Participants stated that ChatGPT also has disadvantages. According to the participants, ChatGPT may misinform patients, cause people to face the problem of being unemployed, sometimes patients and their relatives may become unnecessarily anxious with the information they receive, and they may not be able to provide the necessary explanations as doctors do. Participants stated that artificial intelligence can be used when necessary, but this should not eliminate traditional health communication. As a result, ChatGPT will continue to develop with its advantages and disadvantages in health communication. While benefiting from the benefits of ChatGPT, methods, applications, software and technologies should be developed to alleviate its disadvantages. ChatGPT, whose disadvantages are minimized, can assist people in all transactions and processes, from healthcare professionals to patients.

REFERENCES

-Amanawa Imomoemi, V., Amanawa, D., E. (2024). *"The Application of Artificial Intelligence (AI) in Medicine, with A Focus on Public Health Communication: Prospects for the Nigerian Health Sector"*, International Journal of Academic Health and Medical Research (IJAHMR),Vol. 8 Issue 1 January.

Anand, D., Arulselvi, G., & Balaji, G. N. (2022). A deep convolutional extreme machine learning classification method to detect bone cancer from histopathological images. *Journal of Optoelectronics Laser*, 41(7), 456–468.

Antel, R., Abbasgholizadeh-Rahimi, S., Guadagno, E., Harley, J. M., & Poenaru, D. (2022). The Use of Artificial İntelligence and Virtual Reality in Doctor-Patient Risk Communication: A Scoping Review. *Patient Education and Counseling*, 105(10), 3038–3050. 10.1016/j.pec.2022.06.00635725526

Baltaci, A. (2019). Nitel Araştırma Süreci: Nitel Bir Araştırma Nasıl Yapılır? *Ahi Evran Üniversitesi Sosyal Bilimler Enstitüsü Dergisi*, 5(2), 368–388. 10.31592/aeusbed.598299

Biernacki, P., & Waldorf, D. (1981). Snowball Sampling: Problems and Techniques of Chain Referral Sampling. *Sociological Methods & Research*, 10(2), 141–163. 10.1177/004912418101000205

Butow, P., & Hoque, E. (2020). Using Artificial İntelligence to Analyse and Teach Communication in Healthcare. *The Breast*, •••, 50.32007704

-Bulut H, Kınoğlu NG, Karaduman B. (2024). *"The Fear of Artificial İntelligence: Dentists and the Anxiety of the Unknown"*, Journal of Advanced Research in Health Sciences, 7(1), https://doi.org/. 30.03.2024.10.26650/JARHS2024-1302739

Chow, J. C. L., Sanders, L., & Li, K. (2023). Impact of ChatGPT on medical chatbots as a disruptive technology". *Frontiers in Artificial Intelligence*, 6(1), 1–3. 10.3389/frai.2023.116601437091303

Creswell, J. W. (2021). *A Concise Introduction To Mixed Methods Research*. SAGE publications.

Dave, T., Athaluri, S. A., & Singh, S. (2023). Chatgpt in Medicine: An Overview of İts Applications, Advantages, Limitations, Future Prospects, and Ethical Considerations. *Frontiers in Artificial Intelligence*, 6, 1169595. 10.3389/frai.2023.116959537215063

Duffy, FD, Gordon, GH, Whelan, G, Cole-Kelly, K, & Frankel, R. (2004). Assessing competence in communication and interpersonal skills: The Kalamazoo II report. *Academic Medicine*, •••, 79.15165967

Van Dis, E. A., Bollen, J., Zuidema, W., Van Rooij, R., & Bockting, C. L. (2023). ChatGPT: Five priorities for research. *Nature*, 614(7947), 224–226.

Dwivedi, Y.K. (2023). Opinion Paper: "So What if Chatgpt Wrote İt?" Multidisciplinary Perspectives on Opportunities, Challenges and İmplications of Generative Conversational aI For Research, Practice and Policy. *International Journal of Information Management*. Advance online publication. 10.1016/j.ijinfomgt.2023.102642 26.03.2024

-Else, H. (2023). *"Abstracts Written by Chatgpt Fool Scientists"*, 423-423 Nature, *613* (7944). https://doi.org/.10.1038/d41586-023-00056-7

Golan, R., Reddy, R., & Ramasamy, R. (2024). The Rise of Artificial İntelligence-Driven Health Communication. *Translational Andrology and Urology*, 13(2), 356–358. 10.21037/tau-23-55638481858

- Guba, E. G., Lincoln, Y. S. (1994). "Competing Paradigms In Qualitative Research". Handbook of qualitative research, *2*(163-194), 105.

Heisler, M, Bouknight, RR, Hayward, RA, Smith, DM, & Kerr, EA. (2002). The relative importance of physician communication, participatory decision-making, and patient understanding in diabetes self-management. *Journal of General Internal Medicine*, •••, 17.11972720

Green, N., Rubinelli, S., Scott, D., & Visser, A. (2013). Health Communication Meets Artificial İntelligence. *Patient Education and Counseling*, 92(2), 139–141. 10.1016/j.pec.2013.06.01323866991

Safran, DG, Taira, D, Rogers, WH, Kosinski, M, Ware, JE, & Tarlov, AR. (1998). Linking primary care performance to outcomes of care. *The Journal of Family Practice*, 47(3).9752374

Renzi, C, Abeni, D, Picardi, A, Agostini, E, Melchi, CF, Pasquini, P, Prudu, P, & Braga, M. (2001). Factors associated with patient satisfaction with care among dermatological outpatients". *British Journal of Dermatology*, •••, 145.11703289

Qian, X., & Yuan, S. (2014). AI-Powered Mental Health Communication: Examining the Effects of Affection Expectations on Health Behavioral İntentions. *Patient Education and Counseling*, 122, •••. www.journals.elsevier.com/patient-education-and-counseling38237529

-Radford A., Narasimhan K., Salimans T., Sutskever I. (2018). *"Improving Language Understanding by Generative Pre-Training"*, [Google Akademik], 26.03.2024

-Reed, L. (2022). *"Chatgpt For Automated Testing: From Conversation to Code"*. Sauce Labs. https://saucelabs.com/blog/chatgpt-automated-testing-conversation-to-code Accessed: February 20, 2023.

Hohenstein, J., Kizilcec, R. F., DiFranzo, D., Aghajari, Z., Mieczkowski, H., Levy, K., Naaman, M., Hancock, J., & Jung, M. F. (2023). Artificial Intelligence in Communication Impacts Language and Social Relationships". *Scientific Reports*, 13(1), 5487. 10.1038/s41598-023-30938-937015964

Hu, Y. (2015). Health Communication Research in the Digital Age: A Systematic Review. *Journal of Communication in Healthcare*, 8(4), 260–288. 10.1080/17538068.2015.1107308

Kreps, G. L., & Neuhauser, L. (2013). Artificial intelligence and immediacy: Designing health communication to personally engage consumers and providers. *Patient Education and Counseling*, 92(2), 205–210.

Klenke, K. (2016). *Qualitative Research In The Study Of Leadership*. Emerald Group Publishing Limited.

-Koçyiğit, A., Darı, A.B., (2023), *"Yapay Zekâ İletişiminde ChatGPT: İnsanlaşan Dijitalleşmenin Geleceği"*, Stratejik ve Sosyal Araştırmalar Dergisi, C.7, S.2, S..427-438.

Kumar, K., Kumar, V., Seema, , Sharma, M. K., Khan, A. A., & Idrisi, M. J. (2024). *"A Systematic Review of Blockchain Technology Assisted with Artificial Intelligence Technology for Networks and Communication Systems"*, Hindawi. *Journal of Computer Networks and Communications*, 2024, 9979371. Advance online publication. 10.1155/2024/9979371

Lim, S., & Schmälzle, R. (2023). Artificial İntelligence for Health Message Generation: An Empirical Study Using A Large Language Model (LLM) and Prompt Engineering. *Frontiers in Communication*, 8, 1129082. 10.3389/fcomm.2023.1129082

-Marchetti, D., Lanzola, G., Stefanelli, M. (2001). In S. Quaglini, P. Barahona, & S. Andreassen (Eds.), An AI-Based Approach to Support Communication in Health Care Organizations (pp. 384–394). AIME., LNAI 2101.

-Metz, A. (2022). *"6 Exciting Ways to Use Chatgpt – From Coding to Poetry"*. TechRadar. htt ps://www.techradar.com/features/6-exciting-ways-to-use-chatgpt-from-coding-to -poetry Accessed: 26.03.2024.

Menichetti, J., Hillen, M. A., Papageorgiou, A., & Pieterse, A. H. (2023). How Can Chatgpt be Used to Support Healthcare Communication Research? *Patient Education and Counseling*, 115, 107947. 10.1016/j.pec.2023.107947

Nadarzynski, T., Miles, O., Cowie, A., & Ridge, D. (2019). Acceptability of Artificial İntelligence (AI)-led Chatbot Services in Healthcare: A Mixed-Methods Study. *Digital Health*, 5, 1–12. journals.sagepub.com/home/dhj. 10.1177/2055207619871808314 67682

Sallam, M., Salim, N. A., Al-Tammemi, A. B., Barakat, M., Fayyad, D., Hallit, S., Harapan, H., Hallit, R., & Mahafzah, A. (2023). ChatGPT Output Regarding Compulsory Vaccination and COVID-19 Vaccine Conspiracy: A Descriptive Study at the Outset of a Paradigm Shift in Online Search for Information. *Cureus*, 15(2), e35029. 10.7759/cureus.3502936819954

- Seale, C. (1999). *"The Quality Of Qualitative Research"*. The Quality of qualitative research, 1-224.

Sullivan, LM, Stein, MD, Savetsky, JB, & Samet, JH. (2000). The doctor-patient relationship and HIV-infected patients' satisfaction with primary care physicians". *Journal of General Internal Medicine*, •••, 15.10940132

-Zachariae R, Pederson CG, Jensen AB, Ehrnrooth E, Rossen PB, Von der Maase H. (2003). *"Association of Perceived Physician Communication Style With Patient Satisfaction, Distress, Cancer-Related Self-Efficacy, and Perceived Control Over the Disease"*. Br J Canc,88.

-Yıldız, İ.,İmik Tanyıldızı, N. (2015). *"Türkiye'de 2012 Yılında Sağlık Haberlerinin Ulusal Yazılı Basında Yer Alış Biçimleri Ve Bilgilendirme Düzeyleri (Habertürk, Hürriyet, Posta, Sabah, Sözcü Ve Zaman Gazeteleri Örneği)"*, Sosyal Bilimler Dergisi / The Journal of Social Science / SOBİDER, Yıl: 2, Sayı: 2

-Veisdal, J. (2019). "The birthplace of ai, "Cantor's paradise,", https://www.cantorsparadise.com/the-birthplace-of-ai-9ab7d4e5fb00, View at: Google Scholar

-. (2022). Survey on reinforcement learning for language processing. *Artificial Intelligence Review*, •••, 1–33. 10.1007/s10462-022-10205-5

Salvagno, M., Taccone, F. S., & And Gerlı, A. G. (2023). Can Artificial Intelligence Help For Scientific Writing? *Critical Care*, 27(1).

-Stokel-Walker, C. J. N. (2023). *"Chatgpt Listed As Author On Research Papers: Many Scientists Disapprove."* Nature, *613*, 620–621. 26.03.2024.10.1038/d41586-023-00107-z

-Yağar, S.D., (2023). *"Chatgpt'nin Sağlık Alanındaki Potansiyel Kullanımına İlişkin Çıkarımlar"*, bmij 11 (3): 1226-1240, doi: https://doi.org/10.15295/bmij.v11i3.2264

-Yıldız M.S., Alper A. (2023). *"Potential Functions of Artificial İntelligence Chatbot Chatgpt in Health Management: Scoping Review"*, Turk Hijyen ve Biyoloji Dergisi, 80(4).

Sebetci, Ö. (2024). *Yapay Zeka ile Sağlık Sistemlerden Uygulamalara*. Kodlab Basın Yayın.

Zhang, M., & Li, J. (2021). A commentary of GPT-3 in MIT Technology Review 2021. *Fundamental Research (Beijing)*, 1(6), 831–833. 10.1016/j.fmre.2021.11.011

KEY TERMS AND DEFINITIONS

Artificial Intelligence: A system that can be developed that imitates human intelligence to perform certain tasks and can repeatedly present the information they collect.

Health: Health is not merely the absence of disease and infirmity, but a state of complete physical, mental and social well-being.

Communication: The exchange of feelings, thoughts, information and news between people and their mutual transfer from person to person in all kinds of forms and ways.

Chat GPT: A chat application that responds to questions asked by users.

Health communication: The art and technique of informing, influencing and motivating individuals, institutions and the public about important health problems.

Chapter 7
Federated Learning for Securing Glomeruli Detection in Digital Pathology

Shiva Chaithanya Goud Bollipelly
https://orcid.org/0009-0002-1024-9689
Vellore Institute of Technology, India

ABSTRACT

This chapter addresses the imperative for secure and precise glomeruli detection in histopathological images, crucial for diagnosing renal conditions. Using the YOLOv3 object detection algorithm, it integrates federated learning to ensure data security. A custom dataset, annotated with XML labels from histopathological images of sclerosed and normal glomeruli, is created. Initially, a traditional YOLOv3 model achieved 98.55% accuracy but posed privacy risks with centralized data storage. Federated learning decentralizes data across clients, preserving privacy and achieving 98.79% accuracy. Employing cryptographic techniques for data transmission security, this chapter demonstrates federated learning's robustness in medical image analysis. A comparative analysis with traditional methods highlights federated learning's advantages in data security and collaborative learning, showcasing its transformative potential in digital pathology.

DOI: 10.4018/979-8-3693-3719-6.ch007

INTRODUCTION:

In the realm of digital pathology, the precise detection and classification of glomeruli, particularly distinguishing between sclerosed and normal variants, are critical for diagnosing and managing various renal diseases. This chapter explores an innovative approach to augment both the accuracy of glomeruli detection and the protection of confidential medical data through cutting-edge machine learning techniques.

Traditionally, machine learning algorithms like YOLOv3 have played a pivotal role in glomeruli detection, showcasing robust accuracy rates. However, conventional models often require consolidating extensive medical data into centralized repositories for training, raising significant concerns regarding data privacy and security. Enter federated learning, a paradigm that reshapes model training by distributing it across decentralized nodes, thereby alleviating privacy risks associated with centralized data aggregation.

This project embarks on leveraging federated learning for enhancing glomeruli detection while prioritizing data security. The journey commences with the curation of a meticulously annotated dataset sourced from Bueno et al. (2020), encompassing histopathological images encompassing both sclerosed and normal glomeruli instances. Each image undergoes meticulous labeling using XML annotations, laying the foundation for subsequent model training endeavors.

Initially, the project benchmarks the performance of a traditional YOLOv3 model trained on this curated dataset, achieving a commendable accuracy threshold of 98.55%. Subsequently, the focus shifts to federated learning, where the dataset is partitioned across multiple clients to ensure data privacy while maintaining model accuracy. This innovative approach yields comparable results, with the federated learning model achieving an accuracy rate of 98.79%, underscoring its effectiveness in safeguarding data privacy without compromising model performance.

In essence, this chapter serves as a testament to the transformative potential of federated learning in digital pathology, offering a viable solution to enhance glomeruli detection accuracy while preserving the confidentiality of sensitive medical data. Through an in-depth exploration of implementation strategies, empirical results, and future implications, this chapter aims to illuminate the pathway toward a more secure and efficient healthcare ecosystem.

BACKGROUND:

The literature on glomeruli detection and renal pathology encompasses a diverse array of methodologies and applications aimed at enhancing diagnostic accuracy and efficiency. Kawazoe et al. (2018) introduced a Faster R-CNN-based approach tailored specifically for the detection of glomeruli in multistained whole slide images (WSIs) of human renal tissue sections. Leveraging the state-of-the-art Faster R-CNN framework, the study demonstrated the efficacy of deep learning techniques in automating the detection process, thereby alleviating the burden on pathologists and facilitating quantitative analysis of glomeruli in WSIs. Similarly, Gallego et al. (2018) explored the application of convolutional neural networks (CNNs) for glomerulus classification and detection in digitized kidney slide segments. By training a CNN model to distinguish between glomerulus and non-glomerulus regions, the study showcased the potential of deep learning in streamlining glomerular evaluation while minimizing false positive and false negative detections.

In a related vein, Liu et al. (2020) proposed GLO-YOLO, a dynamic glomerular detection and slicing model tailored for high-resolution whole slide images (WSIs) of human renal biopsy microscope slides. Building upon the YOLO-v3 architecture, GLO-YOLO leveraged dynamic scale evaluation and improved training strategies to achieve state-of-the-art performance in glomerulus detection. The study underscored the utility of deep learning frameworks in augmenting the efficiency and accuracy of glomerular evaluation, thereby facilitating rapid and effective diagnosis of renal pathologies. Complementing these endeavors, Nandhini et al. (2022) investigated the application of federated learning in predicting chronic kidney diseases (CKD), addressing the challenges associated with centralized healthcare data repositories. By harnessing federated learning techniques, the study demonstrated the feasibility of training predictive models on decentralized data sources while preserving data privacy, thereby enhancing diagnostic capabilities in CKD prediction.

Furthermore, Lutnick et al. (2022) delved into the domain of federated training for segmentation models on whole slide images (WSIs), addressing the logistical challenges of data sharing in computational pathology. Through federated learning, the study showcased the potential of collaborative model training across multiple institutions to enhance the generalizability and robustness of segmentation models, offering insights into the scalability and efficacy of federated learning in pathology informatics. Expanding the horizons of federated learning, Rjoub et al. (2021) proposed a federated YOLO CNN learning framework for improving object detection accuracy in adverse weather conditions, with a focus on autonomous vehicle safety. By integrating federated learning with the YOLO object detection approach, the study demonstrated the potential of distributed model training in enhancing real-time detection capabilities under challenging environmental conditions, shedding light on the transformative potential of federated learning across diverse domains.

Collectively, these studies underscore the burgeoning interest and innovation in leveraging deep learning and federated learning techniques to address the myriad challenges in glomeruli detection, renal pathology, and healthcare diagnostics. Through a convergence of cutting-edge methodologies and interdisciplinary collaboration, researchers continue to push the boundaries of computational pathology, paving the way for more accurate, efficient, and scalable solutions in disease diagnosis and treatment.

GLOMERULI:

Glomeruli, pivotal structures within the kidney responsible for blood filtration, play a crucial role in diagnosing renal diseases through histopathological analysis. The accurate identification and classification of glomeruli as either normal or sclerosed are essential for determining renal health and guiding appropriate medical interventions.

Figure 1. Normal Glomeruli

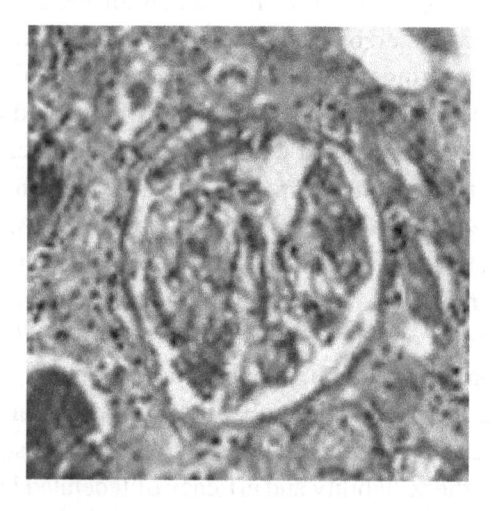

Figure 1 depicts a typical representation of normal glomeruli, characterized by a distinct structure that facilitates efficient filtration of blood components. In digital pathology, the challenge lies in accurately detecting and delineating these structures amidst varying tissue densities and textures. Traditional methods often require intensive manual scrutiny by pathologists, which can introduce subjectivity and variability in diagnostic outcomes.

Figure 2. Sclerosed Glomeruli

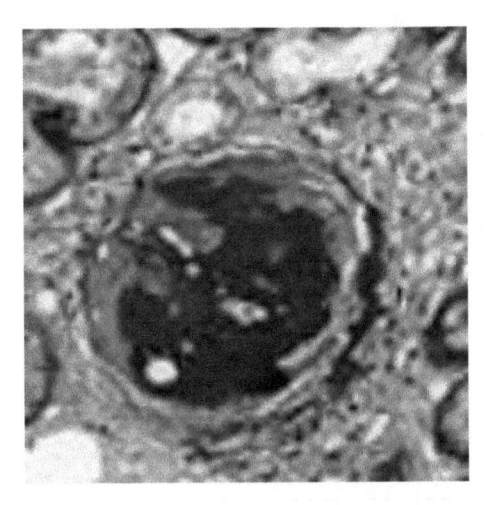

Contrastingly, Figure 2 illustrates sclerosed glomeruli, which exhibit pathological alterations indicative of renal dysfunction. Sclerosis, characterized by the thickening and hardening of glomerular walls, compromises their filtration function and is associated with progressive renal conditions such as glomerulosclerosis. Identifying these pathological changes accurately is crucial for assessing disease severity and planning appropriate treatment strategies.

In our chapter, we explore how artificial intelligence (AI) techniques, specifically the YOLOv3 detection model trained with federated learning, can enhance the accuracy and efficiency of glomeruli detection in digital pathology. By leveraging federated learning, which decentralizes model training while preserving data privacy, we aim to advance diagnostic capabilities while ensuring secure handling of patient information.

FEDERATED LEARNING:

Federated Learning represents a pioneering approach in machine learning aimed at training AI models collaboratively across decentralized devices while preserving data privacy and security. In the context of medical imaging and digital pathology, federated learning offers a robust framework to enhance diagnostic accuracy without compromising sensitive information.

Figure 3. Federated Learning Model Overview

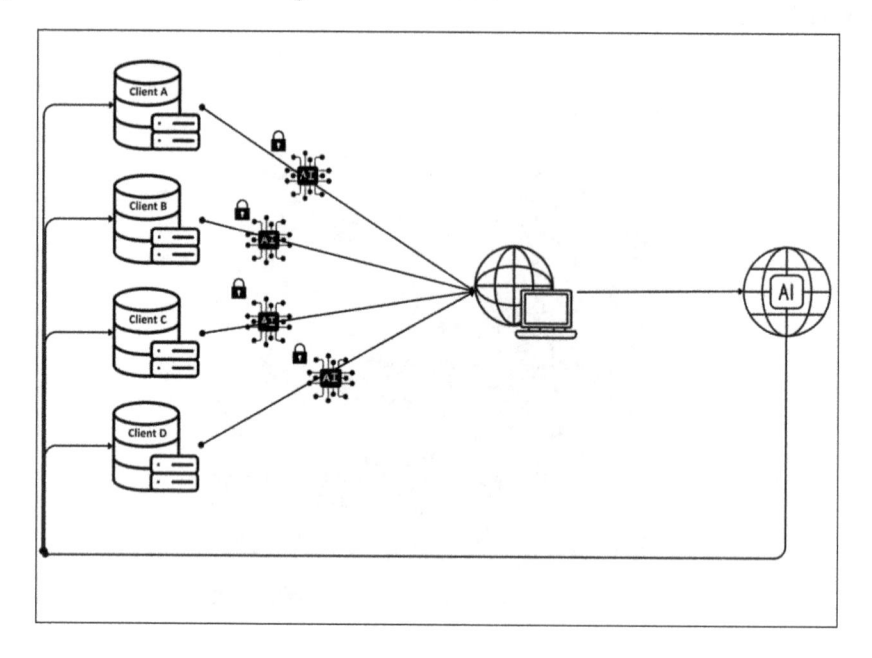

Figure 3 provides a visual representation of the federated learning process adopted in our study. Multiple client devices, representing healthcare institutions or clinics, participate in model training by utilizing their local datasets. Each client independently trains a local AI model using proprietary data and securely transmits model updates to a central server. These updates are aggregated to refine a global AI model, ensuring data privacy by keeping patient information decentralized and under local control.

The rationale behind employing federated learning in our research is twofold. Firstly, it allows for collaborative model improvement across diverse datasets without pooling sensitive medical information. Secondly, by decentralizing data storage and processing, federated learning mitigates privacy risks associated with centralized model training approaches. This approach aligns with ethical principles and instills trust among healthcare providers and patients in AI-driven diagnostic tools.

Our chapter explores how federated learning enhances the detection of glomeruli in digital pathology images, emphasizing its role in advancing diagnostic accuracy while safeguarding patient data. By leveraging this innovative methodology, we aim to contribute to the evolution of healthcare AI applications, ensuring robustness, privacy, and ethical integrity in medical image analysis.

YOLO:

Figure 4 depicts the performance and architecture comparison of YOLOv3, a state-of-the-art object detection algorithm renowned for its speed and accuracy in real-time applications. YOLOv3 surpasses previous versions in processing efficiency, making it highly suitable for tasks requiring rapid and precise object detection, such as glomeruli detection in digital pathology.

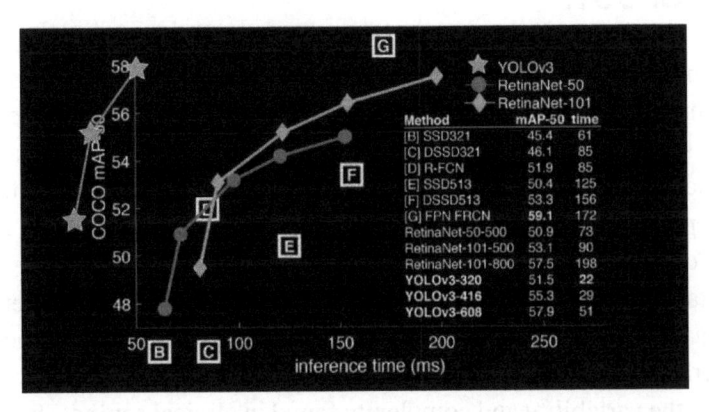

Figure 4. YOLO (You Only Look Once)

Method	mAP-50	time
[B] SSD321	45.4	61
[C] DSSD321	46.1	85
[D] R-FCN	51.9	85
[E] SSD513	50.4	125
[F] DSSD513	53.3	156
[G] FPN FRCN	59.1	172
RetinaNet-50-500	50.9	73
RetinaNet-101-500	53.1	90
RetinaNet-101-800	57.5	198
YOLOv3-320	51.5	22
YOLOv3-416	55.3	29
YOLOv3-608	57.9	51

YOLOv3 is chosen as our object detection algorithm due to its superior performance metrics, particularly in speed. Unlike traditional object detection methods that rely on multiple region proposals and complex computations, YOLOv3 operates by dividing the input image into a grid and predicting bounding boxes and class probabilities directly. This "you only look once" approach enables YOLOv3 to process images faster while maintaining high accuracy, which is crucial for real-time medical imaging applications.

In our project, we adapt YOLOv3 for glomeruli detection within digital pathology images. Although YOLOv3 is originally pretrained on the COCO (Common Objects in Context) dataset, which includes a wide range of object classes, including animals, vehicles, and everyday objects, its versatility allows for fine-tuning on specialized medical datasets. This adaptation involves retraining the YOLOv3 model using annotated images of normal and sclerosed glomeruli, thereby customizing it to excel in medical image analysis.

The integration of YOLOv3 with federated learning further enhances its utility in our research. By decentralizing model training across multiple healthcare institutions, federated learning ensures that the YOLOv3 model can learn from diverse datasets without compromising patient data privacy. This collaborative approach not only improves detection accuracy but also aligns with stringent healthcare data regulations, safeguarding sensitive medical information throughout the training process.

In our chapter, YOLOv3 serves as a cornerstone in our effort to improve the accuracy of glomeruli detection through federated learning. Its exceptional speed, precision, and flexibility render it optimal for real-time analysis of medical images, thereby advancing the field of digital pathology and ensuring the development of secure, efficient diagnostic solutions.

METHODOLOGY:

In our methodology, we undertook a meticulous approach to develop and implement a secure and effective framework for training object detection models in digital pathology, specifically focusing on the detection of sclerosed and normal glomeruli within histopathological images. The methodology began with the critical task of dataset preparation, which involved creating a custom dataset suitable for training our object detection model.

The dataset acquisition phase involved sourcing images from Bueno et al. (2020), providing a foundational set of histopathological images containing glomeruli. These images were chosen based on their relevance and quality, ensuring they adequately represented the variability and complexity found in clinical settings. Each image in the dataset was meticulously annotated using XML format, which included detailed annotations of sclerosed and normal glomeruli regions. This annotation process was essential as it established precise ground truth labels necessary for training the object detection model effectively.

Following dataset preparation, our methodology pivoted towards model training, which employed the YOLOv3 architecture—a state-of-the-art deep learning model renowned for its efficiency and accuracy in object detection tasks. The initial training phase utilized a centralized dataset approach, where the entire dataset was used to train a baseline YOLOv3 model. This phase aimed to establish a benchmark performance for glomeruli detection accuracy under traditional training methods.

To address concerns related to data privacy and security inherent in centralized training approaches, our methodology then embraced federated learning—a decentralized model training paradigm. In federated learning, the dataset was partitioned into distinct subsets, each allocated to different client nodes representing various healthcare institutions. This partitioning ensured that sensitive patient data remained localized within each institution, adhering to strict privacy regulations and ethical guidelines.

The federated learning setup involved establishing a client-server architecture using socket communication protocols, enabling secure and efficient data exchange between client nodes and a central server. Model weights initialized from a pre-trained YOLOv3 model were distributed to client nodes, where local training occurred on their respective dataset subsets. During this local training phase, client nodes iteratively updated the model weights based on their locally stored data, without transmitting raw data outside their respective environments.

Figure 5. XML Labelling

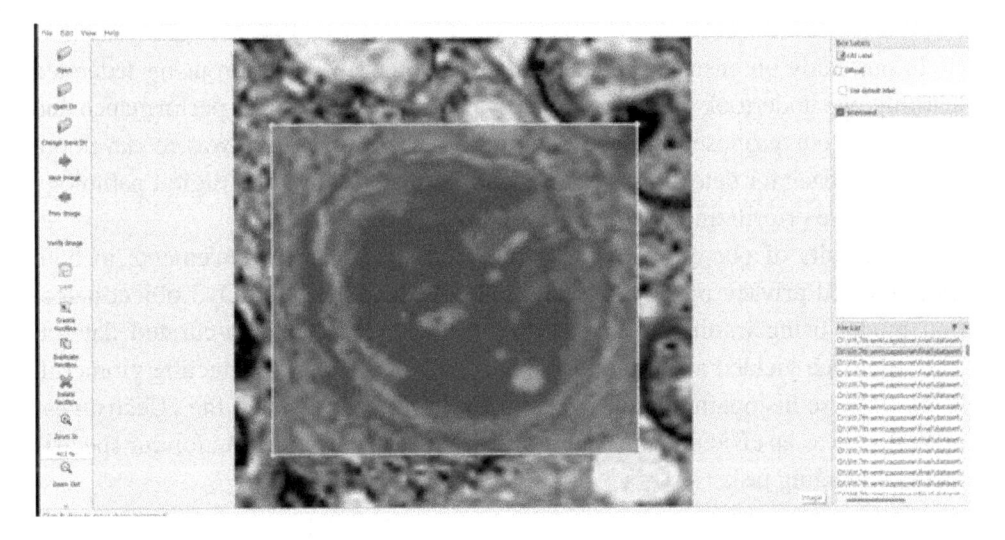

Simultaneously, to streamline and enhance dataset annotation efficiency, we developed a Python-based XML labelling software tailored for pathologists and researchers. This software facilitated the annotation process by providing intuitive tools for labelling glomeruli regions within histopathological images. By integrating this software into our workflow, we aimed to standardize and expedite the dataset annotation process, thereby improving overall dataset quality and usability for model training (Figure 5).

The culmination of our methodology was the evaluation phase, where we rigorously assessed the performance of both traditional centralized training and federated learning approaches. Key metrics such as detection accuracy, computational efficiency, and scalability were meticulously analyzed to compare the effectiveness of each approach in glomeruli detection tasks. The evaluation results provided empirical evidence supporting the superiority of federated learning in achieving comparable or superior model performance while upholding stringent data privacy standards.

In conclusion, our methodology represents a comprehensive and secure approach to training object detection models in digital pathology, specifically tailored for glomeruli detection using federated learning. By combining a custom dataset, YOLOv3 model architecture, federated learning framework, secure data handling protocols, and intuitive XML labelling tools, we have demonstrated a robust methodology that not only enhances diagnostic capabilities but also ensures the confidentiality and privacy of patient data—a crucial consideration in healthcare AI applications.

RESULTS:

In our study on ensuring data security in glomeruli detection using federated learning, we undertook comprehensive evaluations to assess the performance and efficacy of our proposed methodology. The primary objective was to develop a robust approach for detecting sclerosed and normal glomeruli in digital pathology images while prioritizing data privacy and security.

The results of our experiments showcased significant achievements in both accuracy and privacy preservation. Initially, we trained a YOLOv3 object detection model using traditional centralized methods on a custom-curated dataset. This approach yielded a commendable accuracy of 98.55% in detecting glomeruli across diverse histopathological images. These results validated the effectiveness of YOLOv3 as an efficient and accurate object detection algorithm for our specific medical imaging task.

Figure 6. Traditionally Trained Model Output

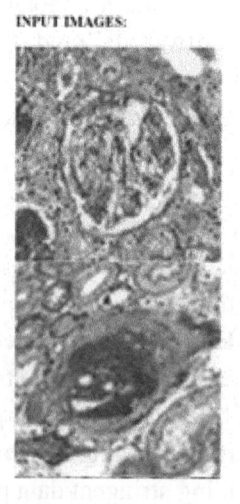

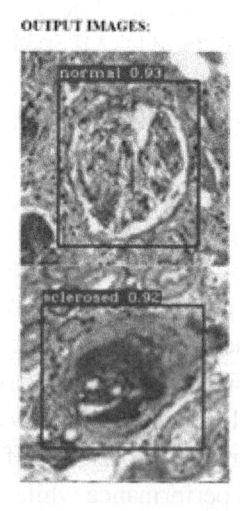

Subsequently, we implemented federated learning to enhance our model's performance while addressing concerns related to data privacy. The federated learning approach decentralized the training process, allowing multiple healthcare institutions (clients) to train the model locally on their respective datasets. Model updates, rather than raw data, were transmitted to a central server for aggregation. This methodology not only maintained patient data confidentiality throughout the training process but also facilitated collaborative model improvement across distributed datasets.

Figure 7. Federated Learning Model Output

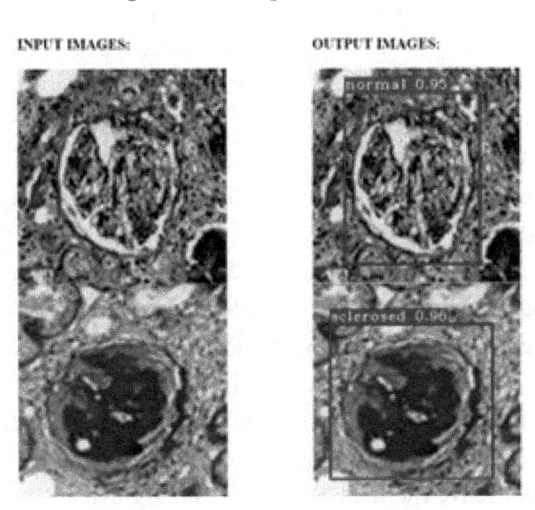

Upon completion of federated learning training rounds, our model achieved an enhanced accuracy of 98.79% in glomeruli detection. This improvement underscored the efficacy of federated learning in leveraging diverse datasets without compromising on detection performance. Moreover, the computational efficiency of federated learning remained comparable to traditional centralized training methods, highlighting its practicality for large-scale medical image analysis.

To summarize, our study has demonstrated the effectiveness of integrating YOLOv3 with federated learning to achieve robust glomeruli detection capabilities while maintaining stringent data security measures. The results underscore the potential of this approach in advancing digital pathology, offering a reliable framework for accurate and privacy-preserving medical image analysis. These findings not only validate the applicability of federated learning in healthcare but also pave the way for future developments in collaborative AI-driven diagnostic tools.

COMPARISON BETWEEN TRADITIONAL MODEL AND FEDERATED LEARNED MODEL:

The comparison between the traditional learning model and the federated learning model offers a comprehensive understanding of the strengths and limitations of each approach in the context of glomeruli detection within digital pathology. Traditional learning models rely on centralized data, where all training data is aggregated into a single location. This method, while effective in many applications, presents significant challenges concerning data privacy, especially in sensitive fields like medical imaging. The centralized approach necessitates the transfer of patient data to a central server, raising concerns about data breaches and unauthorized access.

In our study, the traditional YOLOv3 model was trained using a centralized dataset of histopathological images containing both normal and sclerosed glomeruli. The model achieved a high accuracy of 98.55%, demonstrating its efficacy in detecting glomeruli. Figure 6 shows the output of the traditional model, highlighting its ability to accurately identify and delineate glomeruli in pathology images. However, despite its high accuracy, the traditional model's reliance on centralized data poses inherent risks to data security and patient privacy.

Conversely, the federated learning model offers a decentralized approach to training, addressing the privacy concerns associated with traditional models. In the federated learning setup, data remains on local servers, and only model updates are shared with a central server for aggregation. This method ensures that sensitive patient data does not leave the local environment, significantly enhancing data security. Our federated learning model, trained across multiple decentralized datasets, achieved an accuracy of 98.79%, slightly surpassing the traditional model. Figure 7 illustrates the output of the federated learning model, showcasing its comparable, if not superior, accuracy in detecting glomeruli.

The improvement in accuracy observed in the federated learning model can be attributed to the diverse data sources used during training. The decentralized nature of federated learning not only preserves data privacy but also facilitates collaboration across multiple institutions without the need for data pooling.

Furthermore, federated learning incorporates robust encryption techniques to secure the transmission of model updates between clients and the central server. This additional layer of security ensures that even the transmitted model updates are protected from unauthorized access, reinforcing the overall data security framework.

Figure 8. Comparison between Traditionally Trained Model Output and Federated Learning Model Output

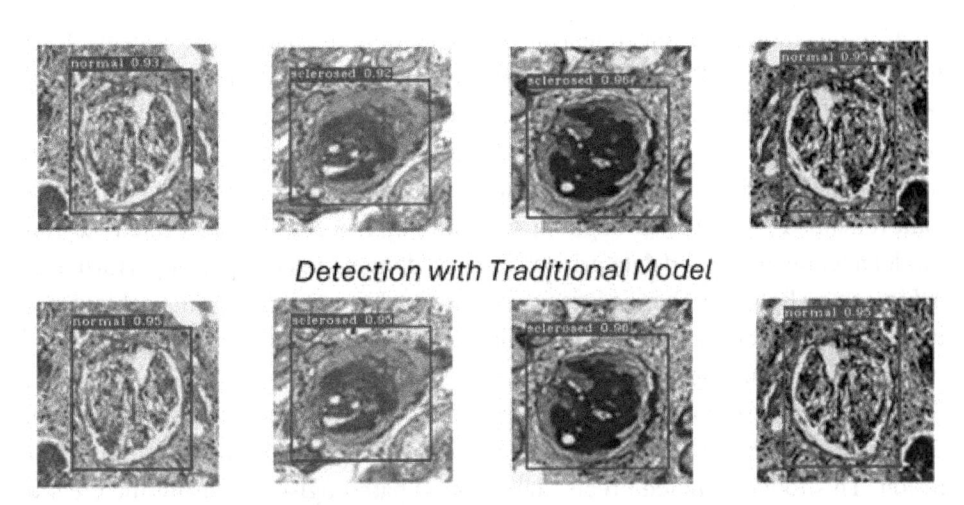

Detection with Traditional Model

Detection with Federated Learning Model

In summary, the comparison between traditional and federated learning models highlights the trade-offs between centralized and decentralized training approaches. While the traditional model offers high accuracy, it does so at the expense of data privacy. On the other hand, the federated learning model achieves comparable, if not better, accuracy while maintaining stringent data security standards. This makes federated learning a highly suitable approach for medical applications where data privacy is paramount. The findings from this comparison underscore the potential of federated learning to revolutionize medical image analysis, offering a secure and effective alternative to traditional centralized models.

CONCLUSION:

The integration of advanced artificial intelligence techniques with digital pathology presents a transformative opportunity to enhance diagnostic accuracy and efficiency in medical imaging. This chapter has explored the development and application of a federated learning approach to detect sclerosed and normal glomeruli in histopathological images, emphasizing data security and patient privacy. Through the meticulous curation and annotation of a custom dataset, the study established a robust foundation for training a YOLOv3 object detection model. The initial phase of traditional model training yielded impressive results, achieving a high accuracy in glomeruli detection. However, the limitations of centralized data processing, particularly concerning data privacy and security, necessitated the exploration of alternative methodologies.

The transition to federated learning addressed these concerns by decentralizing the training process. By distributing model updates to a central server while keeping the data localized, federated learning maintained the integrity and privacy of sensitive medical data. The implementation of cryptographic techniques further fortified the security of the model updates during transmission, ensuring that patient data remained protected throughout the training process. The federated learning model not only preserved data privacy but also demonstrated superior performance, achieving a slightly higher accuracy than the traditional model. This achievement underscores the efficacy of federated learning in leveraging diverse data sources without compromising data security.

The project also introduced an innovative XML labeling software to streamline the annotation process, enhancing the accessibility and usability of dataset preparation. This tool facilitated precise labeling by pathologists, ensuring the creation of high-quality annotated datasets essential for training the YOLOv3 model. The combination of federated learning and advanced labeling techniques showcased a comprehensive methodology for glomeruli detection, addressing critical challenges in medical image analysis.

The results of this study highlight the significant potential of federated learning to revolutionize digital pathology. The comparison between traditional and federated learning models demonstrated the trade-offs between centralized and decentralized approaches, ultimately favoring federated learning for its robust data security measures and collaborative potential. By maintaining patient data privacy and achieving high diagnostic accuracy, federated learning emerges as a viable and effective solution for medical applications.

Looking ahead, the integration of federated learning with other advanced AI techniques holds promise for further enhancing diagnostic capabilities in digital pathology. Continued research and development in this area can lead to more sophisticated models and methodologies, ultimately improving patient outcomes and advancing the field of medical imaging. The findings from this chapter serve as a foundation for future exploration and innovation, paving the way for secure, efficient, and accurate diagnostic tools in healthcare.

FUTURE WORK:

The promising results obtained from integrating federated learning with digital pathology for glomeruli detection open several avenues for future research and development. One key area for future work involves expanding the dataset to include a more diverse range of histopathological images from various sources. This will help in improving the model's generalizability and robustness, ensuring that it performs well across different populations and clinical settings. Additionally, incorporating other pathological features and disease conditions into the dataset can enhance the model's utility in broader diagnostic contexts.

Further exploration into advanced federated learning techniques and frameworks is another critical direction. Techniques such as differential privacy, homomorphic encryption, and secure multi-party computation can be integrated into the federated learning process to bolster data security and privacy. These approaches can provide stronger guarantees against data breaches and unauthorized access, making the methodology even more reliable for clinical applications. Additionally, optimizing the federated learning process for efficiency, including reducing communication overhead and improving convergence rates, will be essential for practical deployment in healthcare environments.

Moreover, enhancing the interpretability and explainability of the AI models used in this context is crucial. Developing methods to visualize and understand how the models make their predictions can aid pathologists in validating and trusting the AI-driven diagnostic tools. Explainable AI techniques can be employed to provide insights into the decision-making process of the models, ensuring that they align with clinical reasoning and pathology expertise.

Another important aspect of future work is the integration of multimodal data. Combining histopathological images with other types of medical data, such as genomic information, clinical records, and laboratory results, can provide a more comprehensive view of a patient's health. This multimodal approach can lead to more accurate and personalized diagnoses, ultimately improving patient care and outcomes. Developing models that can effectively handle and integrate these diverse data types will be a significant advancement in the field.

Collaboration and standardization are also vital for the future success of this approach. Establishing standardized protocols for data sharing, annotation, and model evaluation can facilitate collaboration between different institutions and researchers. Creating open-access repositories and platforms for federated learning in digital pathology can accelerate research progress and innovation. Additionally, involving stakeholders such as healthcare professionals, patients, and regulatory bodies in the development process can ensure that the solutions are ethically sound, clinically relevant, and widely accepted.

Lastly, real-world implementation and validation of the proposed methodologies in clinical settings are imperative. Pilot studies and clinical trials can provide valuable insights into the practical challenges and benefits of using federated learning for glomeruli detection. These studies can help refine the models and methodologies, addressing any limitations and ensuring that they meet the stringent requirements of clinical practice.

While the current work has demonstrated the potential of federated learning in ensuring data security and enhancing diagnostic accuracy in glomeruli detection, there are numerous opportunities for further advancement. By expanding datasets, incorporating advanced security techniques, improving model interpretability, integrating multimodal data, fostering collaboration, and validating in real-world settings, future research can significantly advance the field of digital pathology, ultimately leading to better patient outcomes and more efficient healthcare systems.

REFERENCES:

Al Zorgani, M. M., Mehmood, I., & Ugail, H. (2022). Deep yolo-based detection of breast cancer mitotic-cells in histopathological images. In Proceedings of 2021 International Conference on Medical Imaging and Computer-Aided Diagnosis (MICAD 2021) Medical Imaging and Computer-Aided Diagnosis (pp. 335-342). Springer Singapore. 10.1007/978-981-16-3880-0_35

Babu, G. M., Wong, K. W., & Parry, J. (2022). Federated Learning for Digital Pathology: A Pilot Study. *Procedia Computer Science*, 207, 736–743. 10.1016/j.procs.2022.09.129

Bercea, C. I., Wiestler, B., Rueckert, D., & Albarqouni, S. (2021). Feddis: Disentangled federated learning for unsupervised brain pathology segmentation. arXiv preprint arXiv:2103.03705.

Bueno, G., Gonzalez-Lopez, L., Garcia-Rojo, M., Laurinavicius, A., & Deniz, O. (2020). Data for glomeruli characterization in histopathological images. *Data in Brief*, 29, 105314. 10.1016/j.dib.2020.10531432154349

Gallego, J., Pedraza, A., Lopez, S., Steiner, G., Gonzalez, L., Laurinavicius, A., & Bueno, G. (2018). Glomerulus classification and detection based on convolutional neural networks. *Journal of Imaging*, 4(1), 20. 10.3390/jimaging4010020

Hemmatirad, K., Babaie, M., Afshari, M., Maleki, D., Saiadi, M., & Tizhoosh, H. R. (2022, June). Quality Control of Whole Slide Images using the YOLO Concept. In 2022 IEEE 10th International Conference on Healthcare Informatics (ICHI) (pp. 282-287). IEEE. 10.1109/ICHI54592.2022.00049

Kawazoe, Y., Shimamoto, K., Yamaguchi, R., Shintani-Domoto, Y., Uozaki, H., Fukayama, M., & Ohe, K. (2018). Faster R-CNN-based glomerular detection in multistained human whole slide images. *Journal of Imaging*, 4(7), 91. 10.3390/jimaging4070091

Liu, X., Li, M., Hao, F., Zhang, G., Wang, C., & Zhou, X. (2020, October). GLO-YOLO: a dynamic glomerular detecting and slicing model in whole slide images. In *Proceedings of the 2020 Conference on Artificial Intelligence and Healthcare* (pp. 229-233). 10.1145/3433996.3434038

Lu, M. Y., Chen, R. J., Kong, D., Lipkova, J., Singh, R., Williamson, D. F., Chen, T. Y., & Mahmood, F. (2022). Federated learning for computational pathology on gigapixel whole slide images. *Medical Image Analysis*, 76, 102298. 10.1016/j.media.2021.10229834911013

Lutnick, B., Manthey, D., Becker, J. U., Zuckerman, J. E., Rodrigues, L., Jen, K. Y., & Sarder, P. (2022). A tool for federated training of segmentation models on whole slide images. *Journal of Pathology Informatics*, 13, 100101. 10.1016/j.jpi.2022.10010135910077

Nandhini, J. M., Joshi, S., & Anuratha, K. (2022, November). Federated learning based prediction of chronic kidney diseases. In 2022 1st International Conference on Computational Science and Technology (ICCST) (pp. 1-6). IEEE. 10.1109/ICCST55948.2022.10040317

Rjoub, G., Wahab, O. A., Bentahar, J., & Bataineh, A. S. (2021, August). Improving autonomous vehicles safety in snow weather using federated YOLO CNN learning. In *International Conference on Mobile Web and Intelligent Information Systems* (pp. 121-134). Cham: Springer International Publishing. 10.1007/978-3-030-83164-6_10

Chapter 8
Advances and Strategies in Addressing Plant Health Challenges:
Insights from Recent Research

Sameera Kuppam
Vellore Institute of Technology, India

R. Venkatesan
https://orcid.org/0000-0002-4336-8628
SASTRA University (Deemed), India

Vuppala Balaji
Vardhaman College of Engineering, India

ABSTRACT

This chapter explores the complex issues that contemporary agriculture and natural ecosystems face when it comes to plant health. It starts by going over the several biotic variables that endanger plant productivity and vigor, like pests, invasive species, and diseases. The dynamic aspect of these threats is emphasized, which is made worse by climate change and global trade, which promote the spread and evolution of dangerous species. The chapter also looks at abiotic stresses, such as pollution, soil deterioration, and drought, emphasizing how these factors interact to reduce plant resilience. Sustainable agriculture methods and integrated pest management (IPM) techniques are highlighted as essential solutions to these problems. The chapter also emphasizes the value of sophisticated biotechnology instruments, early detection methods, and the protection of plant health through legislation and education.

DOI: 10.4018/979-8-3693-3719-6.ch008

INTRODUCTION

The stability of ecosystems, economic growth, and global food security all depend on the health of plants. Healthy plants serve as the cornerstone of agricultural systems, ensuring a steady supply of food, fiber, and other necessities. However, because there are so many biotic and abiotic stressors, sustaining plant health is becoming an increasingly difficult task.

Pathogens, pests, and invasive species are examples of biotic factors that pose serious risks to plants and frequently result in major losses in production and quality. Due to increased global trade and climate change, these risks are dynamic and always changing. Modern economies are interconnected, which makes it easier for dangerous pathogens to spread quickly across borders and presents new difficulties for plant defenses due to shifting environmental conditions.

Abiotic factors that further complicate the landscape of plant health include pollution, soil deterioration, and drought. In addition to having a direct impact on plant development and production, these variables can interact with biotic stresses to produce a cumulative effect that can be extremely harmful to both crops and native vegetation. Climate change-related increases in the frequency and severity of extreme weather events intensify these abiotic issues, underscoring the need for resilient agricultural systems.

A comprehensive strategy that incorporates scientific research, technical developments, and workable management techniques is needed to address these complex issues. A crucial tactic that encourages the sustainable application of chemical interventions, cultural practices, and biological controls is integrated pest management, or IPM. Furthermore, new tools for the precise management and early detection of plant health issues are made possible by biotechnology advancements.

Figure 1. Stages of Plant Health Maintenance

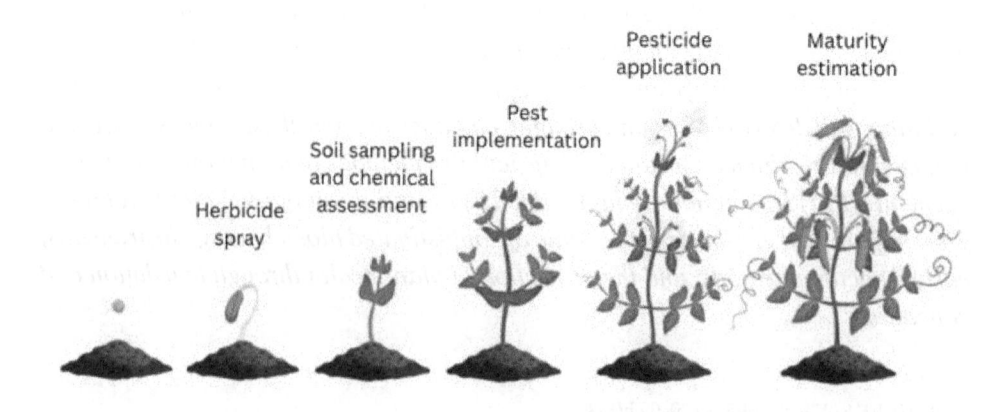

In this quest, policy and education are essential. Improving the understanding of plant health issues and their remedies among farmers, agronomists, and policymakers is crucial for successful execution. Long-term plant health management depends on policies that encourage sustainable farming methods and research funding. Figure 1 depicts the different stages of maintaining plant health throughout its lifecycle.

This chapter attempts to give a thorough overview of the problems facing plant health today, highlighting the intricacy and pressing nature of the matter through case studies and new research. The goal of this chapter is to contribute to a more resilient and sustainable future for agriculture and ecosystems by examining the biotic and abiotic elements that affect plant health and by talking about creative solutions and policies.

LITERATURE SURVEY

Significant progress has been made in the last few years in our understanding of the problems and potential solutions related to plant health. The literature on biotic and abiotic stressors, integrated pest management (IPM), early detection systems, sustainable agricultural practices, biotechnological tools, and the function of policy and education is reviewed in this survey.

In their assessment on the emergence of novel fungal pathogens in crops, (Figueroa et al., 2021) highlight the contribution of global trade and climate change to the spread of these diseases. Early SMV detection with hyperspectral imaging to prevent yield losses was proposed in (Venkatesan et al., 2024).

The effects of invasive insect pests on international agriculture and the efficacy of biological management methods are examined in a recent study by (Desneux et al., 2020). (Appe et al., 2023) proposed an improved YOLOv5 model to detect and classify the dense tomatoes by adding the coordinate attention mechanism and bidirectional pyramid network for the detection and classification of dense tomato fruits.

In their revised meta-analysis on the ecological effects of invasive plant species, (Pyšek et al., 2020) address the most recent management approaches and their efficacy. (Simberloff et al., 2021) stress the significance of international collaboration and policy frameworks and stress the necessity of early detection and quick reaction to invasive species.

In their overview of recent developments in drought-tolerant crop varieties, (Daryanto et al., 2021) place particular emphasis on the application of genetic engineering and conventional breeding techniques to increase water use efficiency. (Leng et al., 2019) talk about how plants react physiologically to drought stress and how plant growth-promoting rhizobacteria (PGPR) may be able to lessen these effects.

In order to reduce soil erosion and enhance soil health, (Keesstra et al., 2019) study looks at sustainable soil management techniques including conservation tillage and cover crops. (Delgado et al., 2020) investigate how soil microbiomes support plant growth and preserve soil health in a variety of stressful environments.

PLANT NUTRITION MANAGEMENT FOR HUMAN HEALTH

Unfortunately, estimates indicate that up to two-thirds of the world's population may be at danger of insufficiency in one or more important mineral elements (Huang et al., 2020 and Mena et al., 2020). Mineral malnutrition is a widespread issue in both industrialized and developing nations. One of the biggest problems facing humanity is nutrient deficiency, which affects millions of individuals. At least 25 mineral elements are probably necessary for human health, according to (Brevik et al., 2020), and plants are the primary source of most of these nutrients. The minerals that humans are most lacking in are iron (Fe), zinc, iron, selenium, calcium, magnesium, and copper (Stein et al., 2010). Edible plants may not contain adequate mineral components for human sustenance for a variety of reasons. The genetics of plant species with low concentrations of specific mineral elements, variations in crop phytoavailability (e.g., Cu, Fe, and Zn in alkaline or calcareous soils), and plant anatomy, including limited phloem mobility of elements in edible portions like seeds, fruits, and tubers at low concentrations, may be some of these explanations (White et al., 2010). As a result, it is imperative to grow edible plants that are appropriately nourished for human consumption. This can be done in a number of ways, most notably through the use of biofortification techniques (Szerement et al., 2022). Biofortification is the process of applying nutrients to cultivated plants; it can be accomplished through nanobiofortification, agronomic and genetic biofortification, and other methods.

In addition to folate and vitamins, the biofortification method is successful in adding nutrients including Fe, Cu, Mn, Ca, and Zn to a variety of crops, primarily staples (Kumar et al., 2022, Kumar et al., 2022, Schiavon et al., 2020 and Sharma et al., 2017). Fortification is the addition of necessary or important nutrients to meals. Combating hidden hunger, which arises from ingested meals lacking in important vitamins and micronutrients like Fe, Cu, and Zn, particularly in sub-Saharan Africa and South Asia, is the primary goal of biofortification (Mishra et al., 2022). As a result, food fortification has a long history worldwide and includes the use of vitamins in milk, margarine, butter, and sugar as well as salt (fluoride and iodine). The notion of biofortification (1950–1990), its reality through research (1990–2000), and the production of biofortified crops (2001–2020) may be considered the historical background of biofortification.

One of the most significant worldwide issues facing human life is managing plant nutrition, which calls for responsible plant nutrition and an all-encompassing strategy (Dobermann et al., 2022). Using this method as a new paradigm that primarily relies on the food system and circular economy to fulfill many environmental, social, and health objectives, the future of plant nutrition and its obstacles can be highlighted. Like (Dobermann et al., 2022), these questions could be used to introduce this new paradigm for regulating plant nutrients:

1. How can agricultural productivity be doubled globally, given the current state of the global nutrient imbalance?
2. How can the world ensure that this output will double or triple, especially in developing nations like those in Africa with uneven access to human nutrition?
3. How can farmers embrace more precise nutrient management systems faster if they use smart or precision farming?
4. What are the long-term ways to cut down on nutrient losses so that the wastes they produce are cut in half throughout the entire agri-food chain?
5. How much can be done to close the nutrient cycles in crop and livestock farming?
6. What are the most important steps to maintain and enhance soil health?
7. What is the primary function of mineral nutrition in various crops and how does it alter with climate change?
8. How much can fertilizers that are applied help cut greenhouse gas emissions?
9. What part do cropping systems play primarily in the production of nutrient-dense and high-quality crops?
10. How well can we keep an eye on nutrients in order to apply 4R nutrient stewardship?

Thus, the following goals will help to achieve sound plant nutrition management: (1) raising farmer income and crop productivity; (2) increasing the recovery of nutrients and their recycling from wastes; (3) improving and sustaining soil health and quality; (4) improving human health through the use of specially formulated nutritious crops; and (5) minimizing greenhouse gas emissions, nutrient pollution, and biodiversity loss. The next subsections demonstrate how, with an emphasis on plant bioactive chemicals, some of the issues facing plant nutrition—such as pollution, problematic soil, and climate change conditions—can be controlled in a few chosen case studies.

CHALLENGES

Plant health management has a number of significant obstacles, as the literature review has shown. These difficulties include the introduction of novel pathogens and pests, the effects of climate change, the emergence of pest and pathogen resistance, limitations in terms of money and resources, the intricacies of managing and interpreting data, problems with soil fertility and health, the lack of public knowledge and education, and ethical and regulatory issues. For plant health management strategies to be more sustainable and successful, each of these difficulties offers particular hurdles that need to be overcome.

New Insects and Pathogens Emerging:

New pests and diseases appear frequently, and their evolution frequently outpaces our ability to identify them and apply preventative measures (Desneux et al., 2020).

Changes in Climate:

The distribution and behavior of pests and plant diseases are altered by changing climatic circumstances, making it challenging to anticipate and control epidemics (Chaloner et al., 2021).

Development of Resistance:

CExcessive dependence on chemical pesticides or singular approaches may result in pathogen and pest resistance (Srinivasan et al., 2021).

Resource and Economic Restraints:

It can be expensive and resource-intensive to implement and maintain advanced plant health management techniques (Mahlein et al., 2021).

Handling and Interpreting Data:

Large volumes of data are produced by cutting-edge technologies like precision farming and remote sensing, which can be difficult to handle and analyze.

Healthy Soils and Fertility:

It is difficult to maintain soil fertility and health while controlling pests and plant diseases. Integrated methods are needed (Keesstra et al., 2019).

Public Education and Awareness:

Farmers and other stakeholders must embrace best practices and have broad knowledge in order to maintain plant health effectively.

Regulatory and Moral Concerns:

Regulatory obstacles and ethical considerations frequently arise when biotechnology techniques and novel chemical agents are used (Zhang et al., 2020).

Addressing these challenges requires a multi-faceted approach, integrating technology, policy, and practical management strategies to effectively combat plant health issues.

STRATEGIES

A multifaceted approach is necessary to properly handle the issues in plant health management. Rapid diagnostic technology and improved worldwide monitoring networks can be used to combat emerging infections and pests. This entails creating sophisticated instruments for early detection and keeping up-to-date global databases in order to quickly identify and address emerging risks. Simultaneously, it is imperative to modify farming methods in response to climate change. To better manage shifting climatic circumstances, this entails developing crop types that are tolerant to climate change and applying precision agriculture methods. By integrating these strategies, we can adjust to changing climatic trends and proactively manage the ever-changing dangers posed by both new and old pests and diseases.

Integrated pest management (IPM) solutions can help reduce the enormous challenge of resistance development in pests and pathogens. The development of resistance can be halted by combining crop rotation, biological management, and sparing chemical application. By maximizing the use of technology and establishing public-private partnerships to encourage the adoption of cutting-edge techniques, resource and budgetary constraints can be overcome. Examples of ways to lessen the financial strain on farmers and promote the adoption of creative solutions are affordable remote sensing technologies and financial incentives for sustainable farming techniques.

Using modern data analytics and machine learning methods can help solve issues related to data management and interpretation. Large volumes of data from multiple sources can be handled by these systems, giving managers of plant health useful insights. Furthermore, long-term fertility and resilience depend on preserving soil health through sustainable methods like crop rotation and organic additions. Using digital platforms and focused outreach activities to raise public awareness and educate the public will improve best practices' adoption and knowledge. Lastly, resolving ethical and regulatory concerns entails coordinating laws and interacting with the public to foster confidence in emerging technology. We can manage plant health issues in a more robust and sustainable way by putting these strategies into practice.

CONCLUSION

In conclusion, resolving issues with plant health is critical to maintaining sustainable agriculture and global food security. A comprehensive and integrated approach is necessary to manage new infections, adjust to climate change, and prevent resistance. We can effectively tackle these difficulties by improving global surveillance systems, creating crop types that are tolerant to climate change, and implementing integrated pest control measures. More efficient plant health management techniques will also be supported by promoting public-private collaborations, enhancing data management, and maximizing resource utilization through technology improvements. Agricultural systems will become more resilient through sustainable soil management and raising public awareness via education. Lastly, resolving ethical and regulatory issues through open policy and public participation will encourage the adoption of creative solutions. Together, these initiatives will contribute to the development of a stronger and more long-lasting framework for controlling plant health, which will strengthen food systems and increase agricultural output.

REFERENCES

Appe, S. N., Arulselvi, A., & Balaji, G. N. (2023). Detection and Classification of Dense Tomato Fruits by Integrating Coordinate Attention Mechanism With YOLO Model. In *Handbook of Research on Deep Learning Techniques for Cloud-Based Industrial IoT* (pp. 278–289). IGI Global., 10.4018/978-1-6684-8098-4.ch016

Brevik, E. C., Slaughter, L., Singh, B. L., Steffan, J. J., Collier, D., Barnhart, P., & Pereira, P. (2020). Soil and Human Health: Current Status and Future Needs. *Air, Soil and Water Research*, 13. Advance online publication. 10.1177/1178622120934441

Chaloner, T. M., Gurr, S. J., & Bebber, D. P. (2021). Plant pathogen infection risk tracks global crop yields under climate change. *Nature Climate Change*, 11(8), 710–715. Advance online publication. 10.1038/s41558-021-01104-8

Daryanto, S., Wang, L., & Jacinthe, P. A. (2016). Drought effects on root and tuber production: A meta-analysis. *Agricultural Water Management*, 176, 122–131. 10.1016/j.agwat.2016.05.019

Delgado-Baquerizo, M., Guerra, C. A., Cano-Díaz, C., Egidi, E., Wang, J. T., Eisenhauer, N., Singh, B. K., & Maestre, F. T. (2020). The proportion of soil-borne pathogens increases with warming at the global scale. *Nature Climate Change*, 10(6), 550–554. 10.1038/s41558-020-0759-3

Desneux, N., Wajnberg, E., Wyckhuys, K. A., Burgio, G., Arpaia, S., Narváez-Vasquez, C. A., González-Cabrera, J., Ruescas, D. C., Tabone, E., Frandon, J., Pizzol, J., Poncet, C., Cabello, T., & Urbaneja, A. (2010). Biological invasion of European tomato crops by Tuta absoluta: Ecology, geographic expansion and prospects for biological control. *Journal of Pest Science*, 83(3), 197–215. 10.1007/s10340-010-0321-6

Dobermann, A., Bruulsema, T., Cakmak, I., Gerard, B., Majumdar, K., McLaughlin, M., Reidsma, P., Vanlauwe, B., Wollenberg, L., Zhang, F., & Zhang, X. (2022). Responsible plant nutrition: A new paradigm to support food system transformation. *Global Food Security*, 33, 100636. Advance online publication. 10.1016/j.gfs.2022.100636

Figueroa, M., Hammond-Kosack, K. E., & Solomon, P. S. (2018). A review of wheat diseases—A field perspective. *Molecular Plant Pathology*, 19(6), 1523–1536. 10.1111/mpp.1261829045052

Huang, S., Wang, P., Yamaji, N., & Ma, J. F. (2020). Plant Nutrition for Human Nutrition: Hints from Rice Research and Future Perspectives. *Molecular Plant*, 13(6), 825–835. 10.1016/j.molp.2020.05.00732434072

Keesstra, S. D., Bouma, J., Wallinga, J., Tittonell, P., Smith, P., Cerdà, A., Montanarella, L., Quinton, J. N., Pachepsky, Y., Putten, W. H., Bardgett, R. D., Moolenaar, S., Mol, G., Jansen, B., & Fresco, L. O. (2016). The significance of soils and soil science towards realization of the United Nations Sustainable Development Goals. *Soil (Göttingen)*, 2(2), 111–128. 10.5194/soil-2-111-2016

Kumar, S., Dikshit, H. K., Mishra, G. P., & Singh, A. (2022). *Biofortification of Staple Crops*. Springer Nature Singapore Pte. Ltd., 10.1007/978-981-16-3280-8

Kumar, S., Dikshit, H. K., Mishra, G. P., Singh, A., Aski, M. & Virk, P. S. (2022). Biofortification of Staple Crops: Present Status and Future Strategies. *Biofortification of Staple Crops*, 1-30. 10.1007/978-981-16-3280-8_1

Leng, G., & Hall, J. (2019). Crop yield sensitivity of global major agricultural countries to droughts and the projected changes in the future. *The Science of the Total Environment*, 654, 811–821. 10.1016/j.scitotenv.2018.10.43430448671

Mahlein, A. K. (2016). Plant disease detection by imaging sensors–parallels and specific demands for precision agriculture and plant phenotyping. *Plant Disease*, 100(2), 241–251. 10.1094/PDIS-03-15-0340-FE30694129

Mena, P., & Angelino, D. (2020). Plant Food, Nutrition and Human Health. *Nutrients*, 12(7), 2157. Advance online publication. 10.3390/nu1207215732698451

Mishra, G. P., & Dikshit, H. K. Priti, Kukreja, B., Aski, M., Yadava, D. K., ... & Kumar, S. (2022). Historical overview of biofortification in crop plants and its implications. In Biofortification of Staple Crops (pp. 31-61). Singapore: Springer Singapore.

Pyšek, P., Hulme, P. E., Simberloff, D., Bacher, S., Blackburn, T. M., Carlton, J. T., Dawson, W., Essl, F., Foxcroft, L. C., Genovesi, P., Jeschke, J. M., Kühn, I., Liebhold, A. M., Mandrak, N. E., Meyerson, L. A., Pauchard, A., Pergi, J., Roy, H. E., Seebens, H., & Richardson, D. M. (2020). Scientists' warning on invasive alien species. *Biological Reviews of the Cambridge Philosophical Society*, 95(6), 1511–1534. 10.1111/brv.1262732588508

Schiavon, M., Nardi, S., Vecchia, F. D., & Ertani, A. (2020). Selenium biofortification in the 21st century: Status and challenges for healthy human nutrition. *Plant and Soil*, 453(1-2), 245–270. 10.1007/s11104-020-04635-932836404

Sharma, D., Jamra, G., Singh, U. M., Sood, S., & Kumar, A. (2017). Calcium Biofortification: Three Pronged Molecular Approaches for Dissecting Complex Trait of Calcium Nutrition in Finger Millet (Eleusine coracena) for Devising Strategies of Enrichment of Food Crops. *Frontiers in Plant Science*, 7. Advance online publication. 10.3389/fpls.2016.0202828144246

Simberloff, D., Martin, J. L., Genovesi, P., Maris, V., Wardle, D. A., Aronson, J., Courchamp, F., Galil, B., García-Berthou, E., Pascal, M., Pyšek, P., Sousa, R., Tabacchi, E., & Vilà, M. (2013). Impacts of biological invasions: What's what and the way forward. *Trends in Ecology & Evolution*, 28(1), 58–66. 10.1016/j.tree.2012.07.01322889499

Stein, A. J. (2010). Global impacts of human mineral malnutrition. *Plant and Soil*, 335(1-2), 133–154. 10.1007/s11104-009-0228-2

Szerement, J., Szatanik-Kloc, A., Mokrzycki, J., & Mierzwa-Hersztek, M. (2022). Agronomic Biofortification with Se, Zn and Fe: An Effective Strategy to Enhance Crop Nutritional Quality and Stress Defense-A Review. *Journal of Soil Science and Plant Nutrition*, 22(1), 1129–1159. 10.1007/s42729-021-00719-2

Venkatesan, R., & Balaji, G. N. (2024). Balancing composite motion optimization using R-ERNN with plant disease. *Applied Soft Computing*, 154, 111288. Advance online publication. 10.1016/j.asoc.2024.111288

White, P. J., & Brown, P. H. (2010). Plant nutrition for sustainable development and global health. *Annals of Botany*, 105(7), 1073–1080. 10.1093/aob/mcq08520430785

Zhang, Y., Malzahn, A. A., Sretenovic, S., & Qi, Y. (2019). The emerging and uncultivated potential of CRISPR technology in plant science. *Nature Plants*, 5(8), 778–794. 10.1038/s41477-019-0461-531308503

Chapter 9
Early Detection of Skin Cancer Using Convolutional Neural Networks

Shukraditya Bose
Vellore Institute of Technology, India

G. Megala
https://orcid.org/0000-0002-8084-8292
Vellore Institute of Technology, India

Raghupathyraj Valluvan
University of Jaffna, Sri Lanka

ABSTRACT

The substantial health risks associated with skin cancer make early detection techniques imperative. In this work, we investigate using convolutional neural networks (CNNs) to identify skin cancer. By utilizing the vast HAM10000 dataset comprising various skin lesion images, we aim to create a robust artificial intelligence model to classify pictures accurately. Our approach preprocesses image data, adjusts the Xception architecture, and uses data augmentation techniques to improve model performance. The model's efficacy is evaluated using accuracy, precision, recall, and F1-score metrics. With possible benefits for bettering patient outcomes and healthcare delivery, this research advances automated diagnostic tools for skin cancer detection.

DOI: 10.4018/979-8-3693-3719-6.ch009

Copyright © 2024, IGI Global. Copying or distributing in print or electronic forms without written permission of IGI Global is prohibited.

I. INTRODUCTION

The substantial health risks associated with skin cancer make early detection imperative. Melanoma is the deadliest type of skin cancer, posing a global public health concern. Early detection is essential for improving patient outcomes. Automated skin cancer detection systems have gained traction in recent years due to their ability to alleviate the workload of health professionals while enhancing clinical diagnosis. Convolutional Neural Networks (CNNs) have shown promise in various image classification tasks, with varied uses and applications in the medical field. This paper presents a CNN-based method for detecting skin cancer by utilizing images of different types of skin lesions from the HAM10000 dataset.

II. BACKGROUND INFORMATION

Skin cancer is a major global health issue, melanoma being the most lethal form. The incidence of skin cancer is steadily on the rise due to increased exposure to ultraviolet radiation and lifestyle changes. Research indicates that early detection of cancer leads to more effective treatment and drastically improves survival rates (Crosby et al., 2022), at times even by up to 95% (Sidoti et al., 2008). Traditional diagnostic methods such as visual examination and dermoscopy heavily rely on the expertise and experience of dermatologists, making the diagnosis prone to human error.

Convolutional Neural Networks(CNNs), a type of deep learning model, have shown exceptional success in recent years in image classification tasks. Spatial hierarchies of features in images are easy to learn using CNNs. This makes CNNs especially well-suited for identifying and extracting complex patterns as features from skin lesion images. Leveraging the well-documented large HAM10000 dataset, CNNs can be trained to distinguish between the different types of skin cancer with a high degree of accuracy.

III. RELATED WORK

The field of skin cancer detection using deep learning and machine learning techniques has seen significant advancements in recent years. This section dives deep into the contributions of notable studies, highlighting their methodologies, findings, and implications of the study.

In a groundbreaking study, Esteva et al. (2017) demonstrated the potential of deep learning in the field of dermatology, achieving exceptional dermatologist-level accuracy in classifying skin cancers. The research utilized a CNN trained on over 129,000 clinical images across 2000 diseases. The model classified skin-lesion images into benign and malignant categories, with the focus being on melanoma. Esteva et al. employed transfer learning from the Inception V3, pre-trained on the ImageNet, and fine-tuned with the dermatoscopic dataset. The results were astounding and showed that CNN could perform on par with experienced dermatologists, thus paving the way for future research in the field of AI in clinical diagnostics.

"A Comparative Study for Classification of Skin Cancer" by Tri Cong Pham et al. (2019) also provided insights into preprocessing techniques and classification algorithms. This research aimed to identify the most effective methods for enhancing the performance of machine learning models. A comparative study of traditional image processing techniques, such as histogram equalization and edge detection with modern deep learning approaches was employed. Additionally, different machine learning classifiers, including support vector machines(SVM), random forests, and deep neural networks were evaluated. The findings indicated that deep learning models, particularly CNNs, outperformed traditional classifiers in terms of accuracy and robustness. The study also emphasized the importance of data pre-processing in improving model performance.

A. Murugan et al. (2020) explored various computer-aided detection methods for skin cancer diagnosis, focusing on the integration of machine learning algorithms with image processing techniques. The study proposed a hybrid approach that combined CNNs with traditional machine learning classifiers to enhance diagnostic accuracy. The methodology involved using CNNs for feature extraction from dermatoscopic images, followed by classification using machine learning algorithms like SVM and k-nearest neighbors (KNN). The hybrid model demonstrated superior performance compared to standalone classifiers, achieving higher precision and recall rates. Murugan et al. concluded that combining deep learning with traditional machine learning techniques could lead to more reliable and accurate skin cancer detection systems.

In a comprehensive review, Kinnor Das et al. (2021) synthesized existing research findings on the application of AI in dermatology. The review covered various machine learning and deep learning techniques used for skin cancer detection, highlighting their strengths and limitations. The authors discussed the evolution of AI models from basic machine learning classifiers to advanced deep learning architectures, such as CNNs and recurrent neural networks (RNNs). The review also addressed challenges in the field, including data scarcity, class imbalance, and the need for large, annotated datasets. Das et al. emphasized the potential of AI to transform dermatology by improving diagnostic accuracy, reducing healthcare costs, and enabling personalized treatment plans.

Cian You et al. (2023) investigated the use of multimodal imaging techniques for skin cancer detection. The study integrated cellular-resolution optical coherence tomography (OCT) with Raman spectroscopy to capture both morphological and biochemical information from skin lesions. Machine learning algorithms were then applied to analyze multimodal data and discriminate between benign and malignant cells. The research demonstrated that combining OCT and Raman spectroscopy significantly improved diagnostic accuracy compared to using either modality alone. The study highlighted the potential of multimodal imaging combined with machine learning to provide more comprehensive and accurate diagnostics, paving the way for advanced, non-invasive skin cancer detection techniques.

IV. PROPOSED METHODOLOGY

A. Dataset Selection

1. *Description of the Dataset*

The dataset utilized in this study is the HAM10000 dataset, which is one of the most comprehensive collections of dermoscopic images available under public license. It was created to be the benchmark for the development and evaluation of skin cancer classification algorithms. The dataset includes images from various sources, including the Department of Dermatology at the Medical University of Vienna, Austria, and the Skin Cancer Practice in Queensland, Australia.

2. *Dataset Characteristics*

The dataset consists of approximately 10,000 images, each labeled with its corresponding lesion type. \ The seven different types of skin conditions exhibited in the dataset are:

1. **Melanocytic nevi (nv)**: Benign moles that are common and usually harmless.
2. **Melanoma (mel)**: A type of skin cancer that can be deadly if not detected early.

3. **Benign keratosis-like lesions (bkl)**: Non-cancerous growths that can appear similar to warts.
4. **Basal cell carcinoma (bcc)**: A type of skin cancer that grows slowly and is typically less aggressive.
5. **Actinic keratoses (akiec)**: Precancerous patches of thick, scaly, or crusty skin.
6. **Vascular lesions (vasc)**: Blood vessel abnormalities, including cherry angiomas and hemangiomas.
7. **Dermatofibroma (pdf)**: Benign fibrous nodules that commonly occur on the skin.

3. *Image Annotations*

Each image is accompanied by metadata that includes the following information:

1. Lesion ID: A unique identifier for each lesion
2. Image ID: A unique identifier for each image
3. Diagnosis: The type of skin condition (one of the seven categories mentioned above
4. Diagnosis code: A standardized code for each diagnosis
5. Age: The age of the patient from whom the image was taken
6. Sex: The gender of the patient male or female
7. Localization: The body part from which the image was taken (e.g., face, back, abdomen).

4. *Class Distribution*

The dataset exhibits class imbalance, with certain classes having a significantly larger number of samples than others. For example, quick exploratory data analysis reveals that melanocytic nevi(nv) and benign keratosis-like lesions(bkl) are more prevalent compared to rare classes such as actinic keratoses(apiece) and dermatofibroma(pdf). This imbalance hints and ensures that we use stratified sampling during the train-test split and utilize data augmentation techniques to ensure that the model learns effectively from all classes, and this counteracts potential overfitting.

5. *Image Quality*

The images in the HAM10000 dataset are high-resolution dermatoscopic photographs that capture visual information about skin lesions. The level of detail is of utmost importance as it allows CNN to extract features more minutely and distinguish between different types of lesions based on subtle visual cues. The images vary in terms of lighting, color, and size, introducing variability and challenges in the classification task.

6. *Ethical Considerations*

The dataset was collected given appropriate ethical considerations and patient consent. The use of such datasets and development aims to advance the field of dermatology as well as machine learning by providing robust tools for early detection and diagnosis, ultimately improving patient outcomes.

B. Data Preprocessing

1. *Image Resizing*

All images in the dataset were resized to a uniform size of 71x71 pixels using OpenCV's cv2.resize() function. This resizing ensures uniformity in input dimensions across all images, facilitating compatibility with the chosen CNN architecture.

2. *Edge Detection*

An edge detection algorithm was applied to the resized images to enhance the visibility of lesion boundaries and features. The algorithm utilizes Sobel operators and morphological operations to detect edges and refine the segmentation of skin lesions.

3. *Image Augmentation*

Data augmentation techniques, including rotation, flipping, and zooming, were applied using TensorFlow's ImageDataGenerator. These image augmentations increase the diversity of the training dataset, enabling the model to generalize better to unseen data and reduce overfitting.

4. *Normalization*

Pixel values of the resized and edge-detected images were normalized to the range [0, 1] by dividing each pixel value by 255. This normalization standardizes the pixel intensity values, promoting faster convergence during model training.

Figure 1. Pre-processed Image Preview after Edge Detection and Normalization

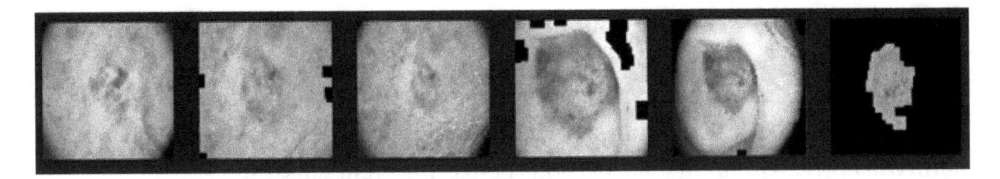

C. Convolutional Neural Network (Cnn) Architecture

1. Description of the Architecture

The CNN model's base architecture is Xception, a deep convolutional neural network pre-trained on the ImageNet dataset. Xception was chosen for its robust feature extraction capabilities and suitability for transfer learning.

2. Pre-trained Models

Transfer learning was employed by initializing the Xception model with pre-trained weights from ImageNet. This initialization allows the model to leverage learned features from a diverse range of images, potentially improving its performance on the skin cancer classification task.

D. Training Procedure

1. Training Process

The CNN model was trained using the Adam optimizer, with a learning rate of 0.001 for 30 epochs and a batch size of 32. These hyperparameters were chosen empirically to optimize model convergence and performance.

2. Optimization Algorithm

The Adam optimizer was utilized for its efficiency in training deep neural networks. The learning rate of 0.001 was selected based on initial experiments to balance convergence speed and stability.

E. Model Evaluation

1. Evaluation Metrics

Model performance was evaluated using accuracy, precision, recall, and F1-score metrics on a held-out validation set. These metrics provide insights into the model's ability to correctly classify skin lesions across different classes.

2. Validation Procedure

The dataset was split into training, validation, and test sets using a stratified approach to ensure class balance across partitions. The validation set was used for hyperparameter tuning and model selection, while the test set was reserved for final performance evaluation.

3. Additional Analyses

Additional analyses, such as confusion matrix visualization and ROC curve analysis, were conducted to assess the model's behavior across different classes and its ability to discriminate between benign and malignant lesions.

V. RESULTS

The performance metrics of the developed skin cancer detection model using Convolutional Neural Networks (CNNs) provide insights into its classification effectiveness across various skin lesion types. The model achieved an overall accuracy of 82.04% on the test set, indicating a reasonable level of performance in correctly identifying the lesions.

The precision, recall, and F1 scores for each class, summarized in Table I, reveal several important aspects of the model's performance. For melanocytic nevi, the model exhibits moderate precision (0.55) and recall (0.52), suggesting a balanced but not highly effective classification for this class. The F1 score of 0.53 further confirms this moderate performance.

Table 1. Performance Metrics of the CNN Model

Class	Precision	Recall	F1-Score
Melanocytic Nevi	0.55	0.52	0.53
Melanoma	0.52	0.67	0.58
Benign Keratosis	0.68	0.63	0.65
Basal Cell Carcinoma	0	0	0
Actinic Keratoses	0.89	0.95	0.92
Vascular Lesions	0.7	0.46	0.55
Dermatofibroma	0.92	0.86	0.89

Melanoma, a critical class due to its severity, shows a higher recall (0.67) compared to precision (0.52), resulting in an F1 score of 0.58. This indicates that while the model is fairly good at identifying actual melanoma cases, it also produces a significant number of false positives.

Benign keratosis and actinic keratoses achieve relatively high-performance metrics, with actinic keratoses displaying the highest precision (0.89), recall (0.95), and F1 score (0.92), indicating robust classification capabilities for these types.

Conversely, the model fails to effectively classify basal cell carcinoma, with precision, recall, and F1 scores all at 0. This points to a need for further training or additional data for this particular class to improve detection.

Vascular lesions and dermatofibroma exhibit varied results. Vascular lesions have a moderate precision (0.70) but a lower recall (0.46), resulting in an F1 score of 0.55, indicating the model's limited ability to recall true positive cases accurately. Dermatofibroma, on the other hand, shows high precision (0.92) and recall (0.86), leading to a strong F1 score of 0.89, reflecting the model's effectiveness in identifying this lesion type.

Additionally, the table summarises the performance metrics of the following studies conducted over the years.

Table 2. Performance Metrics Comparison of Pre-Existing CNN Models

Study	Year	Method	Dataset/Challenge	Classification Type	Reported Accuracy
Yu et al.	2016	CNN with over 50 layers	ISBI 2016 challenge dataset	Malignant melanoma cancer	85.5%
Haenssle et al.	2018	Deep convolutional neural network	Dermatoscopy melanocytic images	Binary diagnostic category	86.6% sensitivity and specificity
Dorj et al.	2019	Pretrained AlexNet	SCC, AK, BCC	Multiclass classification	94.17%
Han et al.	N/A	Deep convolutional neural network	Clinical images of 12 skin diseases	Multiclass classification	96.0% ± 1%

continued on following page

Table 2. Continued

Study	Year	Method	Dataset/Challenge	Classification Type	Reported Accuracy
Mahbod et al.	2018	Pretrained AlexNet, ResNet-18, VGG16	ISIC 2017 dataset	Seborrheic keratosis, melanoma	AUC of 97.55% and 83.83% respectively
Kalouche	2019	Pretrained VGG-16	Lesion images	Melanoma	78%

While 82.04% is lesser than the average benchmark models, the pre-processing method proposed in this paper greatly reduces overfitting, ensuring that the model responds well to unseen data. This approach enhances the robustness of classification results and demonstrates importance of pre-processing in developing machine learning models for skin-cancer detection.

Figure 2. Curves for the Training Loss Compared to Validation Loss and Training Accuracy Compared to Validation Accuracy

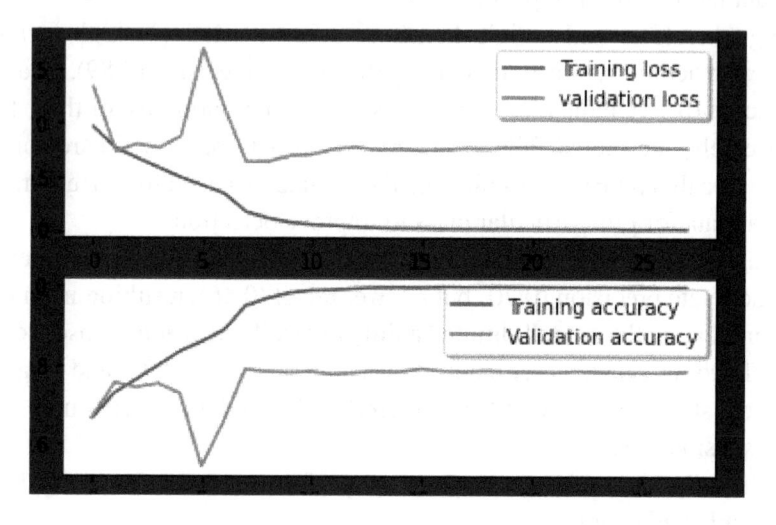

In addition to the performance metrics, it is worth noting that the preprocessing techniques employed in this study significantly reduced the model's runtime and memory usage. By resizing images to a uniform size of 71x71 pixels and applying edge detection, the computational load was minimized, allowing for faster training and inference times. This optimization is crucial for deploying the model in real-world clinical settings where computational resources may be limited.

Figure 3. Confusion Matrix for Model Predictions on the Validation Set

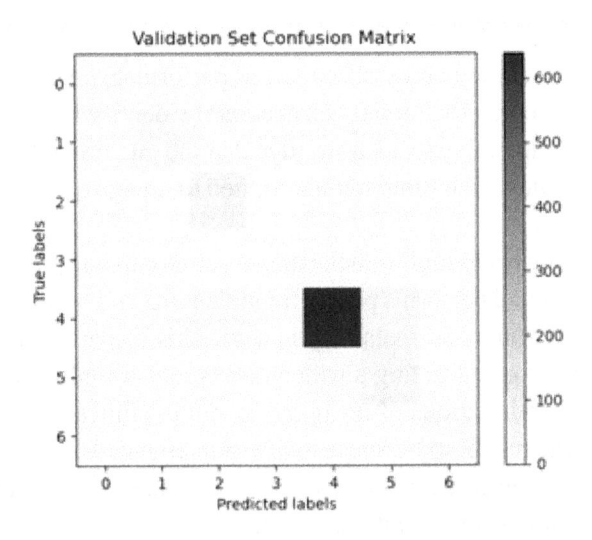

Figure 4. Confusion Matrix for Model Predictions on the Test Set

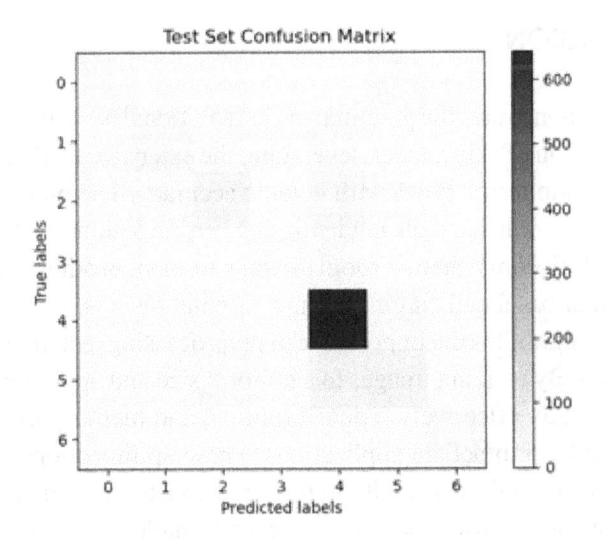

VI. DISCUSSION

The outcomes show how effective the CNN-based method is for detecting skin cancer. The high accuracy and well-balanced performance metrics across various lesion types indicate that the model can accurately identify benign from malignant skin lesions. It is imperative to acknowledge that the outcomes may differ based on the dataset's attributes, including, but not limited to, image quality, lesion diversity, and class imbalance.

The confusion matrices highlight the model's strengths and potential weak points. For example, the model performs poorly for melanoma and basal cell carcinoma but well for dermatofibroma and melanocytic nevi. This disparity might be explained by the difficulties of categorizing a wider variety and complexity of lesion types.

The practical ramifications of using the model in clinical settings must also be considered. For the model to be successfully implemented and adopted by dermatologists and other healthcare professionals, factors like interpretability, scalability, and integration with current healthcare systems must be considered.

Although the CNN-based method appears to improve skin cancer detection potentially, more study is necessary to resolve the issues and improve the model's functionality in various clinical settings.

VII. CONCLUSION

This study demonstrates the potential of Convolutional Neural Networks (CNNs) in the early detection of skin cancer, leveraging the extensive HAM10000 dataset to classify various skin lesion types with notable accuracy. The model's performance metrics reveal that while it excels in identifying certain lesions such as actinic keratoses and dermatofibroma, there is room for improvement in other areas, particularly in the detection of basal cell carcinoma and vascular lesions.

The research highlights the importance of preprocessing techniques in enhancing model efficiency. By resizing images to a uniform size and applying edge detection algorithms, the study effectively reduced runtime and memory usage, making the model more viable for practical applications. These optimizations are essential for real-time diagnostic tools, especially in resource-constrained environments.

However, the study also underscores several challenges and limitations. The model's performance varies significantly across different lesion types, indicating a need for more comprehensive training data and advanced augmentation techniques to address class imbalances. Additionally, the zero scores for basal cell carcinoma suggest that specific attention must be given to this class, potentially by incorporating more targeted data and exploring alternative neural network architectures.

Future research directions should focus on enhancing the model's robustness and generalizability. One promising approach is the integration of multimodal data, such as combining dermatoscopic images with patient metadata (e.g., age, sex, medical history), to provide a more holistic view of each case. This could improve the model's diagnostic accuracy and its ability to differentiate between similar lesion types.

Another critical area for future exploration is the development of interpretable AI models. While CNNs are powerful, their black-box nature can hinder clinical adoption. Techniques such as attention mechanisms and explainable AI (XAI) can help elucidate the model's decision-making process, providing valuable insights to dermatologists and fostering trust in AI-assisted diagnostics.

Collaboration with clinical experts is also vital. Engaging with dermatologists during the model development phase can ensure that the AI system meets clinical needs and adheres to medical standards. Furthermore, clinical trials are necessary to validate the model's efficacy in real-world settings and to gather feedback for iterative improvements.

In conclusion, while this study makes significant strides in utilizing CNNs for skin cancer detection, it also opens the door to numerous avenues for future research. By addressing current limitations and exploring innovative approaches, we can move closer to realizing AI's full potential in improving early skin cancer detection and enhancing patient outcomes.

REFERENCES

Brinker, T. J., Hekler, A., Enk, A. H., Berking, C., Hauschild, A., Ghoreschi, K., & von Kalle, C. (2019). Deep neural networks are superior to dermatologists in melanoma image classification. *European Journal of Cancer*, 119, 11–17. 10.1016/j.ejca.2019.05.02331401469

Codella, N. C., Rotemberg, V., Tschandl, P., Celebi, M. E., Dusza, S., Gutman, D., . . . Halpern, A. (2019). Skin lesion analysis toward melanoma detection 2018: A challenge hosted by the International Skin Imaging Collaboration (ISIC). *arXiv preprint arXiv:1902.03368.*

Crosby, D., Bhatia, S., Brindle, K. M., Coussens, L. M., Dive, C., Emberton, M., Esener, S., Fitzgerald, R. C., Gambhir, S. S., Kuhn, P., Rebbeck, T. R., & Balasubramanian, S. (2022). Early detection of cancer. *Science*. https://doi.org/aay9040

Das, K., Bhattacharya, S., Sinha, R., & Paul, R. R. (2021). Artificial intelligence in dermatology: Recent developments and prospects. *Clinical Dermatology Review*, 5(3), 192–202. 10.4103/cdr.cdr_67_21

Esteva, A., Kuprel, B., Novoa, R. A., Ko, J., Swetter, S. M., Blau, H. M., & Thrun, S. (2017). Dermatologist-level classification of skin cancer with deep neural networks. *Nature*, 542(7639), 115–118. 10.1038/nature2105628117445

Haenssle, H. A., Fink, C., Schneiderbauer, R., Toberer, F., Buhl, T., Blum, A., Kalloo, A., Hassen, A. B. H., Thomas, L., Enk, A., Uhlmann, L., Alt, C., Arenbergerova, M., Bakos, R., Baltzer, A., Bertlich, I., Blum, A., Bokor-Billmann, T., Bowling, J., & Zalaudek, I.Reader Study Level-I Group. (2018). Man against machine: Diagnostic performance of a deep learning convolutional neural network for dermoscopic melanoma recognition in comparison to 58 dermatologists. *Annals of Oncology : Official Journal of the European Society for Medical Oncology*, 29(8), 1836–1842. 10.1093/annonc/mdy16629846502

Jain, A. K., & Farrokhnia, F. (1991). Unsupervised texture segmentation using Gabor filters. *Pattern Recognition*, 24(12), 1167–1186. 10.1016/0031-3203(91)90143-S

Kawahara, J., BenTaieb, A., & Hamarneh, G. (2016). Deep features to classify skin lesions. In 2016 IEEE 13th International Symposium on Biomedical Imaging (ISBI) (pp. 1397-1400). IEEE. https://doi.org/10.1109/ISBI.2016.7493528

Liu, Y., Jain, A., Eng, C., Way, D. H., Lee, K., Bui, P., Kanada, K., de Oliveira Marinho, G., Gallegos, J., Gabriele, S., Gupta, V., Singh, N., Natarajan, V., Hofmann-Wellenhof, R., Corrado, G. S., Peng, L. H., Webster, D. R., Ai, D., Huang, S. J., & Coz, D. (2020). A deep learning system for differential diagnosis of skin diseases. *Nature Medicine*, 26(6), 900–908. 10.1038/s41591-020-0842-332424212

Masood, A., Al-Jumaily, A. A., & Anam, K. (2015). Self-supervised learning model for skin cancer diagnosis. In 2015 7th International IEEE/EMBS Conference on Neural Engineering (NER) (pp. 1010-1013). IEEE. https://doi.org/10.1109/NER.2015.7146798

Nasr-Esfahani, M., Samavi, S., Karimi, N., Najarian, K., & Soroushmehr, S. M. (2016). Melanoma detection by analysis of clinical images using a convolutional neural network. In 2016 38th Annual International Conference of the IEEE Engineering in Medicine and Biology Society (EMBC) (pp. 1373-1376). IEEE. https://doi.org/10.1109/EMBC.2016.7590963

Pham, T. C., Tran, D. H., Dang, T. T., & Nguyen, D. T. (2019). A comparative study for classification of skin cancer. In *2019 International Conference on Advanced Computing and Applications (ACOMP)* (pp. 1-6). IEEE. https://doi.org/10.1109/ICSSE.2019.8823124

Polesel, J., Franceschi, S., Talamini, R., Negri, E., Barzan, L., Montella, M., & La Vecchia, C. (2006). Tobacco smoking and the risk of upper aerodigestive tract cancers: A reanalysis of case-control studies using spline models. *International Journal of Cancer*, 122(10), 2398–2402. 10.1002/ijc.2338518224689

Ren, S., He, K., Girshick, R., & Sun, J. (2017). Faster R-CNN: Towards real-time object detection with region proposal networks. *IEEE Transactions on Pattern Analysis and Machine Intelligence*, 39(6), 1137–1149. 10.1109/TPAMI.2016.257703127295650

Schmidhuber, J. (2015). Deep learning in neural networks: An overview. *Neural Networks*, 61, 85–117. 10.1016/j.neunet.2014.09.00325462637

Sidoti, E., Paolini, G., & Tringali, G. (2008). Skin surveillance attitudes and behaviors about skin checks for early signs of skin cancer in a sample of secondary school students and teachers in Palermo, Western Sicily. *Italian Journal of Public Health*, 5(4). Advance online publication. 10.2427/5818

Tschandl, P., Rosendahl, C., & Kittler, H. (2019). The HAM10000 dataset, is a large collection of multi-source dermatoscopic images of common pigmented skin lesions. *Scientific Data*, 5(1), 180161. 10.1038/sdata.2018.16130106392

Yu, L., Chen, H., Dou, Q., Qin, J., & Heng, P. A. (2016). Automated melanoma recognition in dermoscopy images via very deep residual networks. *IEEE Transactions on Medical Imaging*, 36(4), 994–1004. 10.1109/TMI.2016.264283928026754

Zeiler, M. D., & Fergus, R. (2014). Visualizing and understanding convolutional networks. In *European Conference on Computer Vision* (pp. 818-833). Springer. https://doi.org/10.1007/978-3-319-10590-1_53

Chapter 10
Automatic Screening of Skin Cancer

Singaravelan Shanmugasundaram
 https://orcid.org/0000-0003-4353-2261
PSR Engineering College, India

P. Alwin John
PSR Engineering College, India

M. Vargheese
PSN College of Engineering and Technology, India

P. Gopalsamy
PSR Engineering College, India

D. Pavunraj
Vel Tech Multi Tech Dr. Rangarajan Dr. Sakunthala Engineering College, India

V. Selvakumar
PSR Engineering College, India

D. Arun Shunmugam
 https://orcid.org/0000-0002-1325-9017
PSR Engineering College, India

ABSTRACT

The segmentation of skin lesions plays a crucial role in the prompt and precise detection of skin cancer through computerized systems. Automating the segmentation of skin lesions in dermoscopic images presents a formidable challenge due to obstacles such as artifacts (hairs, gel bubbles, ruler markers), unclear boundaries, poor contrast, and the diverse sizes and shapes of lesion images. Our study introduces an innovative and efficient approach for skin lesion segmentation in dermoscopic images by integrating a deep convolutional neural network with the active contour segmentation algorithm. The technique involves segmenting lesions in dermoscopic images through a five-step process: Pre-processing, identifying lesion location, separating lesion area from the background, ResNet-CNN classification, and Sending automatic notifications via Arduino controller and GSM technology. The proposed approach is expected to yield results similar to existing methods in

DOI: 10.4018/979-8-3693-3719-6.ch010

terms of accuracy, specificity, Dice coefficient, and Jaccard index.

INTRODUCTION

Cancer occurs when cells within the body undergo alterations and proliferate uncontrollably. In order to comprehend the mechanisms involved in cancer development, it is essential to examine the typical functioning of the human body. The human body consists of minuscule units known as cells. These cells typically proliferate in response to the body's requirements and undergo apoptosis when they are no longer necessary.

Cancer comprises of irregular cells that proliferate despite the lack of necessity in the body. Typically, these abnormal cells develop into a lump or mass known as a tumor. With prolonged presence in the body, cancer cells have the potential to invade neighboring regions and metastasize to distant parts of the body.

Skin cancer is a condition that originates in the skin cells, often manifesting as a lesion. It encompasses various types of carcinoma, with melanoma being the most severe, and nonmelanoma skin cancer comprising the rest. These include:

- Basal cell carcinoma
- Squamous cell carcinoma
- Merkel cell carcinoma
- Cutaneous T-cell lymphoma
- Kaposi sarcoma

Basal cell carcinoma and squamous cell carcinoma are overwhelmingly the most prevalent types of skin cancer.

1.1 Understanding The Skin

The skin, being the largest organ of the body, acts as a shield against heat, sunlight, injury, and infection. Furthermore, it has the capacity to store water and fat, and is responsible for the production of vitamin D. The skin is comprised of three layers.

- The outer layer called the epidermis
- The middle layer called the dermis
- The inner layer called the subcutis (subcutaneous)

The epidermis consists of squamous cells, which are flat in shape. Beneath the squamous cells are round basal cells. Melanocytes, which are responsible for producing pigment, are located in the lower part of the epidermis. Exposure to the sun causes these cells to darken the skin.

The dermis contains blood vessels, lymphatic vessels, hair follicles, and glands. Certain glands produce sweat, which aids in regulating body temperature. Other glands produce sebum, an oily substance that prevents the skin from becoming dry. Sweat and sebum are released onto the skin's surface through small openings known as pores.

The subcutaneous tissue, along with the deepest portion of the dermis, creates a meshwork of collagen and adipocytes. This stratum serves to retain heat and provide a protective barrier for the body's internal organs.

1.2 Different Types Of Nonmelanoma Skin Cancer

Basal cell carcinoma

Basal cell carcinoma, or basal cell cancer, is the predominant form of skin cancer. Originating in basal cells located in the deepest layer of the epidermis, this type of cancer typically develops in sun-exposed areas like the face, head, neck, arms, and hands. Characterized by small, raised, shiny, or pearly bumps, basal cell carcinoma can manifest in different forms. Generally, these lesions exhibit slow growth and have a low tendency to metastasize to distant organs.

Squamous cell carcinoma

Squamous cell carcinoma, also referred to as squamous cell cancer, ranks as the second most prevalent form of skin cancer. This type of cancer originates in the flat squamous cells located in the upper layer of the epidermis. Similar to basal cell cancer, squamous cell carcinoma frequently develops in regions of the skin that are regularly exposed to sunlight, including the face, head, neck, arms, and hands. However, it can also manifest in other areas of the body, such as the genital region. Lesions associated with squamous cell carcinoma typically present as rough or scaly reddish patches on the skin that exhibit rapid growth. Nevertheless, they can also display a variety of other appearances.

Merkel cell carcinoma

Merkel cell carcinoma is an uncommon form of skin cancer that originates from Merkel cells located in the epidermis. These specialized cells are situated near nerve endings and play a role in detecting light touch sensations. The development of Merkel cell carcinoma arises when these cells undergo uncontrolled growth. Due to its rapid proliferation, Merkel cell carcinoma poses a significant threat as it can be challenging to manage, especially if it metastasizes beyond the skin.

Merkel cell carcinoma tumors are commonly located on sun-exposed regions of the skin, including the face, neck, and arms. However, they have the potential to develop in any part of the body. Typically, these tumors manifest as solid, glossy skin nodules that are non-painful. The nodules may exhibit red, pink, or blue hues. Moreover, they have a tendency to proliferate rapidly.

Cutaneous T-cell lymphoma

Cutaneous T-cell lymphoma is a form of cancer originating from T-lymphocytes, a type of white blood cell crucial for immune system function. Typically responsible for combating infections within the body, these cells become cancerous and impact the skin, resulting in scaly patches or bumps. Referred to as lymphoma of the skin, this condition falls under the category of non-Hodgkin lymphoma and is characterized by slow growth over an extended period. The most prevalent variations of this cancer include mycosis fungoides and Sezary syndrome.

1.3 Melanoma Skin Cancer

Melanoma is a type of skin cancer that originates in the melanocytes, the cells found in the outer layer of the skin (the epidermis). These cells are responsible for producing melanin, the pigment that gives skin its color and provides protection against the sun's harmful rays. When melanocytes undergo malignant transformation, they become abnormal, grow rapidly, and aggressively invade nearby tissues, leading to the development of melanoma. This type of cancer can be confined to the skin or it can spread to other organs and bones through the blood or lymphatic system.

Melanoma represents the most severe type of skin cancer. When diagnosed and addressed promptly, melanoma can be effectively treated. Nevertheless, if neglected, the vast majority of melanomas tend to metastasize to different areas of the body. Timely identification and surgical intervention for melanoma removal have proven to be highly successful in treating the majority of cases; nonetheless, the disease is seldom curable once it reaches advanced stages.

Melanoma represents around 4% of all newly diagnosed cancers in the United States each year. According to the American Cancer Society, it is projected that around 55,100 new cases of melanoma will be identified in 2004, with approximately 7,910 deaths attributed to this type of cancer in the United States.

Globally, the prevalence of melanoma shows significant variation, with the highest rates observed in countries such as Australia, the United States, Norway, Switzerland, Sweden, Denmark, and Israel, while the lowest rates are found in Japan, the Philippines, China, and India.

Melanoma is frequently diagnosed in individuals who are young or middle-aged, although individuals of all age groups can be affected. Among young adults aged 20-30, it is the most prevalent form of cancer, and it is the primary cause of cancer-related deaths in women aged 25-30. The occurrence of melanoma is notably higher in white populations compared to black and Asian populations; the rate of melanoma in black individuals is roughly 1/20th that of white individuals.

There has been a significant rise in the incidence of melanoma over the past century. In 1935, the lifetime risk of developing melanoma was only 1 in 1500 Americans, while in 2004, it was 1 in 71. The lifetime risk is projected to increase to 1 in 50 Americans by 2010. However, thanks to prevention and early detection measures, melanoma mortality rates have not increased as dramatically and have either remained stable or decreased since the 1990s.

1.4 Types Of Melanoma

The appearance and growth of melanoma will differ depending on the morphologic type:

Superficial spreading melanoma

Superficial spreading melanoma accounts for about 70% of all melanomas and is characterized by a horizontal growth pattern on the skin over a period of years before becoming invasive. Typically, these melanomas present as flat or slightly raised brown lesions with black, blue, or pink discoloration, measuring over 6 mm in diameter and displaying irregular asymmetric borders. They can appear on any part of the body, but are commonly found on the head, neck, and trunk in males, and on the lower extremities in females.

Nodular melanoma

Nodular melanoma accounts for approximately 15% of all melanomas and quickly becomes invasive after its initial onset. It usually resembles a blood vessel growth, appearing as a dark brown-to-black papule or dome-shaped nodule. However, 5% of nodular melanomas are amelanotic. These melanomas are frequently located on various body surfaces, with a higher prevalence on the trunk of males.

Acral-lentiginous melanoma

Acral-lentiginous melanoma accounts for around 8% of all melanomas and is the predominant type of melanoma in individuals with darker skin tones. Among black individuals, acral-lentiginous melanomas make up to 70% of cases, while in Asians, they represent up to 46% of melanomas. This variant can manifest on the palms, soles, and nail beds (subungual). Similar to nodular melanoma, acral-lentiginous melanoma displays high aggressiveness, characterized by swift transition from the radial to vertical growth phase.

Lentigo maligna melanoma

Lentigo maligna melanoma comprises about 5% of all melanomas. It is commonly located on sun-exposed areas of the skin in adults and is strongly associated with sun exposure. There is often a long interval between the initial presentation of this type of melanoma and its invasive stage. The precursor lesion usually exceeds 3 cm in diameter and, upon invasion, exhibits a dark brown to black color or a raised blue-black nodule.

Amelanotic melanoma

Amelanotic melanoma presents a diagnostic challenge due to its rarity and lack of pigmentation. Nevertheless, characteristic features of melanoma, including alterations in size, borders, and symmetry, are still evident in this type of melanoma.

Desmoplastic melanoma

Desmoplastic melanoma is an uncommon form of melanoma, accounting for about 1.7% of all melanomas. This particular type of melanoma exhibits local aggressiveness and poses challenges in terms of clinical and microscopic diagnosis. The majority of these tumors manifest on the head and neck of older patients, with approximately half of them being amelanotic.

1.5 Signs & Symptoms

Alteration in a preexisting mole stands out as the predominant indication of melanoma. Awareness concerning the indicators of early-stage melanoma has been disseminated by utilizing the American Cancer Society's ABCD method of identification, which involves monitoring modifications in specific characteristics of a mole.

Asymmetry

The symmetry of the mole or skin growth is not consistent between its two halves. *Border irregularity* The margins of the mole or skin lesion appear irregular, jagged, or indistinct.

Colour

The growth displays non-uniform pigmentation, with varying shades of tan, brown, and black. Intermittent dashes of red, white, and blue can contribute to a mottled look. It is possible for a section of the mole to experience a loss of color. Alterations in the distribution of color, particularly the extension of color from the border of a mole into the adjacent skin, may manifest.

Diameter

A mole or skin growth that exceeds 6 mm (0.2 in.), or approximately the size of a pencil eraser, should be a cause for concern as its size may rapidly increase.

1.6 Skin Cancer Detection

Melanoma is widely regarded as the most fatal type of skin cancer, stemming from the growth of a malignant tumor in the melanocytes. The aim of the skin cancer detection initiative is to create a system for evaluating and determining the risk of melanoma by analyzing dermatological images captured with a standard consumer-grade camera. The framework for skin cancer detection involves the implementation of innovative algorithms to carry out the following tasks:

- illumination correction pre-processing
- segmentation of the lesion
- feature extraction

The dataset can be found at the bottom of the page, consisting of images sourced from the public databases DermIS and DermQuest, as well as manual segmentations of the lesions.

Correction Preprocessing

The initial stage within the proposed framework involves a preprocessing phase, during which the image undergoes correction to address illumination discrepancies (such as shadows and areas with high brightness). Our strategy for addressing this issue entails the utilization of a multi-stage illumination modeling algorithm. We adopt an illumination-reflectance multiplicative model, wherein every pixel in the Value color channel (within the HSV color space) can be separated into an illumination element and a reflectance element. The primary objective of the algorithm is to initially determine the illumination element and subsequently compute the reflectance element based on the estimated illumination.

The multi-stage illumination modeling algorithm proposed in the VIP lab employs a series of stages to estimate and rectify illumination variation, as illustrated in Figure 1.

Initial Monte Carlo illumination estimate

- Final parametric illumination estimate
- Calculate the reflectance component

Figure 1. Flow Chart Showing the Steps to Correct the Input Image for Illumination Variation

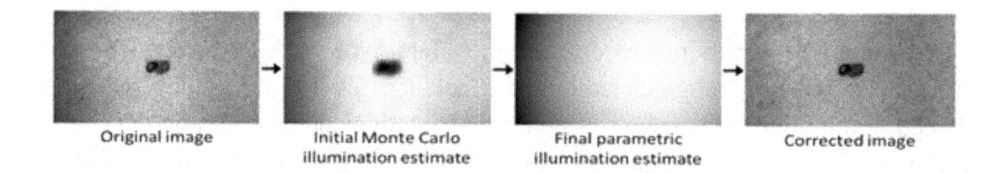

Skin Lesion Segmentation

The primary goal of the skin lesion segmentation process is to accurately identify the boundary of the skin lesion. This step holds significant importance as numerous features utilized in evaluating the risk of melanoma are dependent on the delineation of the lesion border. Our methodology for delineating the lesion border involves a texture distinctiveness-based lesion segmentation approach.

Figure 2. Flow Chart Showing the Steps to Calculate the Texture Distinctiveness of Metric

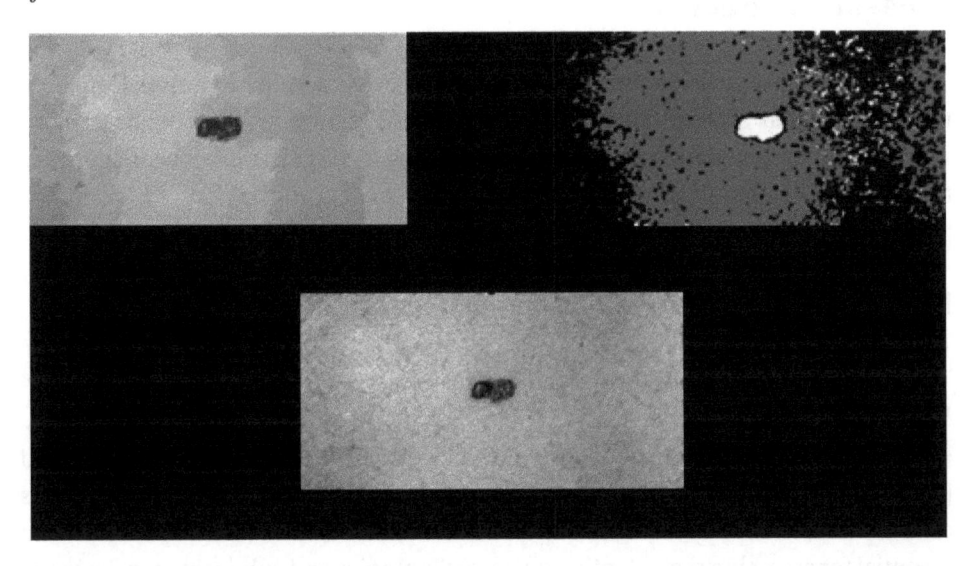

The initial step in the skin lesion segmentation algorithm involves acquiring knowledge of characteristic texture distributions and computing the texture distinctiveness metric for each distribution (as depicted in Figure 2). A texture vector is derived for every pixel within the image. Subsequently, a Gaussian mixture model is utilized to acquire knowledge of the texture distributions using the set of texture vectors. Ultimately, the dissimilarity between a texture distribution and all other texture distributions is assessed, and this is expressed as the texture distinctiveness metric.

Figure 3. Flow Chart showing the Merging of the Texture Distinctiveness Map and Initial Regions. Each Solid Colour in the Image of Initial Regions Corresponds to a Single Region

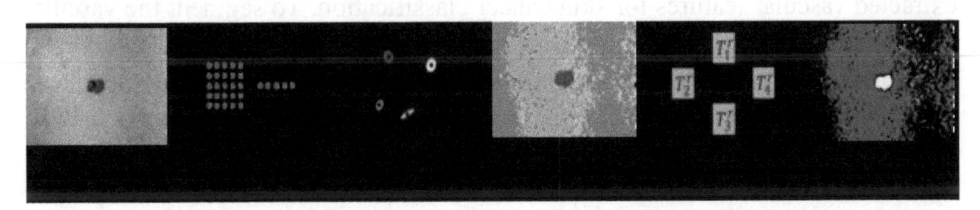

The next phase involves the classification of pixels in the image into either the normal skin or lesion category, as illustrated in Figure 3. This process entails dividing the image into various regions, which are then integrated with the texture distinctiveness map to identify the skin lesion.

1. Feature Extraction

To apply classification methods, the image needs to undergo a transformation to be depicted as a point within an n-dimensional feature space. The dimensions in this feature space correspond to parameters that are significant in characterizing the phenomenon being studied (e.g., malignancy).

LITERATURE SURVEY

Ultrawideband, Stable Normal and Cancer Skin Tissue Phantoms for Millimeter-Wave Skin Cancer Imaging (ACC et al, Green, A., et al., Lee, H. C. et al., 2010).

Amir Mirbeik and colleagues have developed novel skin-equivalent semisolid phantoms that are both stable and broadband, designed to replicate the interactions of millimeter waves with human skin and skin tumors. These realistic phantoms are essential for assessing the potential of new technologies and enhancing the design of millimeter-wave skin cancer detection methods. By utilizing specific combinations of deionized water, oil, gelatin powder, formaldehyde, TX-150, and detergent, normal and malignant skin tissues are effectively simulated. The dielectric properties of these phantoms have been evaluated across the frequency range of 0.5-50 GHz using a slim-form open-ended coaxial probe in conjunction with a millimeter-wave vector network analyzer. The measured permittivity values demonstrate a strong correlation with the permittivity of ex vivo, fresh skin (both normal and malignant) as determined in previous studies conducted by the researchers.

Automated Detection and Segmentation of Vascular Structures of Skin Lesions Seen in Dermoscopy, With an Application to Basal Cell Carcinoma Classification (Aitken, J. F., & et al., She, Z., Liu, Y., et al., 1996).

Pegah Kharazmi and colleagues introduced a new framework for identifying and segmenting cutaneous vasculature from dermoscopy images, and then exploring the extracted vascular features for skin cancer classification. To segment the vascular structures of a lesion from a dermoscopy image, the image is first decomposed using independent component analysis into melanin and hemoglobin components, in order to eliminate the impact of pigmentation on the visibility of blood vessels. The hemoglobin component is then clustered into normal, pigmented, and erythema regions using k-means clustering. Shape filters are subsequently applied to the erythema cluster at different scales.

Water-Based Terahertz Metamaterial for Skin Cancer Detection Application (Fassihi, N., & et al., Havaei, M., et al., 2011).

Afsaneh Keshavarz and colleagues introduced a novel approach for the detection of skin cancer by utilizing a water-based terahertz (THz) metamaterial (MM) along with a semiconductor film. The study employed terahertz pulsed imaging in reflection geometry to investigate skin tissue and various types of cancers. By incorporating different sensing materials into the biosensor design, the refractive index (RI) sensing application of the device was demonstrated. This resulted in a change in the effective RI, enabling the measurement of biosensor sensitivity towards detecting normal skin and basal cell carcinoma. The proposed device exhibited a significantly higher RI figure of merit (FOM) compared to existing sensors that utilize a semiconductor film for biomarker detection in the scientific literature.

Non-invasive Real-Time Automated Skin Lesion Analysis System for Melanoma Early Detection and Prevention (Zikic, I., et al., Urban, B., et al., Pinheiro, P., et al., 2014).

Abuzaghleh and colleagues introduced a non-invasive real-time automated skin lesion analysis system aimed at early detection and prevention of melanoma. The system comprises two main components. The first component involves a real-time alert mechanism designed to assist users in preventing skin burn due to sunlight exposure. This component introduces a unique equation for calculating the time required for the skin to burn. The second component consists of an automated image analysis module, which includes functions such as image acquisition, hair detection and exclusion, lesion segmentation, feature extraction, and classification. The system utilizes the PH2 Dermoscopy image database from Pedro Hispano Hospital for both development and testing purposes. This database consists of a total of 200 dermoscopy images of lesions, encompassing benign, atypical, and melanoma cases.

Synthetic Ultra-High-Resolution Millimetre-Wave Imaging for Skin Cancer Detection (Farabet, C., et al., Brosch, T., et al., Kang, K., & et al., 2013).

Amir Mirbeik and colleagues have introduced a novel millimeter-wave imaging system featuring a "synthetic" ultrawide imaging bandwidth of 98 GHz, aimed at achieving the high resolutions necessary for the early detection of skin cancer. The proposed method involves dividing the required ultrawide imaging bandwidth into four sub-bands, with each sub-band being allocated to a distinct imaging element, specifically an antenna radiator. Each antenna associated with a sub-band is responsible for transmitting and receiving signals within its designated sub-band. Subsequently, the collected signals are amalgamated and processed to generate the image of the target. To cater to each sub-band, a Vivaldi tapered slot antenna, powered by a combination of substrate-integrated waveguide and coplanar waveguide, is meticulously designed and microfabricated. The design strategies outlined also encompass the development of four sub-band antennas with similar shapes, ensuring exceptional impedance matching (S 11 < -10 dB) and nearly consistent gains of 10 dBi across the entire 12-110 GHz bandwidth. The efficacy of the design methodology is confirmed through a comparative analysis between the simulated outcomes and the measurements obtained from the fabricated prototypes.

A New Total Body Scanning System for Automatic Change Detection in Multiple Pigmented Skin Lesions (Long, E. S., et al., Ronneberger, O., et al., 2015).

Konstantin Korotkov et al introduced a photogrammetry-based total body scanning system that utilizes cross-polarized light to capture images of the skin surface. The system is equipped with 21 high-resolution cameras and a turntable, allowing for the automatic acquisition of a series of overlapping images that cover 85%-90% of the patient's skin surface. These images are then used to create maps of pigmented skin lesions (PSLs) and estimate changes between examinations. These maps establish a connection between the images of individual lesions and their specific locations on the patient's body, addressing the challenge of body-to-image and image-to-image correspondence in total body skin examinations (TBSEs). However, the current limitations of the scanner include its suitability for patients with sparse body hair, and the need for manual photography of the scalp, palms, soles, and inner arms for a comprehensive skin examination.

Accessible Melanoma Detection Using Smartphones and Mobile Image Analysis (Huang, J., & et al., Amaral, T., & et al., 2013).

Thanh-Toan Do and colleagues conducted a study on the development of a complete mobile imaging system for the early detection of melanoma. In contrast to previous research, the study also focused on visible light images captured by smartphones. The design of the system aimed to address two main challenges. Firstly, images taken with a smartphone under less controlled environmental conditions may be affected by various distortions, making the detection of melanoma more challenging. Secondly, the processing carried out on a smartphone is limited by computation and memory constraints. The study proposed a detection system that is optimized to operate entirely on the resource-constrained smartphone. This system aimed to localize the skin lesion by combining a lightweight skin detection method with a hierarchical segmentation approach using two fast segmentation methods. Additionally, the study involved an extensive set of image features and introduced new numerical features to characterize a skin lesion. Furthermore, an improved feature selection algorithm was proposed to identify a small set of discriminative features used by the final lightweight system. Moreover, the study also examined the design of the human-computer interface (HCI) to understand the usability and acceptance issues of the proposed system.

In Vitro Dielectric Properties of Rat Skin Tissue for Microwave Skin Cancer Detection (Badrinarayanan, V., et al., 2015).

Cemanur Aydinalp and colleagues have refined the existing measurement methods and instruments in order to enhance their effectiveness in detecting skin cancer. In this research, the authors focus on conducting dielectric property measurements using open-ended coaxial probes with small customized apertures, specifically designed for skin cancer detection.

Detection skin cancer using SVM and snake model (LeCun, Y., & et al., Chang, Y., & et al., 1998).

Prachya Bumrungkun and colleagues conducted the extraction and analysis of features, with image segmentation being a crucial component in the development of an automated skin cancer detection system. The present study introduces an image segmentation approach that relies on Support Vector Machine (SVM) and Snake active contour. The SVM is employed to assist in identifying the suitable parameters for the snake algorithm.

Table 1. Summarized Literature Study

Title of the paper	Methods used	findings
Ultrawideband, Stable Normal and Cancer Skin Tissue Phantoms for Millimeter-Wave Skin Cancer Imaging	Realistic skin phantoms serve as an invaluable tool for exploring the feasibility of new technologies and improving design concepts related to millimeter-wave skin cancer detection methods	Analysis is not compared with existing methods
Automated Detection and Segmentation of Vascular Structures of Skin Lesions Seen in Dermoscopy, With an Application to Basal Cell Carcinoma Classification	It segment vascular structures of the lesion by first decomposing the image using independent component analysis into melanin and haemoglobin components	Its more complex in the skin images extracted form medical diagnostic system
Non-invasive Real-Time Automated Skin Lesion Analysis System for Melanoma Early Detection and Prevention	The component is an automated image analysis module, which contains image acquisition, hair detection and exclusion, lesion segmentation, feature extraction, and classification	It's not analysed in the normal skin cancer images.
Detection skin cancer using SVM and snake model	Image segmentation scheme based on Support Vector Machine (SVM) and Snake active contour	This one of the transitional methods used
A New Total Body Scanning System for Automatic Change Detection in Multiple Pigmented Skin Lesions	It's used for the automated mapping of PSLs and their change estimation between explorations.	It's used for traditional methods used.

SYSTEM ARCHITECTURE

3.1 Existing System

3.1.1 Linear Regression

Real values such as the cost of houses, number of calls, and total sales can be estimated using continuous variables. The relationship between independent and dependent variables is determined by fitting a best line, known as the regression line, which is represented by the linear equation $Y = a*X + b$.

To comprehend linear regression effectively, one can draw parallels with a childhood scenario. For instance, imagine instructing a fifth-grade student to organize their classmates based on weight without directly revealing their weights. In this situation, the child would most likely rely on visual cues such as height and build to make an educated guess and arrange the individuals accordingly. This practical example mirrors the concept of linear regression, where the child intuitively recognizes a correlation between height, build, and weight, akin to the relationship depicted in the equation provided.

In this equation:

- Y – Dependent Variable
- a – Slope
- X – Independent variable
- b – Intercept

The coefficients a and b have been calculated by minimizing the sum of squared differences between the data points and the regression line.

Figure 4. Relation Between Weight & Height

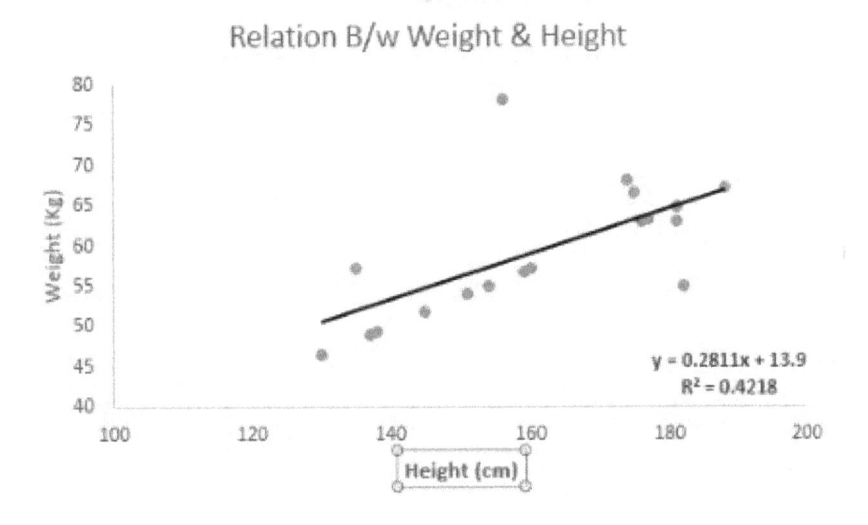

Linear Regression encompasses two primary types: Simple Linear Regression, which involves a single independent variable, and Multiple Linear Regression, which involves multiple independent variables. In the process of determining the optimal fit line, one may opt for a polynomial or curvilinear regression, which are referred to as polynomial or curvilinear regression, respectively.

3.1.2 Logistic Regression

It functions as a classification tool rather than a regression model. This method is employed to predict categorical values (such as binary outcomes like 0/1, yes/no, true/false) using a specified group of independent variables. In essence, it forecasts the likelihood of an event happening by aligning data with a logit function. Consequently, it is commonly referred to as logistic regression. As it deals with probabilities, the resulting values fall within the range of 0 to 1, as anticipated.

3.1.3 Decision Tree

This algorithm is among my preferred ones, and I utilize it regularly. It falls under the category of supervised learning algorithms, primarily employed for classification tasks. Interestingly, it is applicable to both categorical and continuous dependent variables. The algorithm involves dividing the population into two or more homogeneous sets, based on the most significant attributes or independent variables, in order to create distinct groups.

Figure 5. Dependent Variable PLAY

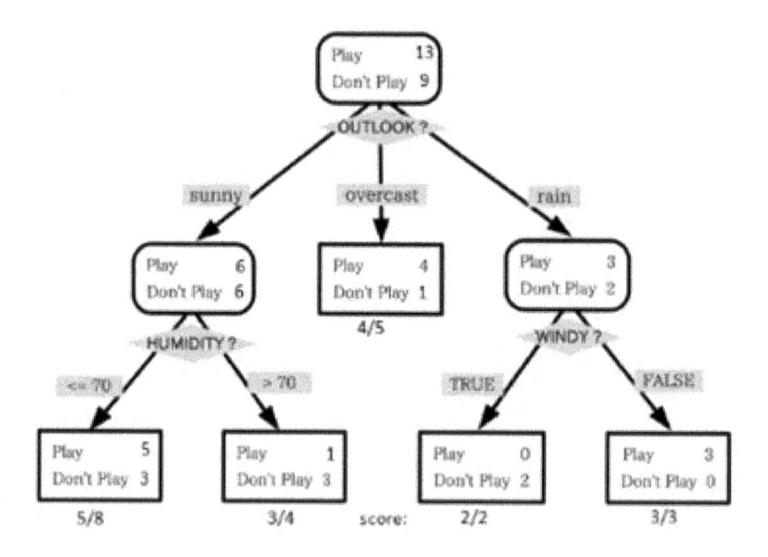

The image depicted above illustrates the categorization of the population into four distinct groups according to several attributes in order to determine their likelihood of playing. Various techniques such as Gini, Information Gain, Chi-square, and entropy are employed to divide the population into different heterogeneous groups.

One effective method to comprehend the functioning of decision trees is by engaging in gameplay of Jezzball, a renowned classic game developed by Microsoft. In this game, players are tasked with strategically placing walls within a room to clear off the maximum area without allowing the balls to collide with the walls. Analogous to this gameplay, decision trees operate by segmenting a population into distinct groups through the process of dividing the data into subsets based on specific criteria.

3.1.4 SVM (Support Vector Machine)

This method involves classifying data by plotting each data item as a point in an n-dimensional space, where n represents the number of features. The value of each feature is then assigned as the value of a specific coordinate within this space.

For instance, in the case of having only two characteristics such as Height and Hair length of a person, the initial step would involve graphing these two attributes in a two-dimensional plane, where each data point is represented by two coordinates (referred to as Support Vectors).

Figure 6. Support Vector Machine Analysis

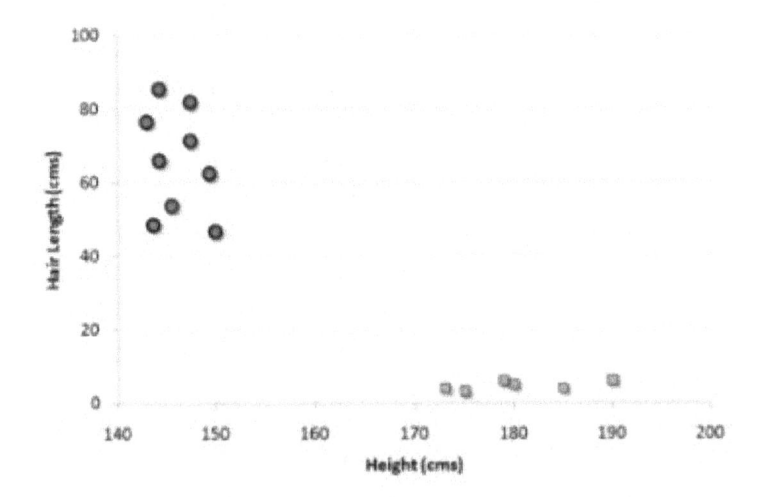

The line identified separates the data into two distinct groups based on classification. It is the line where the distances from the nearest point in each group are maximized.

The line depicted in the illustration above serves as the boundary that separates the data into distinct groups based on classification. This particular line, referred to as the black line, is identified as the classifier due to the fact that the two closest points are situated farthest away from it. Consequently, when testing data falls on either side of this line, it can be classified as new data.

Assume an algorithm as playing JezzBall in n-dimensional space. The tweaks in the game are:

- draw a lines/planes at any angles (rather than just horizontal or vertical as in the classic game)
- The objective of the game is to segregate balls of different colours in different rooms.
- And the balls are not moving.

3.1.5 Naive Bayes

Naive Bayes classification is a method that relies on Bayes' theorem and assumes that predictors are independent of each other. Essentially, this classifier operates under the assumption that the presence of one feature in a class does not affect the presence of another feature. For instance, if a fruit is red, round, and approximately 3 inches in diameter, it may be classified as an apple. Despite potential dependencies between these characteristics, a naive Bayes classifier treats each property as making an independent contribution to the likelihood of the fruit being an apple.

The construction of a Naive Bayesian model is straightforward and proves to be especially advantageous when dealing with extensive data sets. In addition to its simplicity, Naive Bayes has been shown to surpass even the most complex classification techniques.

Bayes theorem provides a way of calculating posterior probability P(c|x) from P(c), P(x) and P(x|c). Look at the equation below:

Figure 7. Naive Bayes

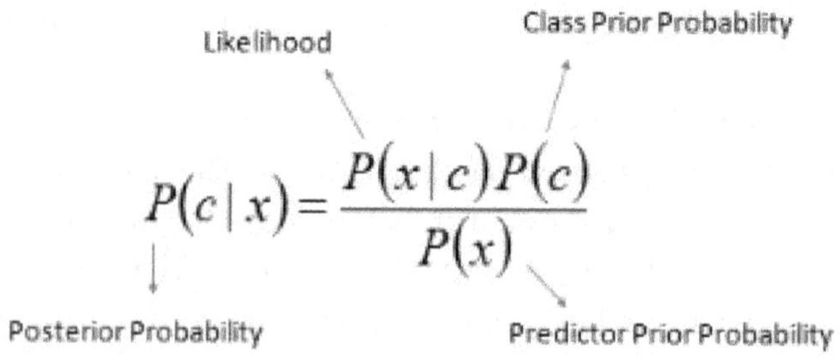

$$P(c|x) = \frac{P(x|c)P(c)}{P(x)}$$

where $P(x|c)$ is the Likelihood, $P(c)$ is the Class Prior Probability, $P(c|x)$ is the Posterior Probability, and $P(x)$ is the Predictor Prior Probability.

$$P(c|X) = P(x_1|c) \times P(x_2|c) \times \cdots \times P(x_n|c) \times P(c)$$

Here,

- $P(c|x)$ is the posterior probability of *class* (*target*) given *predictor* (*attribute*).
- $P(c)$ is the prior probability of *class*.
- $P(x|c)$ is the likelihood which is the probability of *predictor* given *class*.
- $P(x)$ is the prior probability of *predictor*.

kNN (k- Nearest Neighbors)

K nearest neighbors is an algorithm that can be applied to both classification and regression problems, although it is predominantly utilized in the industry for classification purposes. This simple algorithm stores all available cases and categorizes new cases based on the majority vote of its k neighbors. The case is assigned to the class that is most prevalent among its K nearest neighbors, as determined by a distance function.

Various distance metrics such as Euclidean, Manhattan, Minkowski, and Hamming can be utilized in k-nearest neighbors (kNN) modeling. The first three metrics are suitable for continuous variables, whereas the Hamming distance is specifically designed for categorical variables. When K equals 1, the case is straightforwardly assigned to the class of its closest neighbor. However, selecting the appropriate value for K can sometimes pose a challenge during the implementation of kNN modeling.

The K-nearest neighbors (KNN) algorithm can be analogized to our everyday experiences. For instance, when seeking information about an individual with whom we are unfamiliar, we may opt to investigate their social network and affiliations in order to gather insights into their background and characteristics.

Things to consider before selecting kNN:

- KNN is computationally expensive
- Variables should be normalized else higher range variables can bias it
- Works on pre-processing stage more before going for kNN like an outlier, noise removal

3.1.6 K-Means

The algorithm under consideration is categorized as an unsupervised method designed to address clustering issues. Its methodology involves a straightforward approach to categorizing a provided dataset into a specified number of clusters (denoted as k clusters). Within each cluster, data points exhibit both homogeneity and heterogeneity in comparison to other clusters.

Recalling the process of identifying shapes from ink blots? The k-means method bears some resemblance to this activity. One examines the shape and attempts to discern how many distinct clusters/populations are represented.

K-means forms cluster:

1. K-means algorithm selects k centroids to represent each cluster.
2. Data points are then assigned to the cluster with the nearest centroid, resulting in k clusters.
3. The algorithm recalculates the centroids based on the data points in each cluster, creating new centroid positions.
4. This process is iterated by reassigning data points to the closest centroids and updating the centroids until convergence is achieved, meaning that the centroids no longer change.

How to determine value of K:
K-means involves the presence of clusters, with each cluster being associated with its own centroid. The total within sum of square value for a particular cluster is determined by the sum of the squares of the differences between the centroid and the data points within that cluster. Furthermore, the aggregation of the sum of square values for all clusters yields the total within sum of square value for the entire cluster solution.

It is understood that with an increase in the number of clusters, the value of the sum of squared distances decreases. However, upon plotting the results, it becomes apparent that the decrease is more pronounced up to a certain value of k, after which the decrease occurs at a slower rate. This observation allows us to determine the optimal number of clusters.

3.1.7 Random Forest

Random Forest is a proprietary term used to describe a group of decision trees working together. Within the Random Forest model, a set of decision trees, also referred to as a "Forest," is utilized. When classifying a new object based on its attributes, each individual tree provides a classification, effectively casting a "vote" for a particular class. The final classification chosen by the Random Forest is determined by the class receiving the most votes from all the trees within the forest.

Each tree is planted & grown as follows:

1. In the case where the training set consists of N cases, a sample of N cases is randomly selected with replacement to serve as the training set for tree growth.

2. When there are M input variables, a value m<<M is designated to randomly select m variables out of the M at each node. The best split among these m variables is then utilized to split the node, with the value of m remaining constant throughout the forest growing process.
3. Every tree is expanded to its maximum potential without any pruning involved.

3.1.8 Dimensionality Reduction Algorithms

Over the past four to five years, there has been a significant surge in data collection across various stages. Corporations, government agencies, and research organizations have not only introduced new data sources but have also been meticulously capturing data in extensive detail.

E-commerce businesses are gathering extensive information about customers, such as their demographics, browsing history, preferences, purchase behavior, feedback, and more, in order to provide personalized services that go beyond what a local grocery store owner can offer.

When working as a data scientist, the datasets we encounter often contain numerous features. While this can be advantageous for constructing a strong and reliable model, it also presents a challenge. Determining the most significant variables out of a pool of 1000 or 2000 can be a daunting task. In such scenarios, employing dimensionality reduction algorithms becomes essential. These algorithms, such as Decision Tree, Random Forest, PCA, Factor Analysis, and methods based on correlation matrix and missing value ratio, aid in identifying the key variables that have the most impact on the model's performance.

3.2 PROPOSED SYSTEM

3.2.1 Modules

- Preprocessing
- Segmentation
- CNN
- Performance analysis
- Converting Colour to Grayscale

The conversion of a color image to grayscale is not unique, as different weighting of the color channels effectively simulates the effect of shooting black-and-white film with different-colored photographic filters on the cameras. A common approach is to align the luminance of the grayscale image with that of the color image. To transform any color to a grayscale representation of its luminance, one must first obtain the values of its red, green, and blue (RGB) primaries in linear intensity encoding, through gamma expansion. Then, the weights of 30% of the red value, 59% of the green value, and 11% of the blue value are added together. These weights are dependent on the specific choice of the RGB primaries, but are generally typical. Regardless of the scale used, whether it is 0.0 to 1.0, 0 to 255, or 0% to 100%, the resulting number represents the desired linear luminance value, which typically requires gamma compression to return to a conventional grayscale representation. This method differs from the one used to obtain the luma in the Y'UV and related color models, which are utilized in standard color TV and video systems such as PAL and NTSC, as well as in the L*a*b color model. These systems directly calculate a gamma-compressed luma as a linear combination of gamma-compressed primary intensities, rather than using linearization via gamma expansion and compression. To convert a gray intensity value to RGB, all three primary color components (red, green, and blue) are simply set to the gray value, with adjustments made for different gamma if necessary.

3.2.2 Filtering

Image filtering serves various purposes, such as smoothing, sharpening, noise removal, and edge detection. A filter is characterized by a kernel, which is a small array applied to each pixel and its neighboring pixels within an image. Typically, the center of the kernel is aligned with the current pixel, and it is a square with an odd number of elements in each dimension, such as 3, 5, 7, and so on. The process of applying filters to an image is known as convolution, and it can be carried out in either the spatial or frequency domain. In the spatial domain, the initial step of the convolution process involves multiplying the kernel's elements by the corresponding pixel values when the kernel is centered over a pixel. The resulting array, which is the same size as the kernel, is then averaged, and the original pixel value is replaced with this result. The CONVOL function is responsible for executing this convolution process for an entire image. In the frequency domain, convolution can be performed by multiplying the FFT of the image by the FFT of the kernel, and then transforming back into the spatial domain. Prior to applying the forward FFT, the kernel is padded with zero values to expand it to the same size as the image. As filters are fundamental components of numerous image processing techniques, the aforementioned examples demonstrate the application of filters rather than illustrating how a specific filter can be used to enhance a particular image or extract a specific shape. This fundamental overview provides the essential information for carrying out more advanced image-specific processing. Filters can also be utilized to calculate the first derivatives of an image.

Convolutional neural networks (CNNs) are a prominent category within neural networks that excel in tasks such as image recognition and classification. CNNs are extensively utilized in various fields including object detection, facial recognition, and other image-related applications.

CNN image classification involves taking an input image, analyzing it, and categorizing it into specific classes such as Dog, Cat, Tiger, or Lion. Computers interpret an input image as a collection of pixels, with the interpretation varying based on the image's resolution. The image resolution determines how the computer perceives the image, typically represented as h x w x d (where h = Height, w = Width, d = Dimension).

Deep learning CNN models are used for training and testing. In this process, input images are passed through a sequence of convolution layers with filters (Kernals), Pooling, fully connected layers (FC), and the SoftMax function is applied to classify an object with probabilistic values ranging from 0 to 1. The diagram below illustrates the complete flow of CNN for processing an input image and classifying objects based on their values.

Figure 8. Neural Network with many Convolutional Layers

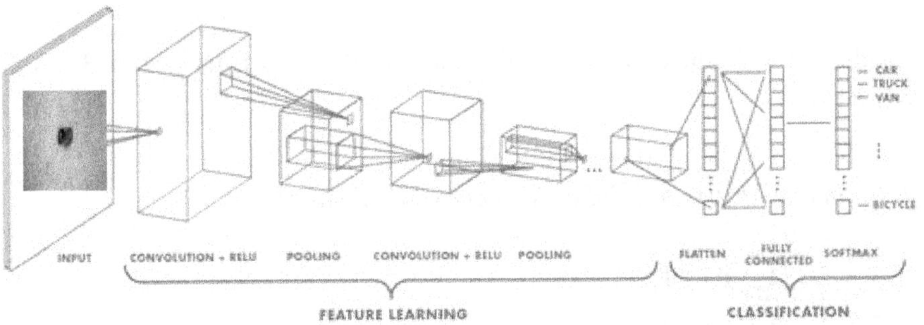

3.2.3 Convolution Layer

The initial step in feature extraction from an input image is convolution. This process maintains the pixel relationships by detecting image features through small input data squares. Convolution involves a mathematical operation that combines two inputs, namely the image matrix and a filter or kernel.

Figure 9. Image Matrix Multiplies Kernel or Filter Matrix

- An image matrix (volume) of dimension **(h x w x d)**
- A filter **(f_h x f_w x d)**
- Outputs a volume dimension **(h - f_h + 1) x (w - f_w + 1) x 1**

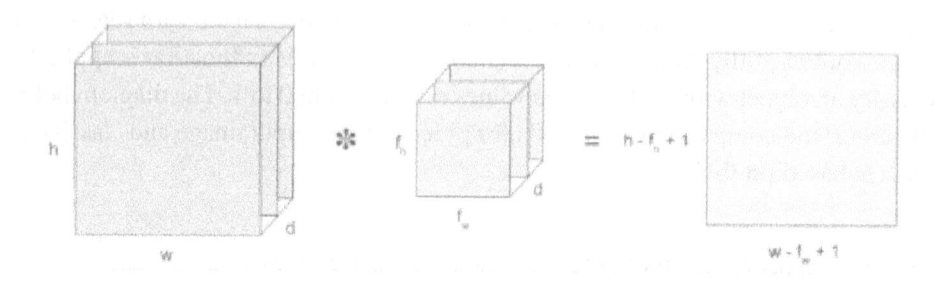

Consider a 5 x 5 whose image pixel values are 0, 1 and filter matrix 3 x 3 as shown in below

Figure 10. Image Matrix Multiplies Kernel or Filter Matrix

1	1	1	0	0
0	1	1	1	0
0	0	1	1	1
0	0	1	1	0
0	1	1	0	0

∗

1	0	1
0	1	0
1	0	1

5 x 5 – Image Matrix **3 x 3 – Filter Matrix**

The 5 x 5 image matrix is convolved with a 3 x 3 filter matrix, resulting in the "Feature Map" displayed below.

Figure 11. 3 x 3 Output Matrix

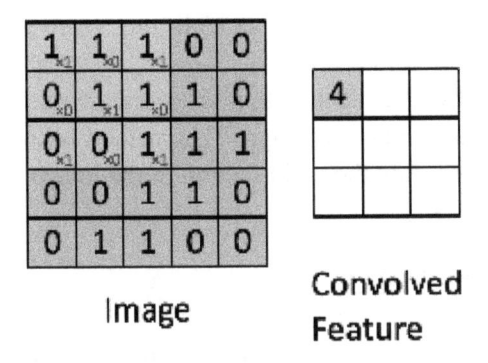

1	1	1	0	0
0	1	1	1	0
0	0	1	1	1
0	0	1	1	0
0	1	1	0	0

Image

4		

Convolved Feature

The application of various filters to an image through convolution can execute tasks like edge detection, blurring, and sharpening.

3.2.4 Strides

The stride refers to the number of pixel shifts across the input matrix. If the stride is set to 1, the filters move one pixel at a time. Conversely, if the stride is set to 2, the filters move two pixels at a time, and this pattern continues for higher stride values. The diagram below illustrates how convolution operates with a stride of 2.

Figure 12. Stride of 2 Pixels

1	2	3	4	5	6	7
11	12	13	14	15	16	17
21	22	23	24	25	26	27
31	32	33	34	35	36	37
41	42	43	44	45	46	47
51	52	53	54	55	56	57
61	62	63	64	65	66	67
71	72	73	74	75	76	77

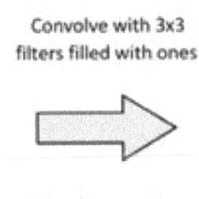

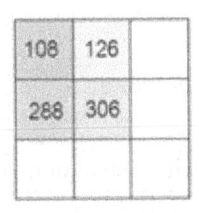

Convolve with 3x3 filters filled with ones ⇒

108	126	
288	306	

3.2.7 Padding

At times, the filter may not align perfectly with the input image. In such cases, there are two possible courses of action:

- One option is to pad the image with zeros (zero-padding) to ensure that it fits the filter dimensions.
- Alternatively, the other option is to discard the portion of the image where the filter does not align. This method is known as valid padding, which retains only the valid section of the image.

3.2.8 Non-Linearity (ReLU)

ReLU, short for Rectified Linear Unit, is utilized as a non-linear operation in neural networks. The function is defined as $f(x) = \max(0, x)$.

The significance of ReLU lies in its ability to introduce non-linearity in ConvNets. This is crucial because real-world data often consists of non-negative linear values, which our ConvNet needs to learn effectively.

Figure 13. ReLU Operation

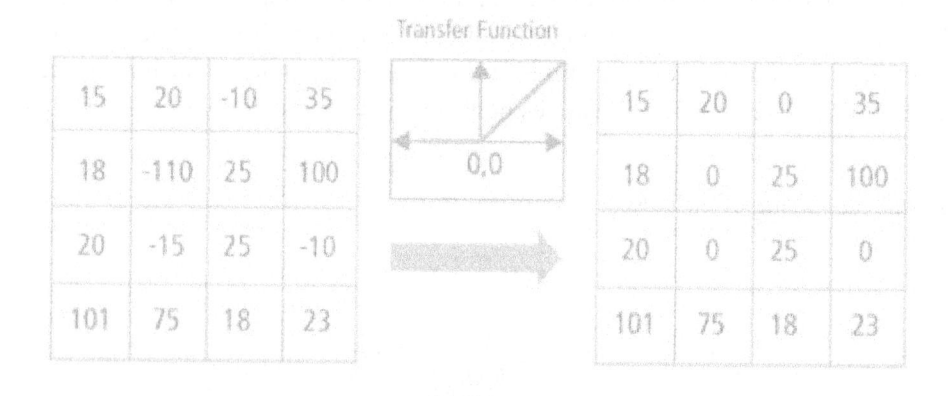

Alternative non-linear functions like tanh or sigmoid can be utilized in place of ReLU. ReLU is commonly preferred by data scientists due to its superior performance compared to the other two options.

3.2.9 Pooling Layer

The pooling layers segment serves to decrease the parameter count in instances where the images are excessively large. Spatial pooling, also known as subsampling or downsampling, aids in diminishing the dimensionality of each map while preserving crucial data. Various types of spatial pooling exist.

- Max Pooling
- Average Pooling
- Sum Pooling

Max pooling selects the maximum value from the rectified feature map, while average pooling calculates the average value. The sum pooling method involves adding up all the elements in the feature map.

Figure 14. Max Pooling

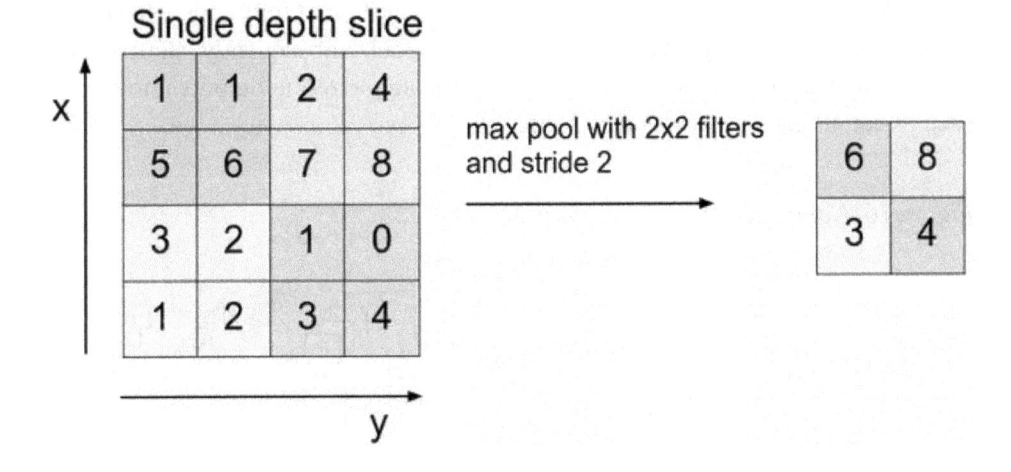

1	1	2	4
5	6	7	8
3	2	1	0
1	2	3	4

Single depth slice

max pool with 2x2 filters and stride 2

6	8
3	4

3.2.10 Fully Connected Layer

The FC layer, also known as the fully connected layer, involves the process of flattening a matrix into a vector before inputting it into a neural network for further processing.

Figure 15. After Pooling Layer, Flattened as FC Layer

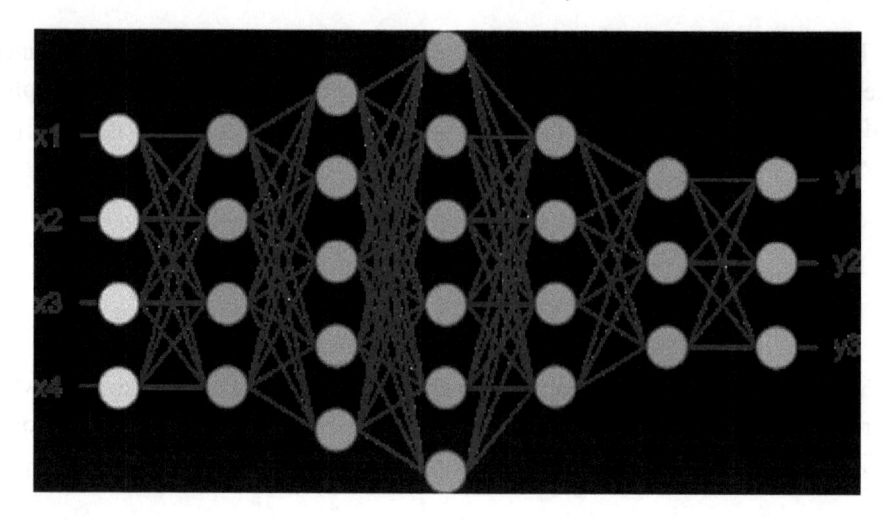

The feature map matrix depicted in the diagram will undergo conversion into a vector denoted as (x1, x2, x3, …). Through the integration of fully connected layers, these features are amalgamated to construct a model. Subsequently, an activation function like softmax or sigmoid is applied to categorize the outputs into classes such as cat, dog, car, truck, and so forth.

Figure 16. Complete CNN Architecture

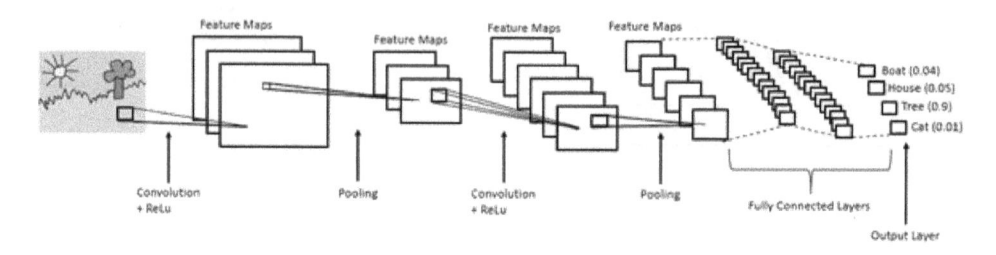

3.2.11 ResNet

ResNet is designed with a variety of different layer numbers, including 34, 50, 101, 152, and even 1202. The popular ResNet50 consists of 49 convolution layers and 1 fully connected layer at the end of the network. The total number of weights and MACs for the entire network are 25.5M and 3.9M respectively. The basic block diagram of the ResNet architecture is depicted in Figure 16. ResNet is a conventional feedforward network with a residual connection. The output of a residual layer can be defined based on the outputs of the (l− 1)th layer, which comes from the previous layer defined as xl-1. The final output of the residual unit is xl, which can be defined with the following equation: $xl = \mathscr{F}(xl\text{-}1) + xl\text{-}1$. (15).

Figure 17. Basic Diagram of the Residual Block

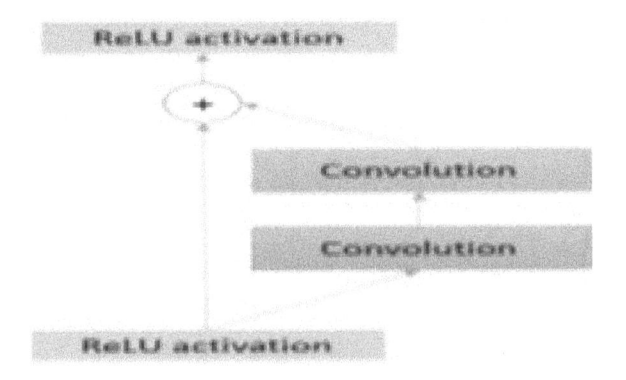

[Diagram: ReLU activation → + → (with branch through Convolution → Convolution) → ReLU activation]

The residual network is composed of multiple fundamental residual blocks. Nevertheless, the operations within the residual block may vary depending on the distinct architecture of residual networks. Zagoruvko et al. introduced a broader version of the residual network, while another enhanced approach to residual networks is the aggregated residual transformation. Recently, additional variations of residual models have been developed based on the Residual Network architecture. Moreover, there are several advanced architectures that integrate Inception and Residual units. The fundamental conceptual diagram of the Inception-Residual unit is depicted below.

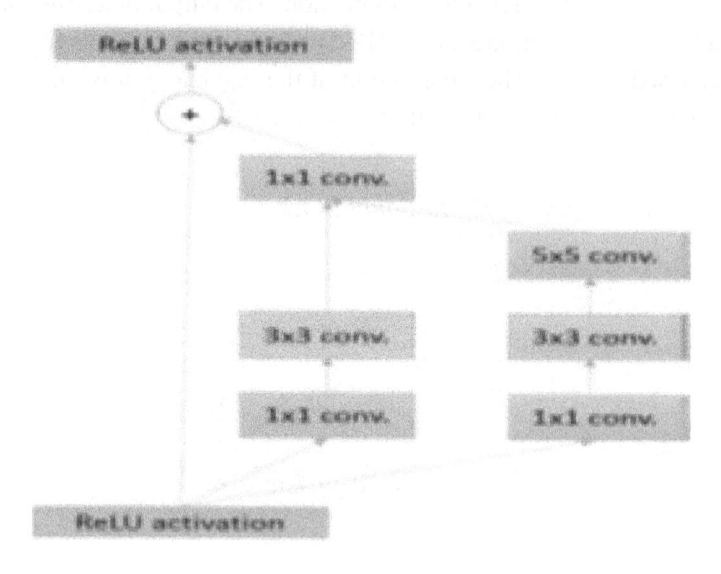

Figure 18. The Basic Block Diagram for Inception Residual Unit

The innovation of the suggested study was incorporated into a convolutional neural network, utilizing a combination of Rectified Linear Unit (ReLu) and ResNet functions, in order to accurately detect skin cancer.

5.4 FUNCTIONAL DIAGRAM:

This study involves the segmentation of skin lesions, followed by the extraction of the peripheral region of the lesion for feature extraction and CNN-based classification to detect melanoma. An active contours method is proposed for segmentation, which utilizes an initial lesion contour and curve fitting to the lesion boundaries. Once the lesion is segmented, its periphery is extracted for melanoma detection using image features trained and classified by a CNN (convolutional neural network).

Figure 19. Functional Diagram

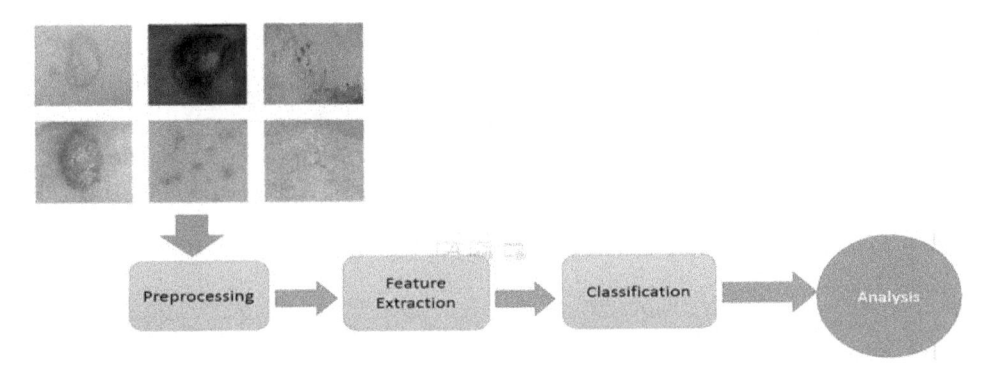

RESULTS

Figure 20. Trained Data Set

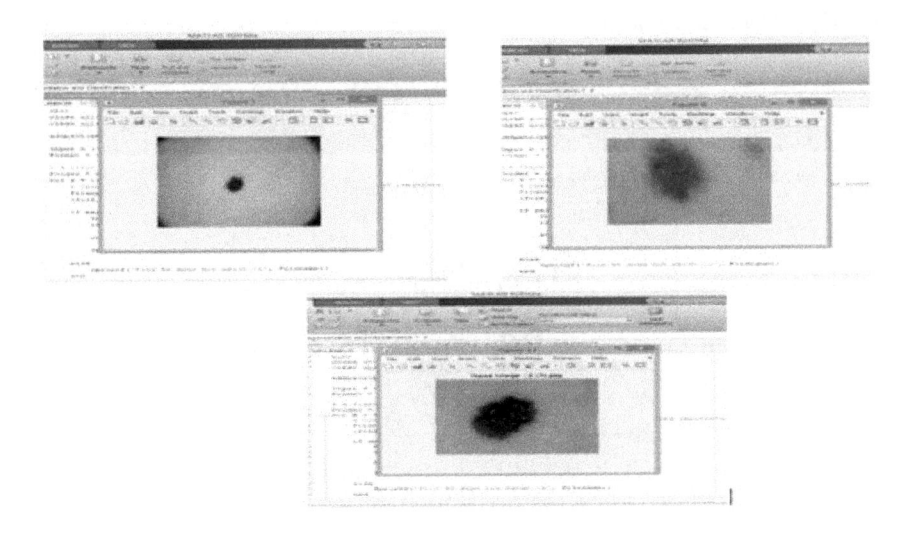

In MATLAB, a trained data set typically refers to a dataset with labelled examples used for training machine learning models. These datasets are essential for developing and evaluating algorithms in fields such as data analysis, image processing, and signal processing.

Figure 21. Input Test Image

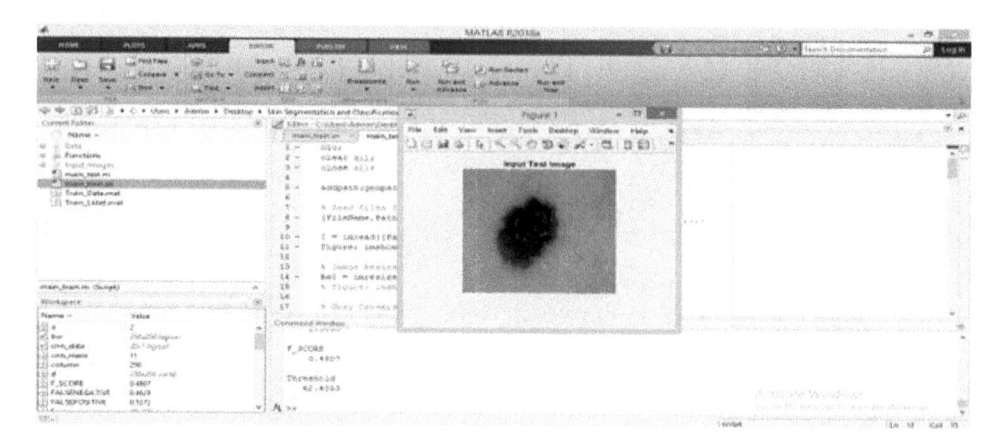

In MATLAB, use the imread function to load a test image for processing and analysis.

Figure 22. Pre-Processed Image

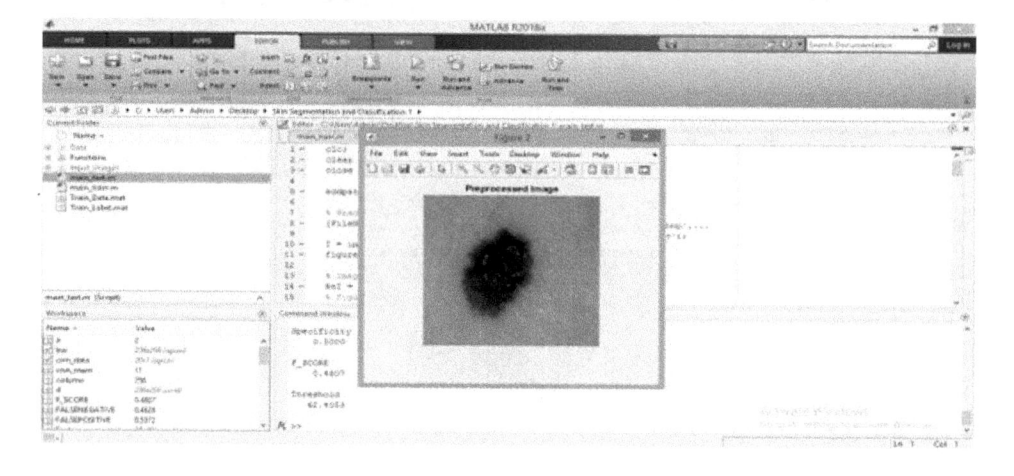

A pre-processed image has undergone various adjustments or enhancements to improve its quality or extract specific features, typically before further analysis or computer vision tasks.

Figure 23. Binary Image

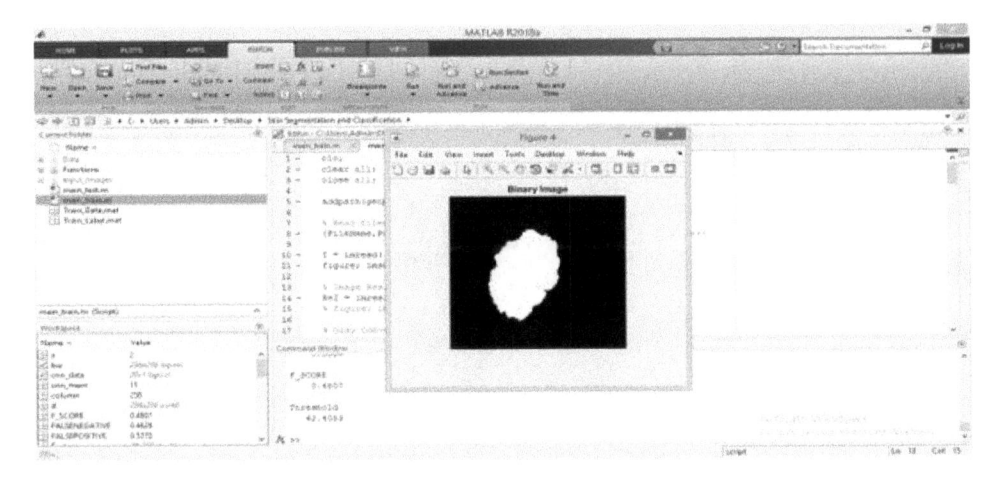

A binary image consists of pixels that are either black (0) or white (1), often used for simple object detection and segmentation in image processing.

Figure 24. Segmented Image by Graph Cut

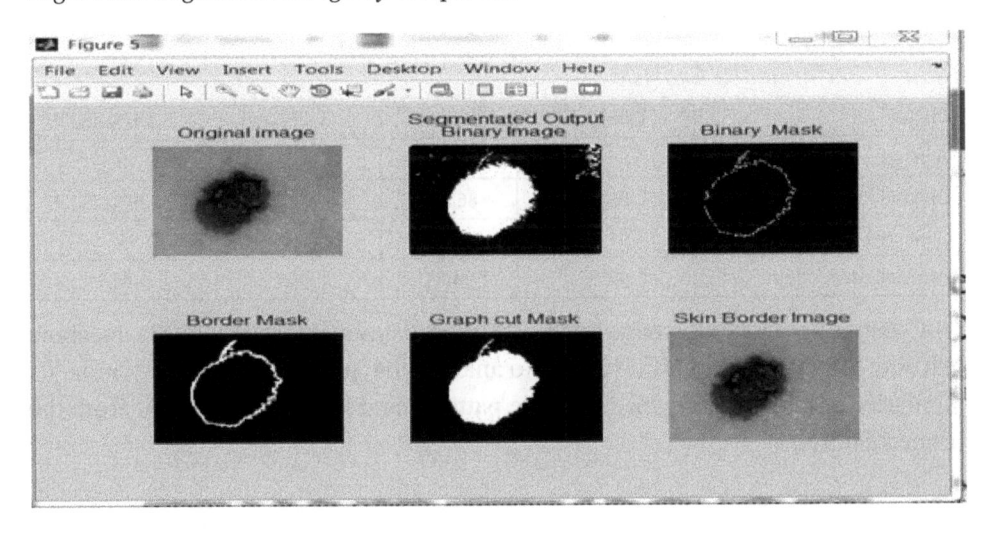

A segmented image by graph cut is the result of a computer vision technique that partitions an image into regions or objects by optimizing an energy function through a graph-based approach, often used for image segmentation tasks.

Figure 25. Comparing Input Image with Trained Data Set

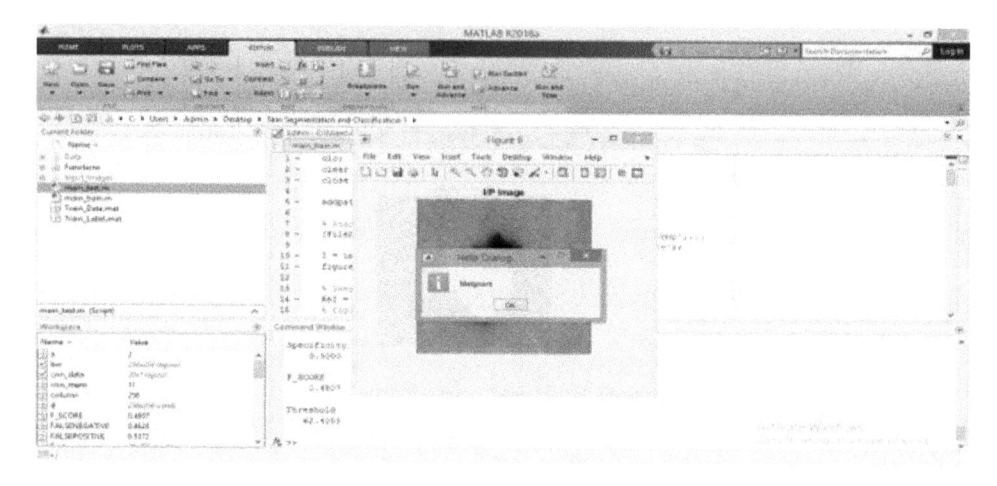

Comparing an input image with a trained dataset involves using a machine learning or pattern recognition model to analyze the input image and determine its similarity or classification based on the patterns and knowledge learned from the trained dataset.

Table 2. Performance Analysis

Models	Precision	Recall	Accuracy	F1-Score
AlexNet	86.51	79.45	86.22	90.33
DarkNet	91.33	86.324	90.78	93.12
ElasticNet	91.32	80.12	85.6	91.75
Proposed Model	97.76	94.78	95.1	98.7

Comparing an input image with a trained dataset involves using a machine learning or pattern recognition model to analyze the input image and determine its similarity or classification based on the patterns and knowledge learned from the trained dataset.

Figure 26. Performance Analysis

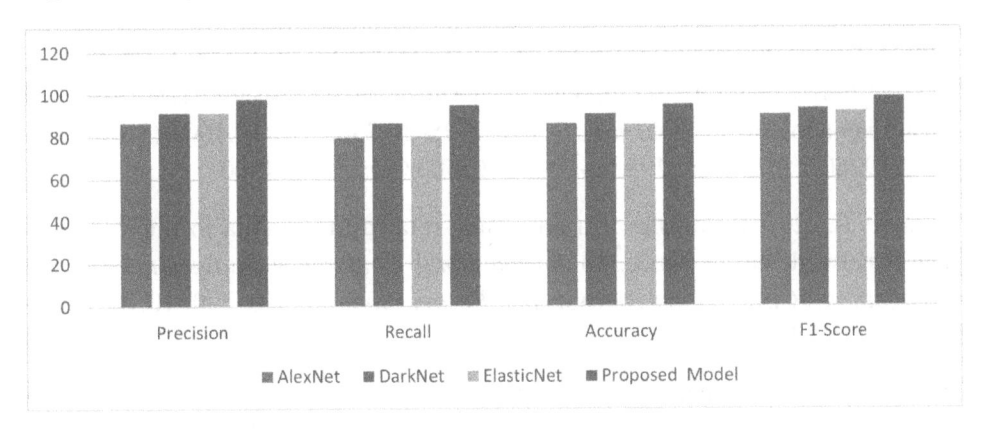

Evaluation of performance through models such as AlexNet, Darknet, or Elastic Net typically includes the assessment of accuracy, precision, recall, and F1 score for tasks like image classification or regression. These metrics play a crucial role in gauging the effectiveness of these models on different datasets and tasks, aiding in the decision-making process regarding their applicability to your specific use case. The selection of a model is contingent upon the nature of the problem at hand.

CONCLUSION

The automatic segmentation of skin melanoma presents a significant challenge due to the variability in lesion size, shape, intensity, and position. Our approach involves the utilization of an active contour segmented CNN neural network structure, which takes the original pixels of the image as input in a hierarchical manner to learn a series of nonlinear transformations that capture the image's contents. The model incorporates local filters, a convolution layer, linear unit activation function, maximization layer, dropout layer, batch normalization layer, merge layer, flatten layer, and sigmoid layer to facilitate effective image feature learning and segmentation testing. To evaluate the performance of our program, we employed the evaluation plan using melanoma test images, compared the results with ground truth, and calculated index parameters. The findings demonstrated that our method achieved higher accuracy than existing architectures in the majority of cases.

REFERENCES

Aitken, J. F., Pfitzner, J., Battistutta, D., O'Rourke, P. K., Green, A. C., & Martin, N. G. (1996). Reliability of computer image analysis of pigmented skin lesions of Australian adolescents. *Journal of Cancer*, 78(2), 252–257. 10.1002/(SICI)1097-0142(19960715)78:2<252::AID-CNCR10>3.0.CO;2-V8674000

Amaral, T.. (2014). Transfer learning using rotated image data to improve deep neural network performance. In *International Conference Image Analysis and Recognition, ICIAR: Image Analysis and Recognition* (pp. 290–300) 10.1007/978-3-319-11758-4_32

Australian Cancer Council. et al. (2010). Cancer Council to launch new research/ failure to monitor highlights cancer risk. Retrieved from http://www.cancer.org.au/cancersmartlifestyle/SunSmart/Skin-cancer-facts-and-figures.htm

Badrinarayanan, V., ... (2015). A deep convolutional encoder-decoder architecture for robust semantic pixel-wise labelling. *arXiv preprint arXiv:1505.07293*.

Brosch, T.. (2015). Deep convolutional encoder networks for multiple sclerosis lesion segmentation. In *International Conference on Medical Image Computing and Computer-Assisted Intervention – MICCAI* (Vol. 9351, pp. 3–11). 10.1007/978-3-319-24574-4_1

Chang, Y., Stanley, R. J., Moss, R. H., & Van Stoecker, W. (2005). A systematic heuristic approach for feature selection for melanoma discrimination using clinical images. *Skin Research and Technology*, 11(3), 165–178. 10.1111/j.1600-0846.2005.00116.x15998327

Farabet, C., Couprie, C., Najman, L., & LeCun, Y. (2013). Learning hierarchical features for scene labeling. *IEEE Transactions on Pattern Analysis and Machine Intelligence*, 35(8), 1915–1929. 10.1109/TPAMI.2012.23123787344

Fassihi, N.. (2011). Melanoma diagnosis by the use of wavelet analysis based on morphological operators. In *Proceedings of the International MultiConference of Engineers and Computer Scientists* (pp. 16–18).

Green, A., Martin, N., Pfitzner, J., O'Rourke, M., & Knight, N. (1994). Computer image analysis in the diagnosis of melanoma. *Journal of the American Academy of Dermatology*, 31(5), 958–964. 10.1016/S0190-9622(94)70264-07962777

Havaei, M.. (2014). Brain tumor segmentation with deep neural networks. In *Proceedings of the BRATS-MICCAI*.

Kang, K., ... (2014). Fully convolutional neural networks for crowd segmentation. *arXiv preprint arXiv:1411.4464*. Retrieved from https://arxiv.org/abs/1411.4464

LeCun, Y., Bottou, L., Bengio, Y., & Haffner, P. (1998). Gradient-based learning applied to document recognition. *Proceedings of the IEEE*, 86(11), 2278–2324. 10.1109/5.726791

Lee, H. C. (1994). *Skin cancer diagnosis using hierarchical neural networks and fuzzy logic*. Department of Computer Science, University of Missouri.

Long, E. S.. (2015). Fully convolutional networks for semantic segmentation. In *Proceedings of the IEEE Conference on Computer Vision and Pattern Recognition (CVPR)* (pp. 3431–3440).

Pinheiro, P.. (2014). Recurrent convolutional neural networks for scene labeling. In *Proceedings of the 31st International Conference on Machine Learning* (pp. 82–90).

Ronneberger, O., ... (2015). U-net: Convolutional networks for biomedical image segmentation. In *Proceedings of the 18th International Conference on Medical Image Computing and Computer-Assisted Intervention (MICCAI)* (p. 8). Huang, J., & et al. (2013). Deep and wide multiscale recursive networks for robust image labeling. *arXiv preprint arXiv:1310.0354*. 10.1007/978-3-319-24574-4_28

She, Z., Liu, Y., & Damatoa, A. (2007). Combination of features from skin pattern and ABCD analysis for lesion classification. *Skin Research and Technology*, 13(1), 25–33. 10.1111/j.1600-0846.2007.00181.x17250529

Urban, B.. (2014). Multi-modal brain tumor segmentation using deep convolutional neural networks. In *Proceedings of the BRATS-MICCAI*.

Zikic, I.. (2014). Segmentation of brain tumor tissues with convolutional neural networks. In *Proceedings of the BRATS-MICCAI*.

Chapter 11
Usage of Machine Learning and Deep Learning for Lung Cancer Detection:
Current Scenario, Challenges and Futuristic Direction

Ishaan Dawar
 https://orcid.org/0000-0003-4217-0182
DIT University, India

Sumedha Bhardwaj
DIT University, India

ABSTRACT

Cancer is a dangerous disease and has been a cause of substantial morbidity and fatality in the world. This chapter provides an exploration of ML and DL techniques used for lung cancer detection between 2019 and 2023. It provides a complete overview of the current methodology, the language used for model implementation, and the results of these models along with the advantages and disadvantages of the studies. It also provides information on the many datasets used to diagnose lung cancer and highlights the unresolved research gaps in the field which can inspire additional research. Furthermore, the chapter outlines futuristic directions, envisioning the integration of emerging technologies such as federated learning, explainable AI, and multimodal data fusion to address existing limitations and enhance the efficacy of lung cancer detection systems. By synthesizing current research findings and identifying key areas for advancement, this chapter serves as a valuable resource

DOI: 10.4018/979-8-3693-3719-6.ch011

for researchers, clinicians, and stakeholders invested in leveraging ML and DL for combating lung cancer.

INTRODUCTION

Cancer is a medical term for the uncontrolled and uneven proliferation of cells in any tissue that develops tumors, nodules, or masses. The development of several genetic abnormalities and epigenetic alterations in the lung region contributes to lung cancer, which causes normal cells to grow in an uncontrolled manner. About 1.6 million people die from cancer-related causes each year worldwide (Barta et al., 2019), and lung cancer is the second most prevalent cancer diagnosis, accounting for 13% of all new cancer cases (Torre et al., 2016). Owing to biological variables such as DNA damage over time and telomere shortening, aging is a risk factor for lung cancer (Galvez-Nino et al., 2020).

Globally, fatal diseases are thought to be cancer-related. Men and women can develop various types of cancer. Various lung conditions affect the thoracic/lung region in various ways. Asthma, COPD, chronic bronchitis, emphysema, acute bronchitis, and cystic fibrosis are some of the lung conditions that affect the airways in the lungs.

Smoking is the primary "agent" in the emergence of lung cancer, and it accounts for approximately 80% of lung cancer-related deaths (Zappa & Mousa, 2016). Men and women who smoke are 23% and 13% more likely to develop lung cancer than non-smokers, respectively (Kanwal et al., 2017). The following symptoms are observed in lung cancer patients: uneasiness, yellow fingers, a raspy voice, weariness, sensitivities, thundering, persistent sickness, wheezing, hacking up blood even in small amounts, bone pain, migraine, difficulty breathing, difficulty gulping, and torment are secondary effects which are used to analyze cellular breakdown in lungs (Ji et al., 2018).

There are two primary histological subtypes of lung cancer: non-small-cell lung cancer (NSCLC) and small-cell lung cancer (SCLC). NSCLC accounts for approximately 85% of lung cancer patients and has a 5-year survival rate of 25% (Zhong et al., 2022). Its two primary histological types, adenocarcinoma and squamous cell carcinoma account for around 40% and 25% of all lung cancers, respectively (Jiang et al., 2022). SCLCs account for 10-15% of all lung malignancies and spread the most rapidly. Patients with this kind of lung cancer had a 5-year survival rate of 7%.

Cancer staging is related to the amount of cancer spread and is usually assessed using a mix of imaging tools and tissue biopsies. Processed CT (Computerized Tomography) and MRI (Magnetic Resonance Imaging) are commonly used to detect early lung cell disintegration. This procedure helps to determine the precise kind of cancer. Staging is critical in determining the prognosis of the disease, allowing healthcare experts to devise appropriate treatment options. Chemotherapy, immunotherapy, radiation therapy, and surgery are all possible therapeutic options, either alone or in combination (Hancock & Magnan, 2019; Sharma et al., 2020). It is vital to remember that when cancer progresses to a more advanced stage, it becomes more aggressive, resulting in a more dangerous state for the patient. The treatments employed on the patients depend on the stage and spread of cancer.

In the past few years, AI-based techniques have been used rapidly in various domains ranging from healthcare to finance, education to environment, etc. Also, fast learning methods for hand-drawn feature extraction, such as the GA or SFF-SA, have helped to produce the highlights to attain the best possible performance. Many clinical image-handling applications have advanced through the usage of AI techniques in the healthcare domain and are being used for the timely detection and diagnosis of cancer.

RT (Radiation Therapy) has made significant growth and is an essential component of lung cancer therapy. Finding cancer foci, eliminating dangerous organs, and avoiding RT-related misconceptions are all necessary for RT to be successful. The General Cancer Volume (GTV) must thus be accurately portioned, and the OARs used in RT treatment must be accurately designed to provide the appropriate portion of GTV (S. Kumar & Raman, 2020; Savic et al., 2021).

Early detection of cancer can reduce mortality significantly. In this context, it is essential to comprehend the significance of technological advancements in automating the diagnosis of cancer. With the progress made in Artificial Intelligence (AI) techniques like Machine Learning (ML) and Deep Learning (DL), it becomes crucial to incorporate them in the automated diagnosis of lung cancer. Considering the availability of numerous training samples, both currently and in the future, deep learning and machine learning prove to be an appropriate approach for the automatic detection of lung cancer. Especially when integrated with the experience of medical practitioners to provide quick and accurate results.

MOTIVATION

The primary goal of this study is to give insights into the function of AI-based ML-DL approaches in the investigation of lung cancer. It will aid in developing a thorough awareness of the current status of research in this area. It outlines the methodology, strategies, language utilized for implementation, benefits and drawbacks, and performance indicators evaluated in existing studies of the last five years. It also explains the datasets used in this domain and their accessibility. Identifying research gaps in previous studies allows future researchers to provide fresh ideas, approaches, or viewpoints through their study.

APPLICATION OF ARTIFICIAL INTELLIGENCE IN LUNG CANCER

Artificial intelligence (AI) is revolutionizing lung cancer diagnosis, detection, and treatment through its ability to analyze vast amounts of medical data with precision and efficiency. In diagnosis, AI algorithms analyze chest X-rays and CT scans to detect subtle abnormalities indicative of lung cancer, assisting radiologists in early detection and accurate interpretation of imaging findings. Moreover, AI-powered computer-aided diagnosis (CAD) systems provide real-time assistance by highlighting suspicious lesions and aiding in differential diagnosis. Beyond detection, AI plays a crucial role in treatment planning and personalization. By integrating patient data, including imaging scans, genomic profiles, and treatment histories, AI models recommend personalized treatment strategies tailored to each patient's unique characteristics and disease stage. Additionally, AI-driven clinical decision support systems assist healthcare providers in selecting optimal treatment options based on evidence-based guidelines and medical literature.

Several critical factors influence the generalizability of findings from AI-based lung cancer research. Patient demographics, including age, gender, ethnicity, and socio-economic status, can significantly impact the applicability of research outcomes, as these variables affect disease prevalence and progression. Disease heterogeneity, which encompasses the genetic, molecular, and histological diversity of lung cancer, further complicates the generalization of AI models trained on specific datasets, potentially limiting their effectiveness across different patient populations. Additionally, variations in healthcare systems, such as differences in diagnostic protocols, treatment standards, and access to medical resources, can influence the performance and reliability of AI models when applied in diverse clinical settings. To enhance generalizability, it is essential to develop and validate AI models on diverse, representative datasets and consider the integration of adaptable and robust algorithms that can accommodate these variations.

Furthermore, AI facilitates the development of targeted therapies by analyzing genomic data to identify genetic mutations and molecular biomarkers associated with lung cancer progression and treatment response. Overall, AI is transforming lung cancer care by enhancing early detection, guiding treatment decisions, and improving patient outcomes. The study contributes to the following areas:

- Exploring the different techniques used to analyze lung cancer.

- Identifying the different datasets that numerous authors have used.
- Open challenges and Futuristic directions in the application of ML and DL for cancer detection.

In this study, 35 articles were considered primary studies. These studies have been categorized based on the year and category of publication, as shown in Figure 1. This review article includes 35 research articles, of which 27 papers are from the journals category, six papers are from the conferences category, and one paper each is from the doctoral and book chapter category.

Various databases like Springer, Elsevier, IEEE Xplore, Taylor & Francis, and Google Scholar were used to find the studies. The graph given below presents a year-wise distribution of the various works considered in this literature review. The highest number of publications are from 2022(10), followed by 2020(9) and 2021(8).

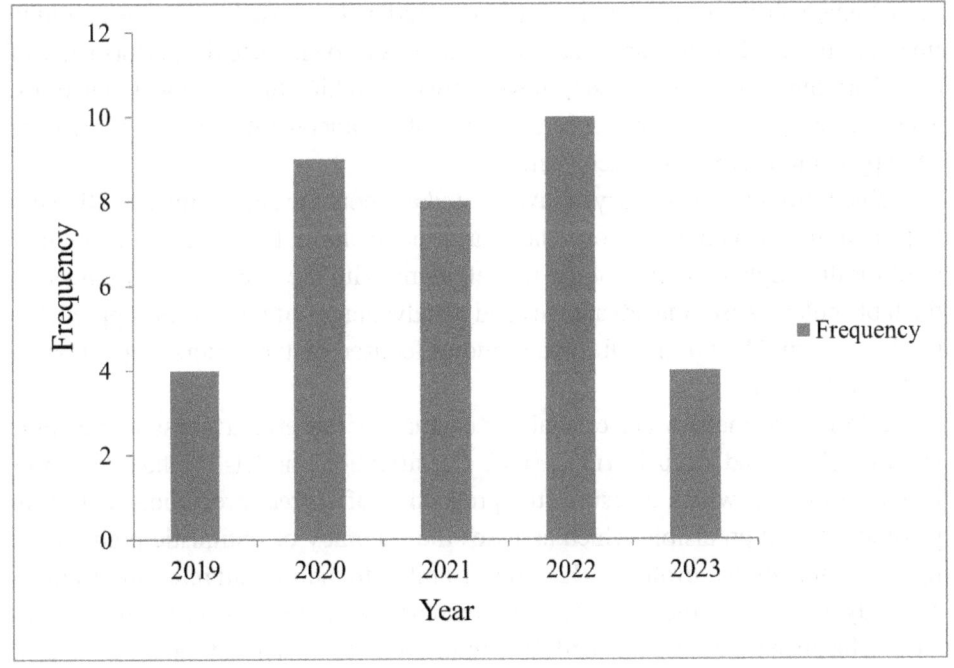

Figure 1. Categorization of Articles for Each Year

DEEP LEARNING TECHNIQUES FOR LUNG CANCER

Deep learning (DL) has emerged as a transformative tool in cancer research and treatment, revolutionizing various aspects of the oncology field. By leveraging DL algorithms, researchers and clinicians can analyze complex datasets such as medical images, genomic profiles, and clinical records with unprecedented accuracy and efficiency. DL excels in tasks like tumor detection, classification, and segmentation in medical imaging, enabling early diagnosis and precise treatment planning. Moreover, DL models can unravel intricate patterns in genomic data, identifying genetic mutations associated with cancer development and guiding the discovery of targeted therapies. Beyond diagnostics, DL facilitates personalized medicine by predicting patient outcomes, optimizing treatment strategies, and stratifying individuals based on their risk profile. The integration of DL into cancer care holds tremendous promise for improving detection rates, treatment efficacy, and patient survival, marking a significant step forward in the fight against cancer. The identification, segmentation, and classification of pulmonary nodules to assess their benign or malignant character are the main tasks covered by DL-based approaches for lung imaging studies. The primary focus of researchers is to enhance the performance of deep learning models by devising novel network architectures and loss functions. These techniques have experienced significant advancements, with new methods and applications emerging each year.

Table 1 provides a summary of diverse studies about the employment of DL techniques for lung cancer detection. The year of publication, technique, and language used for the implementation of the model, along with the results, are discussed in the table below. Also, the advantages and disadvantages of the various approaches used are given. Most of the DL model studies focused on the tumors' segmentation and classification.

Performance metrics are crucial for evaluating the effectiveness of machine learning (ML) and deep learning (DL) classification models. Standard metrics include accuracy, which measures the proportion of correct predictions out of all predictions, and precision, which assesses the accuracy of optimistic predictions. Recall, or sensitivity, evaluates the model's ability to identify all relevant instances correctly. In contrast, the F1 score, the harmonic mean of precision and recall, provides a balanced measure for models with uneven class distribution. Additionally, the area under the receiver operating characteristic curve (AUC-ROC) offers insight into the model's ability to distinguish between classes, and confusion matrices provide a detailed breakdown of true positives, false positives, true negatives, and false negatives. Other metrics, such as Matthews correlation coefficient (MCC) and Cohen's kappa, are used for more nuanced evaluations, especially in imbalanced datasets. These metrics collectively help comprehensively assess the performance, robustness, and reliability of ML-DL classification models in various applications. The highest accuracy obtained was 100%. The focus of improvement has been improving the performance using a balanced dataset and reducing the computation time.

Table 1. Summary of Existing Works on Deep Learning Techniques for Lung Cancer

Article	Year	Method	Technique	Language	Merits	Demerits	Performance Metrics
(Alshmrani et al., 2023)	2023	For the multi-class classification of COVID-19, lung opacity, tuberculosis (TB), lung cancer, and pneumonia, a DL architecture was proposed.	VGG19+CNN	Python	Model performed better than existing models to identify and treat patients more effectively.	-	Accuracy:96.48%, Recall:93.75%, Precision: 96.75%, F1 score; 95.62%, AUC: 99.82%
(Mamun et al., 2023)	2023	A DL-based model using the CNN framework was used for early detection of lung cancer using CT scan images.	Inception V3, Xception, and ResNet-50	Python	Outperformed other existing models	-	Accuracy: 92%, AUC: 98.21%, Recall: 91.72%
(Z. Li et al., 2022)	2022	(MGTA), a DL framework-based mask-guided attention mechanism, was used to predict lung cancer	MGTA	Python	Improved the feature detection of small tumors.	-	AUC:0.822, Sensitivity:0.753, Specificity: 0.743.
(Kanwal et al., 2017)	2020	An effective CNN (EFFI-CNN) based model was used for the detection of lung cancer.	CNN	Python	Reduced detection time.	Annotating large numbers of medical pictures is expensive and time-consuming.	Accuracy:87.02%, Recall:98%, Precision: 81%
(Shandilya & Nayak, 2022)	2022	Developed a CAD method to distinguish between benign lung tissue, lung squamous cell carcinoma, and lung adenocarcinoma in three different types of histopathological pictures.	CNN, MobileNet, VGG-19, ResNet 101, DenseNet 121, DenseNet 169, Inception V3, InceptionResNet V2, and MobileNetV2	Python	-	-	ResNet101 Accuracy: 98.67%
(Maalem et al., 2022)	2022	Detected and classified lung cancer images using DL.	CNN-Fast-RCNN	CAD, Python	High accuracy	Consideration of privacy using security techniques and approaches.	Accuracy:100%

continued on following page

Table 1. Continued

Article	Year	Method	Technique	Language	Merits	Demerits	Performance Metrics
(F. Wang et al., 2022)	2022	ML methods were combined with medical experiments to identify (NSCLC)-related biomarkers.	LASSO Regression, SVM-RFE	R	Identified new potential biomarkers for diagnosing and treating NSCLC.	-	P-value<0.05 and |logFC|≥1
(Zhong et al., 2022)	2022	The predictive accuracy and bio-logic underpinnings of the DL signature were examined in an external cohort.	DNN	-	Accurately predicted N2 illness and predicted prognosis.	Postoperative chemotherapy did not improve survival in low- and moderate-risk patients.	(Changed danger proportion, 2.9; 95% CI: 1.2, 6.9; P = .02) and repeat free endurance (changed risk proportion, 3.2; 95% CI: 1.4, 7.4; P = .007).
(Ibrahim et al., 2021)	2021	The classification model was created to recognize lung cellular degeneration, pneumonia, and coronavirus.	ResNet, CNN, RNN	Python	High performance in comparison to existing studies	The number of images and training epochs in the used datasets is less	Accuracy: 98.05%.
(Ashhar et al., 2021)	2021	Classified lung images into malignant and benign categories using DL techniques.	Google Net, Squeeze Net, Dense Net, Shuffle Net, MobileNetV2	MATLAB	Reliability of results	-	GoogleNet: Accuracy:94.53%, Specificity: 99.06%, Sensitivity: 65.67%, AUC: 86.84%.
(Yang et al., 2021)	2021	Analyzed immunologically stained pathological images to identify and treat lung cancer.	CNN based DLRHE	Python	DL improved illness prognosis by providing targeted treatment.	-	AUC: 87%.
(Sori et al., 2021)	2021	Addressed image label unbalancing for cancer identification.	CNN, DFD-Net	MATLAB	Reduced visual noise balanced receptive field size, and provided more	-	Accuracy:0.878 Recall: 0.874 Speciificity:0.891
(V. Kumar & Bakariya, 2021)	2021	Identification of lung nodules within a region of interest (ROI) by DL-based model.	AlexNet, GoogLeNet, DNN, CNN	MATLAB	Offered accurate and prompt diagnosis for highly skilled medical practitioners.	More studies are needed on the maximum DCM (LIDC-IDRI) dataset using various methodologies.	Alexnet's sensitivity, performance, precision, and specificity: 100% at a zero false rate.

continued on following page

Table 1. Continued

Article	Year	Method	Technique	Language	Merits	Demerits	Performance Metrics
(Jawarkar et al., 2021)	2021	Unambiguous strategy for seeing lung patients in a difficult stage. The shape and surface elements of the CT channel were considered utilizing the ML-DL approach.	CNN	-	Better results than another classifier for this dataset.	NSCLC A quick end is necessary due to stage demand. The foundation of the previous narrative was essentially depicting lung cell disintegration. There would be no stage information.	CNN Precision: 96.88%,
(Yeh et al., 2021)	2020	Models were used for: (1) Nodule detection systems (2) False positive reduction systems	CNN, U-Net, VGG, ResNet, ImageNet, GoogLeNet, AlexNet	-	High Performance	The data was unbalanced. Better results can be obtained with a more balanced dataset.	Accuracy:88.83%.
(Bharati et al., 2020)	2020	X-beam images combined with DL techniques are used to identify lung cancer.	CNN, VNN, VGG, X-Ray, AlexNet, VDSNet, GoogLeNet, ResNet-5, U-Net	-	Reduced clinical expenses.	-	VDSNet Accuracy: 73%
(She et al., 2020)	2020	Evaluated the predictive capabilities of DeepSurv, a DL-based neural network, in comparison to a tumor, node, and metastasis staging system for survival prediction, and examined the effectiveness of individual treatment through reliability testing.	DeepSurv	Python	Useful analytical tool for treatment in patients with NSCLC	Computationally expensive to train and validate	(C statistic=0.742; 95% CI, 0.709-0.775)
(Kriegsmann et al., 2020)	2020	Detected the subtype of lung cancer	VGG16, InceptionV3,	Python	Less training time	Misclassification of ADC and SqCC occurred when trained over 20 epochs	Imaging and QC cutoffs increased accuracy to 100% regardless of the subgroup.
(Kalaivani et al., 2020)	2020	Predicted the lung cancer using CT and DL approach	CT, CNN	Python	-	Content stored on the website can be removed.	Accuracy: 90.85%.

continued on following page

Table 1. Continued

Article	Year	Method	Technique	Language	Merits	Demerits	Performance Metrics
(Bhatia et al., 2019)	2019	Images were used from the dataset of lung cancer for observation symbols, whereas the types of cancer have been states of the system that have created the dataset.	CNN	MATLAB	The performance and effectiveness of the system demonstrated the usefulness of learning and enhancing the medical industry.	-	Precision:89.3%, Recall:72%. Specificity: 98.2%
(J. Wang et al., 2019)	2019	Developed a model utilizing DL techniques in the diagnosis and classification of lung nodules through CT imaging.	CAD, CT, CNN	-	Improved image feature extraction.	-	Accuracy: 86.5% to 91.1%.
(Serj et al., 2018)	2019	Improved the quality of lung images and detected lung cancer by avoiding misclassification.	DNN	MATLAB	-	-	Accuracy: 98.42%

HYBRID TECHNIQUES FOR LUNG CANCER:

Like DL, ML is the superset of DL and finds its application in cancer detection. Machine learning (ML) has become a powerful tool in the fight against cancer, offering innovative solutions across various stages of the disease. ML algorithms analyze vast amounts of data from diverse sources, including medical imaging, genomics, and patient records, to extract valuable insights and support clinical decision-making. In cancer diagnosis, ML models enhance the accuracy and efficiency of tumor detection and classification, aiding in early detection and treatment planning. Additionally, ML techniques contribute to the identification of biomarkers and genetic signatures associated with cancer subtypes and prognosis, facilitating personalized treatment approaches. ML algorithms also play a crucial role in drug discovery and development by predicting drug response and toxicity, accelerating the identification of novel therapies. Furthermore, ML-based predictive models help clinicians anticipate disease progression and patient outcomes, enabling proactive management strategies. Overall, the integration of ML into cancer research and clinical practice holds immense potential to improve patient care, outcomes, and our understanding of this complex disease.

Hybrid methods integrating ML and DL techniques are frequently used to identify lung cancer. The thorough study done in this field is summarized in Table 2. The procedure generally involves several pre-processing stages to extract pertinent characteristics from various input sources, primarily pictures, using statistical techniques and pre-trained convolutional neural networks (CNNs) along with other ML techniques like SVM, KNN, etc. The categorization of various lung cancer tasks is therefore made more accessible by using these extracted characteristics as input into numerous machine learning algorithms. Examples include classifying normalized biological data points into carcinogenic and non-cancerous categories or differentiating between malignant and benign lung nodules.

Table 2. Summary of Existing Works on Machine Learning and Deep Learning Techniques for Lung Cancer

Article	Year	Method	Technique	Language	Merits	Demerits	Performance Metrics
(Pradhan et al., 2023)	2023	The suggested model utilizes RNN to create an ensemble learning model, incorporating the proposed BF-SSA. It assigns five sets of features to each stage of classification, enabling accurate lung cancer classification.	PCA, CNN (t-SNE)	MATLAB	The hybrid optimization method improved feature selection performance.	Each approach is utilized independently, gaining dependability and more uniform results is more complicated.	Performed better by 8.79% by existing models.
(Rajput & Subasi, 2023)	2023	Different DL models and techniques detected lung cancer using histopathological images.	ResNet + SVM	Python	High Accuracy and Less Training Time.	-	Accuracy: 98.57%
(Mamun et al., 2022)	2022	Lung cancer prediction using ML and EL	XGBoost, LightGBM, Bagging, and AdaBoost by k-fold 10 cross-validation	Python	Increased the predictability of predictions made by classifiers.	-	Accuracy:94.42%, Precision:95.66%, Recall: 94.46%, AUC: 98.14%.
(Jiang et al., 2022)	2022	CT images of lung cancer were used with a DL-based model, and effectiveness is verified in the accurate prediction of lung disease.	U-Net, RNN, CNN, AlexNet, ImageNet, ResNet, SVM, RF	-	Anti-interference performance was improved by the 3D U-Net structure to a certain extent.	-	A nodule is detected in 0.5 seconds. FROC: 0.883

continued on following page

Table 2. Continued

Article	Year	Method	Technique	Language	Merits	Demerits	Performance Metrics
(Khademi et al., 2023)	2022	A hybrid transformer-based framework, referred to as the CAET-SWin, was proposed to predict adenocarcinoma subsolid nodules and the invasiveness of lung accurately and reliably from non-thin 3D CT scans	CAE, SWin	-	Reduced computation complexity	-	Accuracy:82.65%, Sensitivity:83.66%, Specificity: 81.66%
(Rahman, 2021)	2022	The approach involved expanding the dataset through information augmentation techniques and employing CNN to eliminate connected highlights in the dataset for lung cancer detection.	CNN, KNN	Python	100% Recall rate	Feature selection technique was not applied.	Accuracy: 90%
(Hashemzadeh et al., 2021)	2022	Cell-line images were divided into six groups, five of which represented various disease cell lines.	CNN, KNN, ResNet18, AlexNet, GoogLeNet, ImageNet	MATLAB	Reduced the requirement for significant human involvement and enabled precise and reliable processing of vast volumes of data.	-	ResNet18: Accuracy:98.37%, F1-score: 97.29%
(Doppalapudi et al., 2021)	2021	Patients with cellular breakdowns in the lungs were the subjects in this work. Models using DL techniques were built to address the problems of disease endurance grouping and relapse.	ANN, CNN, RNN, SVM, DT, RF	-	Results contributed to the development of an early diagnosis of a cancer patient.	-	ANN Accuracy:71.18% CNN RMSE: 13.50% R2 value: 50.66% in regression technique.
(Chaunzwa et al., 2021)	2021	Developed DL-based solid radionics models to aid in the identification of clinically significant NSCLC subtypes by predicting cellular breakdown in lung histology.	CNN, KNN, SVM, ImageNet	-	Reduce reader variability	Small dataset	AUC:0.71

continued on following page

Table 2. Continued

Article	Year	Method	Technique	Language	Merits	Demerits	Performance Metrics
(Lai et al., 2020)	2020	The 5-year endurance status of NSCLC patients was predicted by researchers using biomarkers and clinical data.	DNN, CT, KNN, RF, SVM,	-	Detected non-small lung cancer with high accuracy.	Works for 5-year survival only.	AUC:0.8163, Accuracy: 75.44%
(Subramanian et al., 2020)	2020	DL model using AlexNet was developed to differentiate lung CT images properly.	Alexnet, SVM, KNN, CNN	Python	A consistent and sustainable model for diagnosis of Lung cancer.	-	Accuracy: 99.52%
(B. Li et al., 2020)	2020	DL restored the drug based on transcriptomic and chemical data properties were developed.	DNN, RF	-	-	Building large-scale drug-transcriptomic datasets has proved difficult.	In the 6-point division, DNN and RF performed at a score of F1 of 0.41 and 0.35 points, respectively.
(X. Wang et al., 2019)	2019	A thorough and accurate diagnosis is essential for therapeutic care, and FCN and CNN can be used to generate discriminative zones and DL features.	X-Ray, CT, MRI, CNN, RF, SVM, GoogLeNet, AlexNet, VGG-16, ImageNet	Python	Helped in improving lung cancer image quality.	The WSI classification task is substantially more difficult because only image-level labels are typically provided.	Accuracy: 97.3%, AUC with 85.6% in public data from TCGA.

DATASET DESCRIPTION

The presence of datasets is vital for automating the detection and classification of lung cancer nodules. To achieve accurate performance outcomes through computational methods, having a dataset is an essential prerequisite. Table 3 represents various datasets along with their availability or accessibility, and their diversity in terms of samples and characteristics which have come into view while exploring the works of different researchers. Some researchers built their datasets or gathered data directly from hospitals, while others relied on datasets from Kaggle and other sources.

The table below contains the multiple datasets utilized in the original research, as well as the dataset description and accessible status (public or private). The bulk of the datasets utilized are publicly available, with the LIDC-IRDI dataset being the most popular among academics. Many privately accessible datasets, such as those stated in (Alshmrani et al., 2023) and (She et al., 2020), show that ML-DL approaches may be used in real-world clinical settings to increase early diagnosis rates. However, the dataset used determines the generalizability and reliability of ML and DL models for lung cancer detection. The dataset used for training, validation, and testing directly affects how well the model performs in real-world scenarios.

The quality and accuracy of the dataset influence the performance of the model. Inaccurate or noisy data can lead to incorrect model predictions and reduced reliability. Ensuring high-quality, reliable data is critical. Also, the size of the dataset matters for model generalizability. A dataset that is too small might result in overfitting; hence a more extensive dataset may be suited for better generalizability. Imbalanced datasets can also lead to biased model predictions. For example, if the dataset has a higher proportion of benign cases than malignant cases, the model might perform well for benign cases but poorly for detecting malignancies.

Addressing data-related challenges in lung cancer detection using machine learning can be approached through practical strategies like data augmentation techniques and collaborative data-sharing initiatives. Data augmentation, including methods such as image transformations, synthetic data generation, and oversampling of minority classes, can enhance the diversity and size of training datasets, thereby improving model robustness and accuracy. Collaborative data-sharing initiatives, such as multi-institutional partnerships and federated learning frameworks, facilitate the pooling of diverse and comprehensive datasets while preserving patient privacy. These collaborations enable the development of more generalizable and reliable models by incorporating a wide range of patient demographics and disease variations. By leveraging these strategies, researchers can overcome data limitations and advance the effectiveness of AI-driven lung cancer detection.

Table 3. Datasets used in the Previous Works Considered

Dataset	Article	Dataset Description	Accessibility
CXR dataset from the National Library of Medicine Shenzhen No.3 Hospital	(Alshmrani et al., 2023)	326 standard cases and 336 patients with TB symptoms were found in 662 CXRs.	Public
Lung Cancer Dataset	(Mamun et al., 2023)	960 7 CT scan pictures. The dataset comprises four different sorts of classes: adenocarcinoma, big cell carcinoma, squamous cell carcinoma, and regular (not lung cancer).	Public
DM dataset	(Z. Li et al., 2022)	There are 2814 lung cancer patients, 1845 of whom are diagnosed without distant metastasis, and 969 of whom are diagnosed with this complication.	Public
LIDC-IDRI and Mendeley data sets.	(Kanwal et al., 2017)	LIDC-IRDI: 1,018 low-dose lung CTs from 1010 lung patients.	Public

continued on following page

Table 3. Continued

Dataset	Article	Dataset Description	Accessibility
Publicly Available Dataset	(Shandilya & Nayak, 2022)	15,000 examples of histological images of benign lung tissue, lung squamous cell carcinoma, and lung adenocarcinoma from three distinct types.	Public
Kaggle	(Maalem et al., 2022)	1097 chest X-rays from three collaborating centers, of which 416 were routine exams, 561 had cancerous lung nodules, and 120 had benign nodules that CT later verified.	Public
Microarray Dataset	(F. Wang et al., 2022)	Combined data on cancer cases from (GSE18842, GSE32863, and GSE21933) from the Gene Expression Omnibus (GEO)	Public
Clinical Dataset	(Zhong et al., 2022)	Review of CT scans and clinical information from patients at Shanghai Pulmonary Hospital who underwent surgery for clinical stage I NSCLC between January 2011 and December 2013	Public
Multiple Source Dataset	(Ibrahim et al., 2021)	33,676 images included. The Italian Society of Medical and Interventional Radiology (SIRM), the Radiological Society of North America (RSNA), and Radiopaedia all contributed to the production of these materials.	Public
LIDC-IRDI	(Ashhar et al., 2021; Bhatia et al., 2019; Jiang et al., 2022; V. Kumar & Bakariya, 2021; J. Wang et al., 2019)	LIDC-IRDI: 1,018 low-dose lung CTs from 1010 lung patients.	Public
TCGA	(Yang et al., 2021)	180 images	Public
Kaggle Data Science Bowl 2017 challenge (KDSB) and LUNA 16.	(Sori et al., 2021)	Kaggle Data Science Bowl dataset: 2,101 labeled data. LUNA16: 1,186 lung nodules annotated in 888 CT scans.	Public
DICOM	(Jawarkar et al., 2021)	1693 CT, MRI, PET, and digital X-ray images	Public
Taiwan National Health Insurance Research Database	(Yeh et al., 2021)	2 million participants who got care between 1999-2013.	Public
NIH Dataset	(Bharati et al., 2020)	112,000 X-rays of the chest from over 30,000 different patients	Public
Population study	(She et al., 2020)	1182 individuals with newly discovered stages I to IV NSCLC between January 2010 and December 2015	Private

continued on following page

Table 3. Continued

Dataset	Article	Dataset Description	Accessibility
-	(Kriegsmann et al., 2020)	SCLC (n = 80), ADC (n = 80), and SqCC (n = 80) as well as skeletal muscle (n = 30) as a control, were compiled from the Institute of Pathology, University Clinic Heidelberg's archive with the aid of the Tissue Biobank of the National Centre for Tumour Diseases (NCT).	Public
CT SCAN IMAGE, EM, CNN	(Kalaivani et al., 2020)	To forecast cancer pictures, the CNN model is utilized, which is embedded with the Gaussian Mixture model and the EM algorithm to predict essential characteristics from the CT scan and estimate the percentage of cancer that spreads to the extremities by markers. A set of CT Scan images was used to conduct the tests	Public
Kaggle Data Science Bowl 2017 challenge (KDSB)	(Serj et al., 2018)	2101 labeled data images.	Public
-	(Jawarkar et al., 2021)	-	Public
Survey Dataset	(Mamun et al., 2022)	308 people.	Private
-	(Khademi et al., 2023)	Pathologically proven SubSolid Nodules (SSNs) of 114 samples.	Private
SPIE- American Association of Physicists in Medicine (AAPM) and National Cancer Institute (NCI)	(Rahman, 2021)	60 CT scans	Public
Cell culture Sample	(Kriegsmann et al., 2020)	Research Institute of Molecular Pathology (IMP), Technical University of Vienna (TU Wien), and Ludwig Boltzmann Institute for Cancer Research, Vienna, Austria	Public
Surveillance, Epidemiology, and End Results (SEER)	(Doppalapudi et al., 2021)	It is population-based because local registries from 18 states provide data on all cancer cases within a given region and a particular racial/ethnic population.	Public
-	(Chaunzwa et al., 2021)	311 patients with early-stage NSCLC who had surgical treatment at Massachusetts General Hospital (MGH).	Private
E-MTAB-923, Gene Expression Omnibus (GEO) database, STRING	(Lai et al., 2020)	The initial set of E-MTAB-923 patients (n = 90) with (51 survivors, and 39 fatalities). The information was given by the National Centre for Biotechnology Information (NCBI).	Public
-	(Subramanian et al., 2020)	100 images, with 50 as cancer images and 50 as regular images.	Public

Dataset	Article	Dataset Description	Accessibility
MESH dataset	(B. Li et al., 2020)	75 medicines were connected to 6 MeSH-derived therapeutic categories. Vasodilator agents, anti-dyskinesia agents, anticonvulsants, hypolipidemic agents, anti-asthmatic agents, and antineoplastic medicines are among the six therapeutic use groups.	Public
The Cancer Genome Atlas (TCGA) Dataset	(X. Wang et al., 2019)	Over 11000 primary cancer sample cases were molecularly characterized and sequenced as part of a cancer genomics program.	Public

RESULTS AND DISCUSSION

This section discusses the findings of the statistical overview of 35 papers that are considered in this survey. It discusses the category to which the paper belongs, different ML and DL techniques used for lung cancer detection, keyword frequency, and the programming languages used to employ ML and DL.

Type of Articles

This review paper comes from numerous journals and conferences. As the primary source for authoring reviews, 35 papers were examined: 27 papers from various journals, 6 from conferences, 1 from a book chapter, and 1 doctoral thesis. Figure 3 demonstrates that 78% of the papers used in the primary research were journal articles, 16% were conference papers, 3% were book chapters, and 3% were doctoral dissertations, as illustrated in Figure 2.

Figure 2. Percentage of Publications from Journals, Conferences, Doctoral, and Book Chapters Utilized in Research

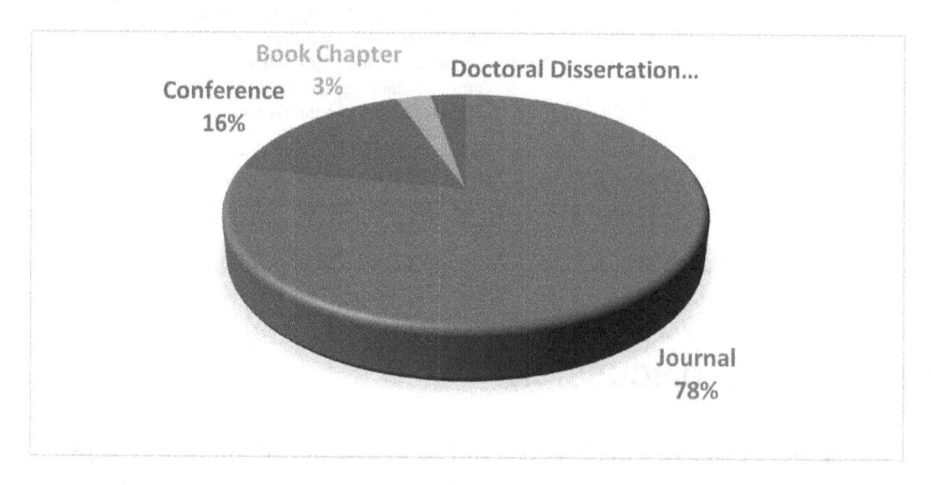

Keywords

Word Cloud is an easy way to find out what common themes and keywords are used in the headings shown to find out the most popular phrases. In Figure 3, the most frequently used words are highlighted in large, bold font, whereas the less commonly used phrases are highlighted in smaller, more common words.

Figure 3. Word Cloud for most Frequently used Keywords

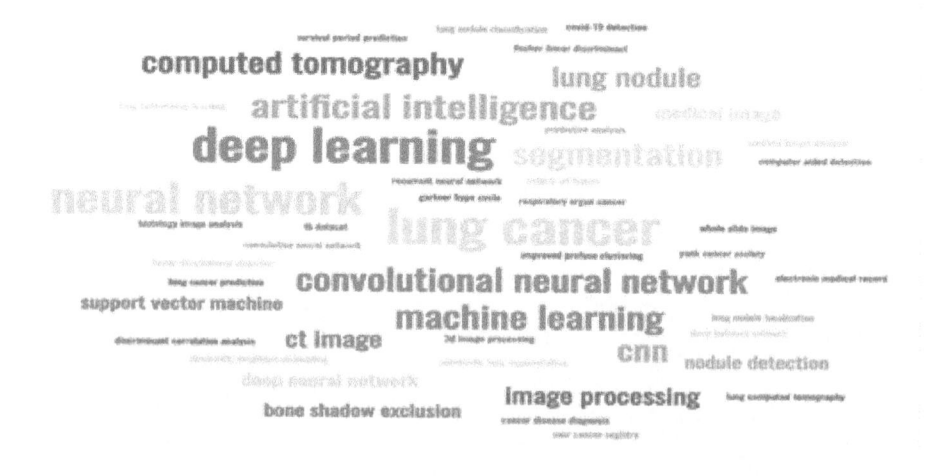

Programming Language

Researchers have used a variety of languages to develop their models for lung cancer screening. Python is the most widely used planning language, as shown in Figure 4. Python is the language of choice for 57% of researchers, followed by MATLAB (36%) and R (3%).

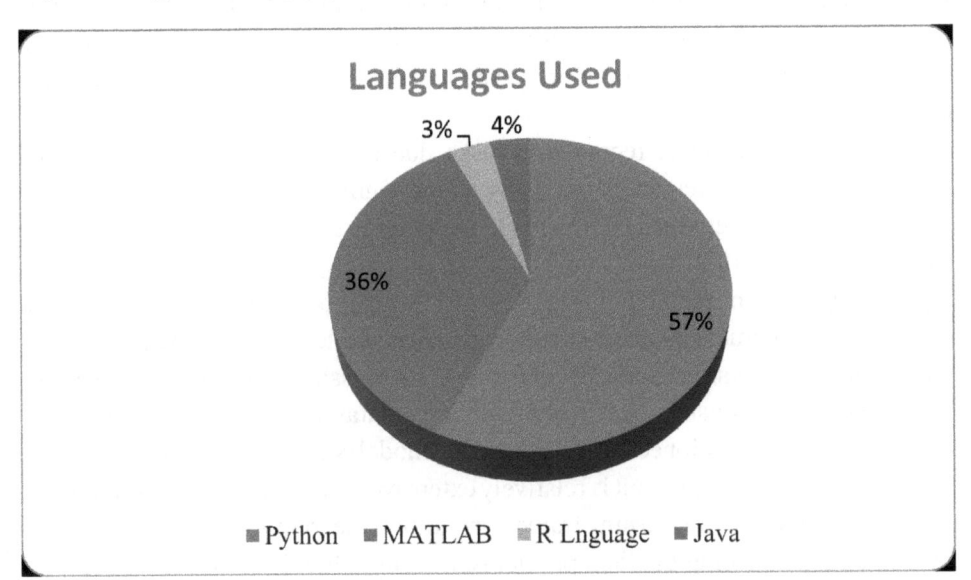

Figure 4. Different Languages used to Develop the Models

Various techniques used by different researchers

The various methods utilized in the research publications are described in this section in Figure 5. The graph was made using fundamental studies to identify lung cancer. The graph's Y-axis displays the number of publications, while the X-axis displays the various methodologies utilized in the research report. Out of 35 different types of algorithms, the top 10 algorithms are highlighted below in the graph. This graph shows that CNN is the methodology many first researchers most frequently employed. Followed by SVM and AlexNet. As observed from this analysis, the usage of neural networks is gaining popularity for lung cancer detection.

As observed, CNNs have emerged as the cornerstone technique for lung cancer detection and treatment owing to their exceptional performance in medical image analysis. CNNs are particularly adept at automatically learning and extracting intricate features from radiographic images, such as chest X-rays and CT scans, enabling highly accurate detection of suspicious nodules or lesions indicative of lung cancer. Their hierarchical architecture allows for the detection of subtle abnormalities and precise localization of lesions, which is crucial for early diagnosis and effective treatment planning. Moreover, CNNs can be trained on large datasets of annotated medical images, enabling them to improve their performance and generalize well to unseen data continually. Additionally, the interpretability of CNNs facilitates their integration into clinical workflows, providing radiologists and oncologists with valuable insights for decision-making. With their proven efficacy, adaptability, and scalability, CNNs continue to drive advancements in lung cancer detection and treatment, offering promise for improved patient outcomes and enhanced healthcare delivery.

CNN excels in image recognition tasks due to its ability to capture spatial hierarchies, but they require large datasets and significant computational power. Recurrent Neural Networks (RNNs) are effective for sequential data, such as time series or text, but suffer from vanishing gradient issues, making training challenging for long sequences. KNN is simple and intuitive, performing well with small datasets, but becomes computationally expensive and less effective with more extensive, high-dimensional data. SVM is robust for classification with clear margins between classes but can be inefficient with large datasets and complex, non-linear problems. AlexNet, a pioneering deep learning model, significantly advanced image classification performance but is relatively extensive and computationally intensive. ResNet, with its residual learning framework, allows the training of intense networks by mitigating vanishing gradient problems, making it highly effective for complex tasks. However, it requires substantial computational resources and careful design to avoid overfitting.

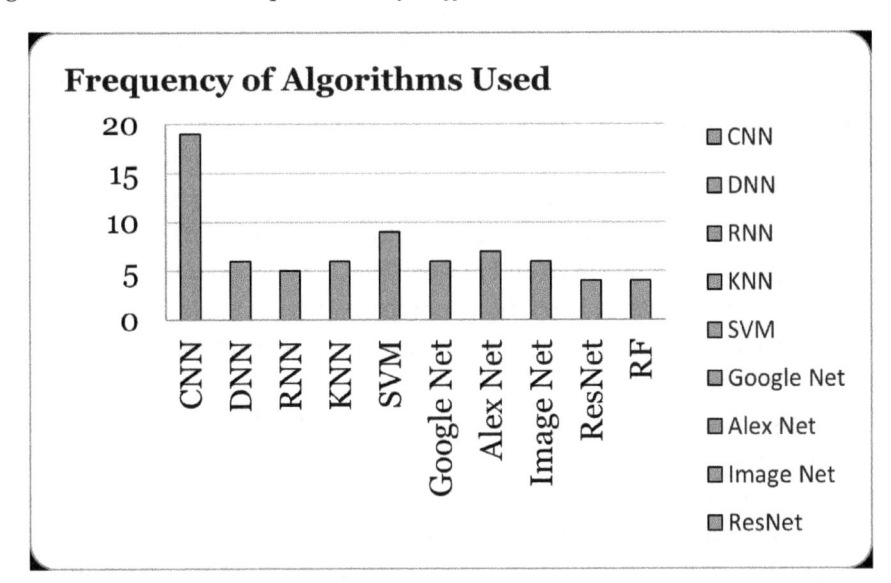

Figure 5. Various Techniques used by Different Researchers

[Bar chart titled "Frequency of Algorithms Used" showing frequencies for CNN, DNN, RNN, KNN, SVM, Google Net, Alex Net, Image Net, ResNet, RF]

OPEN CHALLENGES AND FUTURISTIC DIRECTIONS

After a thorough study of the available literature, numerous research gaps and challenges are identified as follows:

The performance of existing models can be enhanced by extending training sessions, adding images to the datasets, and utilizing more advanced learning strategies like GAN in both additions and divisions.

(V. Kumar & Bakariya, 2021; X. Wang et al., 2019) Further, advanced hybrid approaches or intelligent machines can be utilized to improve the accuracy of models. Immunotherapy, a new concept in cancer treatment, can be explored since it is highly efficient.

(Bharati et al., 2020) proposed more techniques can be utilized to enhance image data, such as color space augmentations, kernel filters, feature space augmentations, etc. A limited amount of accessible coarse annotations can help achieve even higher accuracy levels (J. Wang et al., 2019). Variables that influence the development of lung cancer in humans can be identified by employing similar features (Subramanian et al., 2020). To broaden the use of ML/DL approaches, it is recommended that models for various illnesses and medical imaging should be used in the future

DFD-Net is easily adaptive to fluctuations in nodule size, as well as other medical image identification tasks, even with denoised data that has lost certain information during the denoising process (Sori et al., 2021). DNNs with federated learning algorithms can be utilized to identify additional health conditions, such as respiratory ailments, via lung sounds, cancer detection, heart failure prediction, and other diseases (Mamun et al., 2022). Deep neural networks with federated learning algorithms are utilized to identify additional health issues, such as respiratory ailments via lung sounds, cancer detection, heart failure prediction, and others. More cancer kinds might be expected, as stated in (Hashemzadeh et al., 2021) and (Doppalapudi et al., 2021); advanced integration extraction approaches with AI calculations, together with the usage of the large dataset were suggested by (Chaunzwa et al., 2021; Lai et al., 2020; Mamun et al., 2023).

Other challenges include the integration of AI technologies into clinical practice, which faces several limitations and challenges. Workflow disruptions are a significant concern, as implementing AI systems often requires changes to existing procedures and can initially slow down clinical processes. There is also resistance from healthcare providers, stemming from skepticism about the reliability of AI tools and concerns over job displacement. Additionally, issues such as the need for extensive training, the potential for biases in AI algorithms, data privacy concerns, and the interoperability of AI systems with existing electronic health records further complicate integration. Ensuring that AI tools are user-friendly, transparent, and aligned with clinical workflows is essential to overcoming these challenges and achieving successful adoption in healthcare settings.

Furthermore, to obtain more accurate and fast results, XAI techniques and more real-time datasets may be used for real-time cancer analysis and its early prediction for timely analysis. Lung cancer diagnosis has significantly benefited from technological improvements, notably in the areas of ML and DL. These developments have increased lung cancer detection's precision, effectiveness, and early diagnosis, thereby improving patient outcomes. Medical imaging analysis has been transformed by ML and DL approaches, enabling automated interpretation. The interpretability and explainability of ML-DL models for medical imaging using XAI approaches can be improved through research. These methods aid in improving the clarity and interpretability of ML-DL models for doctors. It may be possible to increase the clinical utility and acceptance of these models by devising techniques to display and comprehend the features learned by them.

Telemedicine platforms can incorporate ML-DL models for remote monitoring and diagnosis. For patients who live in remote or underserved locations, this is especially important. They can investigate continuous data streams and wearable technology for real-time monitoring. It would be beneficial to create models that can adjust to changes in patient conditions and send timely signals to medical personnel.

A more comprehensive understanding of lung cancer is possible by combining data from many sources, including patient records, medical pictures, and genetic data. This combination can enhance the accuracy of the diagnosis and treatment planning.

By doing this, many different sources of data can be brought together, making predictions more reliable and valid. Secondly, this method is helpful because it explains how decisions are arrived at by complex ML and DL models to increase trust among users, such as doctors who need to interpret diagnostic outcomes. In the same breath, the integration of explainable AI methods enhances clarity and confidence by providing insights into the decision-making process of intricate ML and DL models. This helps doctors understand and confirm diagnostic results. At the same time, a new possibility emerges with the use of combined data from different sources.

ETHICAL CONSIDERATION AND REGULATIONS

The application of ML and DL techniques in healthcare, particularly for tasks like lung cancer detection, comes with several ethical considerations that need to be carefully addressed. Privacy and Data Security is one issue where patient data used to train and test ML/DL models must be treated with the utmost privacy and security. Another issue is that obtaining informed consent from patients whose data is being used for training and validation is crucial. Patients should be fully informed about how their data will be used and the potential implications of the research. These models can aid in decision-making and early detection, but they should not replace human judgment entirely. There should be a balance between automated systems and the expertise of medical professionals to make the best use of the latest technologies.

The regulatory landscape governing AI applications in healthcare is evolving rapidly, with various jurisdictions introducing guidelines and standards to ensure the safety, effectiveness, and ethical use of AI-driven diagnostic tools. Organizations such as the FDA in the United States and the European Commission have published frameworks outlining the requirements for the development, validation, and deployment of AI-based medical devices. These guidelines emphasize the importance of transparency, accountability, and clinical validation in the development process, aiming to promote trust and confidence in AI technologies while safeguarding patient safety and privacy.

REFERENCES

Alshmrani, G. M. M., Ni, Q., Jiang, R., Pervaiz, H., & Elshennawy, N. M. (2023). A deep learning architecture for multi-class lung diseases classification using chest X-ray (CXR) images. *Alexandria Engineering Journal*, 64, 923–935. 10.1016/j.aej.2022.10.053

Ashhar, S. M., Mokri, S. S., Abd Rahni, A. A., Huddin, A. B., Zulkarnain, N., Azmi, N. A., & Mahaletchumy, T. (2021). Comparison of deep learning convolutional neural network (CNN) architectures for CT lung cancer classification. *International Journal of Advanced Technology and Engineering Exploration*, 8(74), 126–134. 10.19101/IJATEE.2020.S1762126

Barta, J. A., Powell, C. A., & Wisnivesky, J. P. (2019). Global epidemiology of lung cancer. *Annals of Global Health*, 85(1), 8. 10.5334/aogh.241930741509

Bharati, S., Podder, P., & Mondal, M. R. H. (2020). Hybrid deep learning for detecting lung diseases from X-ray images. *Informatics in Medicine Unlocked*, 20, 100391. 10.1016/j.imu.2020.10039132835077

Bhatia, S., Sinha, Y., & Goel, L. (2019). Lung cancer detection: a deep learning approach. *Soft Computing for Problem Solving: SocProS 2017, Volume 2*, 699–705.

Chaunzwa, T. L., Hosny, A., Xu, Y., Shafer, A., Diao, N., Lanuti, M., Christiani, D. C., Mak, R. H., & Aerts, H. J. W. L. (2021). Deep learning classification of lung cancer histology using CT images. *Scientific Reports*, 11(1), 5471. 10.1038/s41598-021-84630-x33727623

Doppalapudi, S., Qiu, R. G., & Badr, Y. (2021). Lung cancer survival period prediction and understanding: Deep learning approaches. *International Journal of Medical Informatics*, 148, 104371. 10.1016/j.ijmedinf.2020.10437133461009

Galvez-Nino, M., Ruiz, R., Pinto, J. A., Roque, K., Mantilla, R., Raez, L. E., & Mas, L. (2020). Lung cancer in the young. *Lung*, 198(1), 195–200. 10.1007/s00408-019-00294-531773258

Hancock, M. C., & Magnan, J. F. (2019). Level set image segmentation with velocity term learned from data with applications to lung nodule segmentation. *ArXiv Preprint ArXiv:1910.03191*.

Hashemzadeh, H., Shojaeilangari, S., Allahverdi, A., Rothbauer, M., Ertl, P., & Naderi-Manesh, H. (2021). A combined microfluidic deep learning approach for lung cancer cell high throughput screening toward automatic cancer screening applications. *Scientific Reports*, 11(1), 9804. 10.1038/s41598-021-89352-833963232

Ibrahim, D. M., Elshennawy, N. M., & Sarhan, A. M. (2021). Deep-chest: Multi-classification deep learning model for diagnosing COVID-19, pneumonia, and lung cancer chest diseases. *Computers in Biology and Medicine*, 132, 104348. 10.1016/j.compbiomed.2021.10434833774272

Jawarkar, J., Solanki, N., Vaishnav, M., Vichare, H., & Degadwala, S. (2021). Multistage lung cancer detection and prediction using deep learning. *International Journal of Scientific Research in Science, Engineering and Technology*, •••, 54–60. 10.32628/IJSRSET218217

Ji, X., Bossé, Y., Landi, M. T., Gui, J., Xiao, X., Qian, D., Joubert, P., Lamontagne, M., Li, Y., Gorlov, I., de Biasi, M., Han, Y., Gorlova, O., Hung, R. J., Wu, X., McKay, J., Zong, X., Carreras-Torres, R., Christiani, D. C., & Amos, C. I. (2018). Identification of susceptibility pathways for the role of chromosome 15q25. 1 in modifying lung cancer risk. *Nature Communications*, 9(1), 3221. 10.1038/s41467-018-05074-y30104567

Jiang, W., Zeng, G., Wang, S., Wu, X., & Xu, C. (2022). Application of deep learning in lung cancer imaging diagnosis. *Journal of Healthcare Engineering*, 2022, 2022. 10.1155/2022/610794035028122

Kalaivani, N., Manimaran, N., Sophia, S., & Devi, D. D. (2020). Deep learning based lung cancer detection and classification. *IOP Conference Series. Materials Science and Engineering*, 994(1), 012026. 10.1088/1757-899X/994/1/012026

Kanwal, M., Ding, X., & Cao, Y. (2017). Familial risk for lung cancer. *Oncology Letters*, 13(2), 535–542. 10.3892/ol.2016.551828356926

Khademi, S., Heidarian, S., Afshar, P., Naderkhani, F., Oikonomou, A., Plataniotis, K. N., & Mohammadi, A. (2023). Spatio-Temporal Hybrid Fusion of CAE and SWin Transformers for Lung Cancer Malignancy Prediction. *ICASSP 2023-2023 IEEE International Conference on Acoustics, Speech and Signal Processing (ICASSP)*, 1–5.

Kitchenham, B. (2004). Procedures for performing systematic reviews. *Keele, UK, Keele University, 33*(2004), 1–26.

Kitchenham, B., Brereton, O. P., Budgen, D., Turner, M., Bailey, J., & Linkman, S. (2009). Systematic literature reviews in software engineering–a systematic literature review. *Information and Software Technology*, 51(1), 7–15. 10.1016/j.infsof.2008.09.009

Kriegsmann, M., Haag, C., Weis, C.-A., Steinbuss, G., Warth, A., Zgorzelski, C., Muley, T., Winter, H., Eichhorn, M. E., Eichhorn, F., Kriegsmann, J., Christopoulos, P., Thomas, M., Witzens-Harig, M., Sinn, P., von Winterfeld, M., Heussel, C., Herth, F., Klauschen, F., & Kriegsmann, K. (2020). Deep learning for the classification of small-cell and non-small-cell lung cancer. *Cancers (Basel)*, 12(6), 1604. 10.3390/cancers1206160432560475

Kumar, S., & Raman, S. (2020). Lung nodule segmentation using 3-dimensional convolutional neural networks. *Soft Computing for Problem Solving: SocProS 2018, Volume 1*, 585–596.

Kumar, V., & Bakariya, B. (2021). Classification of malignant lung cancer using deep learning. *Journal of Medical Engineering & Technology*, 45(2), 85–93. 10.1080/03091902.2020.185383733448905

Lai, Y.-H., Chen, W.-N., Hsu, T.-C., Lin, C., Tsao, Y., & Wu, S. (2020). Overall survival prediction of non-small cell lung cancer by integrating microarray and clinical data with deep learning. *Scientific Reports*, 10(1), 4679. 10.1038/s41598-020-61588-w32170141

Li, B., Dai, C., Wang, L., Deng, H., Li, Y., Guan, Z., & Ni, H. (2020). A novel drug repurposing approach for non-small cell lung cancer using deep learning. *PLoS One*, 15(6), e0233112. 10.1371/journal.pone.023311232525938

Li, Z., Wang, S., Yu, H., Zhu, Y., Wu, Q., Wang, L., Wu, Z., Gan, Y., Li, W., Qiu, B., & Tian, J. (2022). A novel deep learning framework based mask-guided attention mechanism for distant metastasis prediction of lung cancer. *IEEE Transactions on Emerging Topics in Computational Intelligence*, 7(2), 330–341. 10.1109/TETCI.2022.3171311

Maalem, S., Bouhamed, M. M., & Gasmi, M. (2022). A deep-based compound model for lung cancer detection. *2022 4th International Conference on Pattern Analysis and Intelligent Systems (PAIS)*, 1–4.

Mamun, M., Farjana, A., Al Mamun, M., & Ahammed, M. S. (2022). Lung cancer prediction model using ensemble learning techniques and a systematic review analysis. *2022 IEEE World AI IoT Congress (AIIoT)*, 187–193.

Mamun, M., Mahmud, M. I., Meherin, M., & Abdelgawad, A. (2023). Lcdctcnn: Lung cancer diagnosis of ct scan images using cnn based model. *2023 10th International Conference on Signal Processing and Integrated Networks (SPIN)*, 205–212.

Pradhan, K. S., Chawla, P., & Tiwari, R. (2023). HRDEL: High ranking deep ensemble learning-based lung cancer diagnosis model. *Expert Systems with Applications*, 213, 118956. 10.1016/j.eswa.2022.118956

Rahman, Md. M. (2021). *A Deep Learning Approach to Detect Lung Cancer Using Alexnet and kNN*. Daffodil International University.

Rajput, A., & Subasi, A. (2023). Lung cancer detection from histopathological lung tissue images using deep learning. In *Applications of Artificial Intelligence in Medical Imaging* (pp. 51–74). Elsevier. 10.1016/B978-0-443-18450-5.00008-6

Savic, M., Ma, Y., Ramponi, G., Du, W., & Peng, Y. (2021). Lung nodule segmentation with a region-based fast marching method. *Sensors (Basel)*, 21(5), 1908. 10.3390/s2105190833803297

Serj, M. F., Lavi, B., Hoff, G., & Valls, D. P. (2018). A deep convolutional neural network for lung cancer diagnostic. *ArXiv Preprint ArXiv:1804.08170*.

Shandilya, S., & Nayak, S. R. (2022). Analysis of lung cancer by using deep neural network. *Innovation in Electrical Power Engineering, Communication, and Computing Technology: Proceedings of Second IEPCCT 2021*, 427–436.

Sharma, S., Fulzele, P., & Sreedevi, I. (2020). Hybrid model for lung nodule segmentation based on support vector machine and k-nearest neighbor. *2020 Fourth International Conference on Computing Methodologies and Communication (ICCMC)*, 170–175. 10.1109/ICCMC48092.2020.ICCMC-00034

She, Y., Jin, Z., Wu, J., Deng, J., Zhang, L., Su, H., Jiang, G., Liu, H., Xie, D., Cao, N., Ren, Y., & Chen, C. (2020). Development and validation of a deep learning model for non–small cell lung cancer survival. *JAMA Network Open*, 3(6), e205842–e205842. 10.1001/jamanetworkopen.2020.584232492161

Sori, W. J., Feng, J., Godana, A. W., Liu, S., & Gelmecha, D. J. (2021). DFD-Net: Lung cancer detection from denoised CT scan image using deep learning. *Frontiers of Computer Science*, 15(2), 1–13. 10.1007/s11704-020-9050-z

Subramanian, R. R., Mourya, R. N., Reddy, V. P. T., Reddy, B. N., & Amara, S. (2020). Lung cancer prediction using deep learning framework. *International Journal of Control and Automation*, 13(3), 154–160.

Torre, L. A., Siegel, R. L., & Jemal, A. (2016). Lung cancer statistics. *Lung Cancer and Personalized Medicine: Current Knowledge and Therapies*, 1–19.

Wang, F., Su, Q., & Li, C. (2022). Identidication of novel biomarkers in non-small cell lung cancer using machine learning. *Scientific Reports*, 12(1), 16693. 10.1038/s41598-022-21050-536202977

Wang, J., Lin, L., Zhao, S., Wu, X., & Wu, S. (2019). Research progress on computed tomography image detection and classification of pulmonary nodule based on deep learning. *Sheng Wu Yi Xue Gong Cheng Xue Za Zhi= Journal of Biomedical Engineering= Shengwu Yixue Gongchengxue Zazhi*, 36(4), 670–676.

Wang, X., Chen, H., Gan, C., Lin, H., Dou, Q., Tsougenis, E., Huang, Q., Cai, M., & Heng, P.-A. (2019). Weakly supervised deep learning for whole slide lung cancer image analysis. *IEEE Transactions on Cybernetics*, 50(9), 3950–3962. 10.1109/TCYB.2019.293514131484154

Webster, J., & Watson, R. T. (2002). Analyzing the past to prepare for the future: Writing a literature review. *Management Information Systems Quarterly*, xiii–xxiii.

Yang, Y., Yang, J., Liang, Y., Liao, B., Zhu, W., Mo, X., & Huang, K. (2021). Identification and validation of the efficacy of immunological therapy for lung cancer from histopathological images based on deep learning. *Frontiers in Genetics*, 12, 642981. 10.3389/fgene.2021.64298133633793

Yeh, M. C.-H., Wang, Y.-H., Yang, H.-C., Bai, K.-J., Wang, H.-H., & Li, Y.-C. J. (2021). Correction: Artificial Intelligence–Based Prediction of Lung Cancer Risk Using Nonimaging Electronic Medical Records: Deep Learning Approach. *Journal of Medical Internet Research*, 23(10), e33519–e33519. 10.2196/3351934653015

Zappa, C., & Mousa, S. A. (2016). Non-small cell lung cancer: Current treatment and future advances. *Translational Lung Cancer Research*, 5(3), 288–300. 10.21037/tlcr.2016.06.0727413711

Zhong, Y., She, Y., Deng, J., Chen, S., Wang, T., Yang, M., Ma, M., Song, Y., Qi, H., Wang, Y., Shi, J., Wu, C., Xie, D., & Chen, C. (2022). Deep learning for prediction of N2 metastasis and survival for clinical stage I non–small cell lung cancer. *Radiology*, 302(1), 200–211. 10.1148/radiol.202121090234698568

KEY TERMS AND DEFINITIONS

Artificial Intelligence: The theory governing the development of computer systems that can perform tasks that normally require human intelligence, such as visual perception, speech recognition, decision-making.

Deep Learning: A part of a broader family of machine learning methods based on learning data representations.

Lung Cancer: A type of cancer that begins in the lungs, characterized by uncontrolled cell growth in lung tissue, which can spread to other body parts.

Machine Learning: A field of artificial intelligence that uses statistical techniques to give computer systems the ability to learn.

Smart Healthcare: Integrating advanced technologies to improve medical diagnosis, treatment, and patient care efficiency.

Chapter 12
Efficient Brain Tumor Classification With Optimized Hybrid Deep Neural Networks

V. Sanjay
 https://orcid.org/0000-0002-6383-3793
Vellore Institute of Technology, India

G. Megala
 https://orcid.org/0000-0002-8084-8292
Vellore Institute of Technology, India

Vuppala Balaji
Vardhaman College of Engineering, India

ABSTRACT

Segmentation is an important stage in the processing of images. Following pre-processing, segmentation methods are used to isolate the tumor region from the MRI images. It's one of the most crucial CAD procedures from the perspective of medical imaging. The challenges in segmenting the tumor area is overcome by using the semantic segmentation method, in which each pixel in an image receives a name or classification. It is used to recognize collections of pixels that stand in for different categories. Semantic Segmentation is proposed which is used to separate the tumor region and then the deep learning classification is done using Augmented Radial Basis Function Network (ARBFNs) based deep learning, Long Short Term Based Recurrent Neural Network (LSTM-RNN) methodology and Regularized Convolutional Neural Network with Dimensionally Reduction Module (RCNN-DRM) architecture.

DOI: 10.4018/979-8-3693-3719-6.ch012

The proposed algorithm providing 95% accuracy on training data.

INTRODUCTION:

Brain tumor is a source of mortality and morbidity for which diagnosis and treatment require extensive resource allocation and sophisticated diagnostic and therapeutic technology. A group of abnormal cells located within the skull results in brain tumor. The skull, which is highly rigid, protects the brain. Any expansion within such a tiny area can present difficulties. Tumors are classified as benign or malignant. When tumors grow inside the skull, they might result in an increase in pressure. This can cause brain damage, which is potentially fatal. Brain tumors are distinguished as Benign and Malignant (NCI, 2014). Brain tumors that are benign do not contain cancer cells. They grow slowly; they are frequently reversible; and they rarely spread to surrounding brain tissue. They can cause complications if they press against specific areas of the brain. They can be life-threatening, depending on which section of the brain they affect. Following deep learning's success, research on brain tumor early detection offers promising, highly accurate medical imaging options. It is also a crucial technique for upcoming uses in the medical field. Automated brain tumor recognition in magnetic resonance imaging (MRI) is a challenging task because of the heterogeneity in size and location. This study suggests using deep learning CNN-based methods to process MRI brain image data in order to detect tumors. The results produced by this approach will increase the accuracy and reduce the number of iterations and complexity of the task. The proposed approach contains fine information of texture from MRI images that contains texture properties like size, shape, color and brightness that helps to detect texture feature extraction.

In many medical image applications, segmentation of brain tumors is one of the most challenging and critical tasks. Patients' mobility, short acquisition times, and soft tissue boundaries can all contribute to artefacts that are difficult to distinguish. Among the many tumor kinds, there is a wide range of both shape and size. They can emerge in a variety of shapes and sizes, as well as with varying levels of intensity. Some of them may also have an effect on the surrounding structures that alter the tumor's imaging intensity. It is estimated by the WHO that roughly 4,00,000 persons in the world have been diagnosed with a brain tumor and that 1,20,000 people died from the disease in the preceding year (Shen D., 2016) (12). Medical professionals must first confirm the tumor's limits and areas and pinpoint its specific location and affected area before treating it with chemotherapy, radiation, or brain 17 operations. Using an automated or semi- automatic brain tumor segmentation tool can aid in the evaluation of the cancer's side effects, and it also serves as a pre-requisite step for medical practitioners to detect the brain tumor prior to surgery.

LITERATURE SURVEY

Several types of image processing and computer-aided diagnosis techniques for the identification of brain tumors were examined. Additionally, various techniques for segmenting brain tumors are investigated, along with feature extraction, tumor classification, and deep learning algorithms. An attempt was made to examine and evaluate the state of knowledge regarding the efficient segmentation approach for automatic brain tumor identification. This literature has addressed the significance of accuracy and tumor classification in great detail. This overview examines several research efforts on brain tumor detection using different efficient image classifiers.

Devkota et al. (2018), have proposed computer-aided detection to examine the brain tumor at an early stage using Mathematical Morphological Reconstruction (MMR). To reduce noise and artefacts, the image is pre-processed and then segmented to identify regions of interest with potential tumors. Poornachandra & Naveena (2017) have proposed pre-processing algorithms for MRI brain imaging, which is the first and most important step in achieving superior glioma segmentation. Jaffar & Choi (2014) Saraswat & Kalra (2021), have intended an automatic reliable scheme for the brain tumor identification. It had been a multi-stage scheme for diagnosing the brain tumor and extracting the tumor region.

Joris et al. (2018) have proposed a more conventional and information driven technique, which depends on the possibility of pre processing using specific intensity measures. Initially a method was applied to evaluate those intensity measures taken from a single image or a group of images. The analyzed results are then compared utilizing an assortment of uses including both homo and heteroscedastic CT and MR images. Vallabhaneni et al. (2006) reported that the clamour system has a image-based tumor detection method that they developed. Edge Adaptive Total Variation De-noising is approved for the image's denoising (EATVD). During the process of removing the commotion from the image, the framework is employed to protect the edges.

C-means cascaded algorithm for brain tumor segmentation was implemented by Laszlo Szilagyi et al. (2015). There are two steps to this process: In the first stage, normal brain tissue is removed, and in the second stage, the tumor-containing tissues are removed. A hybrid technique was demonstrated by Praveen et al. (2015). Also, similar work by G.N. Balaji et. al.(2024) Region-based and texture-based techniques work together to detect and classify brain tumors, respectively. This algorithm begins by segmenting the tumor in order to isolate the skull from the rest of the image.

Ursula Perez et al. (2016) developed a strategy for detecting brain metastases that has been validated. It was possible to extract and process brain shape characteristics as well as energy contrast characteristics for different regions of the brain. Finally, the tumor region is classed with its individual feature values based on the features that were retrieved from it.

PROPOSED METHOD:

A Convolutional Neural Network is used to classify brain tumors, and the process is divided down into two phases: training and testing as shown in Figure 1. For example, several categories are created for brain scans based on tumor and non-tumor status. Preprocessing the input image, removing features from it, and classifying the result is done during the training stage in order to create a prediction model. Naming and identifying the pictures in the training set is the first stage. Images that are preprocessed are scaled to change their dimensions. We then apply convolution neural networks to automatically categorize brain tumors.

Figure 1. Overview of the Proposed Method

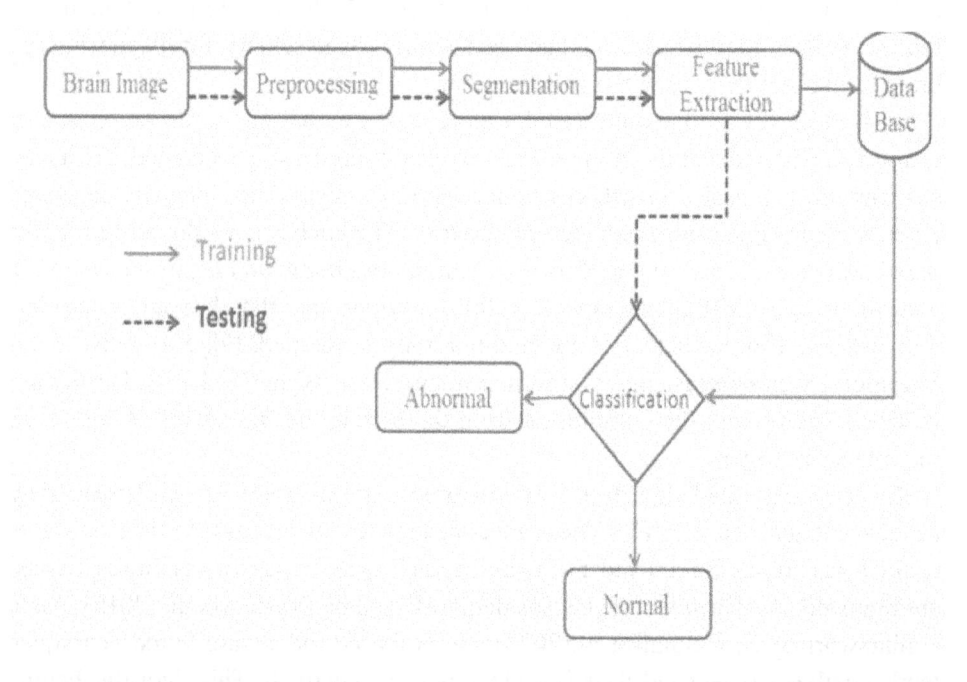

At first, image acquisition is done and subjected to pre-processing. After the grayscale images were first converted to RGB images and subsequently to HSV, image enhancement is done during the pre-processing stage. Following local histogram equalization, the images were once again transformed to RGB format. The second phase involves applying morphological operations to these improved images. The last stage of pre-processing for the suggested framework is segmentation, which is done next. Features are extracted from the post-processing module and a ROI (Region of Interest) is identified. From there, the features can be classified into many categories, such as shape, size, and color features. As seen in Figure 2, images of the detected ROIs were then superimposed over the original test image to verify the outcomes. By calculating several performance indicators with both traditional and suggested classifiers, the results were further confirmed. CNN is considered in the context of the deep machine learning methodology. The same set of data as in the traditional machine learning method is employed here. This method applies the image collection to a model that has already been trained (vgg16). Conv2d, or the convolutional layer, is applied in the following step with a filter size of 32. In terms of train versus validation accuracy for each epoch, as well as the Confusion Matrix, filter sizes 40, 28, and 16 did not yield the best results. An activation function was used in this design. ReLu did not produce the best results when used as an activation function; instead, Sigmoid produced the best outcomes. Max Pooling is utilized in the following step. In this case, 4x4 Max Pooling produced the best results while 2x2 Max Pooling did not. This uses a 50% dropout rate. It was shown that when the percentage of dropouts increased, the number of nodes in the layers increased, whereas the computational intensity increased when the percentage of dropouts decreased. The flatten layer was then put into practice. Using Softmax as the activation function in the dense layer did not yield the best results; instead, using Sigmoid produced the best results.

Figure 2. Sample, Preprocessed and Segmented Image

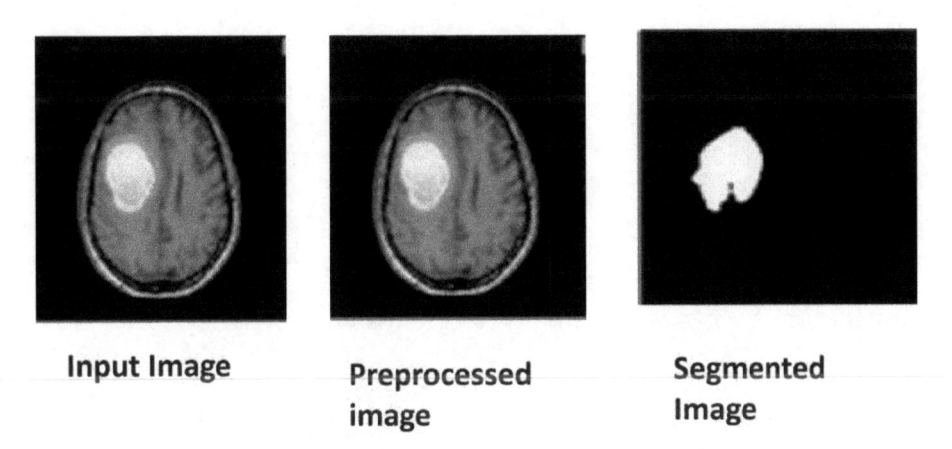

Input Image   **Preprocessed image**   **Segmented Image**

Deep leaning classifiers are used to classify the sample images in this section. It classifies the cancerous image, determining if the area has a benign or malignant brain tumor. The classification is performed by the following three proposed techniques. Augmented Radial Basis Function Network (ARBFNs) based deep learning, Long Short Term Based Recurrent Neural Network (LSTM-RNN) methodology Regularized Convolutional Neural Network (ERCNN) based dimensionally reduction nodule by segmented-PCA.

CONCLUSION:

95 percent of the time, the RCNN-DRM classifier correctly detects the tumor images. Efficiency is influenced by sensitivity, specificity, accuracy, precision, and error value, among other things. When the aforementioned classifier outputs are finally compared, Deep learning produces the best results. this is the minimum time to process compared to the existing model. In future, the proposed approach will extend to achieve the maximum accuracy and it can be extended for various types of brain images.

REFERENCES:

Ain, Q., Jaffar, M. A., & Choi, T. S. (2014). „Fuzzy Anisotropic Diffusion Based Segmentation and Texture based Ensemble Classification of Brain Tumor. *Applied Soft Computing*, 21(8), 330–340. 10.1016/j.asoc.2014.03.019

Devkota, A. A., B, Prasad, PWC, Singh, AK & Elchouemi, A 2018, „Image Segmentation for Early Stage Brain Tumor Detection using Mathematical Morphological Reconstruction", Int. Conference on Smart Computing and Communications, Procedia Computer Science vol. 125, pp. 115–123. 10.1016/j.procs.2017.12.017

Joris, P., Develter, W., Van De Voorde, W., Suetens, P., Maes, F., Vandermeulen, D., & Claes, P. (2018). „PreProcessing of Heteroscedastic Medical Images". *IEEE Access : Practical Innovations, Open Solutions*, 6(2), 26047–26058. 10.1109/ACCESS.2018.2833286

Perez-Ramirez, U., Arana, E., & Moratal, D. (2016). „Brain Metastases Detection on MR by means of Three-Dimensional Tumor Appearance Template Matching". *Journal of Magnetic Resonance Imaging*, 44(3), 642–652. 10.1002/jmri.2520726934581

Poornachandra, S., & Naveena, C. (2017). *Pre-processing of MR Images for Efficient Quantitative Image Analysis using Deep Learning Techniques"*, *Recent Advances in Electronics and Communication Technology*. ICRAECT.

Praveen, G. B. & Anita Agarwal 2015, „Hybrid Approach for Brain Tumor Detection and Classification in Magnetic Resonance Images", International Conference on Communication, Control and Intelligent Systems (CCIS). Balaji, G. N., & Parthasarathy, G. (2024, March). A modified convolutional neural network for tumor segmentation in multimodal brain magnetic resonance images. In *AIP Conference Proceedings* (Vol. 2919, No. 1). AIP Publishing.

Saraswat, M. A., & Kalra, B. (2021). Identification and classification of brain tumors with optimized neural network and canny edge detection algorithm. *Annals of the Romanian Society for Cell Biology*, •••, 5651–5660.

Szilagyi, L. Laszlo Lefkovits & Balázs Benyo 2015, „Automatic Brain Tumor Segmentation in multispectral MRI vol.s using a fuzzy c means cascade algorithm", *12th International Conference on Fuzzy Systems and Knowledge Discovery (FSKD)*, DOI: . 2015. 7381955.10.1109/FSKD

Vallabhaneni, R. B., & Rajesh, V. (2018). „Brain tumor detection using mean shift clustering and GLCM features with edge adaptive total variation denoising technique". *Alexandria Engineering Journal*, 57(4), 2387–2392. 10.1016/j.aej.2017.09.011

Chapter 13

Enhancing Brain Cancer Detection and Localization Using YOLOv8 Object Detection:
A Deep Learning Approach

Seetharam Nagesh Appe
https://orcid.org/0009-0009-9751-6612
CVR College of Engineering, India

G. Arulselvi
Annamalai University, India

G. N. Balaji
https://orcid.org/0000-0002-5346-0989
Vellore Institute of Technology, India

ABSTRACT

Brain cancer poses a significant challenge to patient survival, necessitating early detection. Recent advancements in computer-aided diagnosis systems, leveraging magnetic resonance imaging (MRI), offer promising solutions for detecting brain tumors. This study introduces a transfer learning approach using deep learning to detect malignant brain tumors from MRI scans. Leveraging the YOLO (You Only Look Once) object detection framework, specifically YOLOv8, known for its efficiency in computational architecture, we present a deep learning-based approach for brain tumor identification and classification. By leveraging MRI analysis, our method

DOI: 10.4018/979-8-3693-3719-6.ch013

aims to enhance detection and precise localization to improve patient prognosis and treatment outcomes. Employing the YOLOv8 model, we achieve a precision of 0.894 and a recall of 0.915 in brain cancer detection and an mAP_0.5 of 0.938 in brain cancer localization, demonstrating the effectiveness of the proposed model.

INTRODUCTION

Brain cancer is a devastating disease with significant morbidity and mortality rates worldwide. Among the various types of brain tumors, malignant gliomas, particularly glioblastoma, pose significant challenges due to their aggressive nature and limited treatment options. Early detection and accurate diagnosis of brain tumors are crucial for improving patient outcomes and guiding appropriate treatment strategies (Karuna & Joshi, 2013).

In recent years, advances in medical imaging, particularly magnetic resonance imaging (MRI), have revolutionized the diagnosis and management of brain tumors. MRI provides detailed anatomical information, allowing for the visualization of tumor morphology, location, and extent. However, the manual interpretation of MRI scans by radiologists is time-consuming and subject to inter-observer variability, highlighting the need for automated and accurate image analysis methods.

Deep learning-based approaches have emerged as powerful tools for medical image analysis, offering the potential to assist clinicians in the detection and classification of brain tumors (Rehman et al., 2019). In particular, the You Only Look Once (YOLO) object detection framework has gained widespread popularity for its real-time detection capabilities and high accuracy.

In this study, we propose a novel approach for brain tumor detection and classification using YOLOv8, an advanced version of the YOLO framework. YOLOv8 incorporates state-of-the-art object detection techniques and architectural improvements, resulting in enhanced performance and efficiency compared to previous versions.

The primary objective of our research is to develop a deep learning-based model capable of accurately identifying malignant brain tumors from MRI scans (Anand et al., 2024). We leverage transfer learning techniques (Balaji et al., 2023) to fine-tune the pre-trained YOLOv8 model on a large dataset of annotated MRI images.

Our research aims to address several key challenges in brain tumor detection, including the detection of subtle tumor features, the differentiation of malignant tumors from benign lesions, and the localization of tumor boundaries. By harnessing the capabilities of YOLOv8, we seek to develop a robust and accurate model that can assist clinicians in the early diagnosis and treatment planning of brain tumors.

In the following sections, we present the methodology employed in our study, the experimental results obtained, and a discussion of the implications of our findings. Through this research, we aim to contribute to the advancement of automated brain tumor detection methods and ultimately improve patient outcomes in the field of neuro-oncology.

LITERATURE REVIEW

For the diagnosis of brain tumors, various deep learning models have been employed, showcasing the versatility and efficacy of machine learning techniques in medical imaging analysis. However, it's worth noting that while deep learning has seen extensive use in this domain, object detection methods have been relatively less explored.

Indeed, the field of brain tumor classification has seen numerous valuable contributions aimed at providing robust and accurate solutions. The (Kavin Kumar et al., 2018; Shrot et al., 2019; Zacharaki et al., 2009) likely represent significant studies or papers that have made notable advancements in this area. These contributions may encompass a range of methodologies, including traditional machine learning techniques and deep learning approaches, each with its strengths and limitations.

(Soltaninejad et al., 2016) employs an automated approach to recognise and categorise MRI images. This method uses the Super Pixel Technique and classifies each Super Pixel. The extreme randomised trees (ERT) classifier is compared with SVM is used to classify each super pixel as either cancer or normal. This approach uses two datasets: 19 MRI FLAIR images and BRATS 2012 dataset. The results show that this method's use of the ERT classifier yields good results.

(Deepak & Ameer, 2019) the proposed classification system employs deep transfer learning, utilizing a pre-trained GoogLeNet to extract features from brain MRI images. These features are then fed into proven classifier models to perform the final classification. It addresses the significant problem of brain tumor classification in computer-aided diagnosis (CAD) for medical applications. Specifically, it focuses on a 3-class classification task aimed at distinguishing among glioma, meningioma, and pituitary tumors, which are three prevalent types of brain tumors

(Asif et al., 2023) employs several popular deep learning architectures, including Xception, DenseNet201, DenseNet121, ResNet152V2, and InceptionResNetV2, for the task of brain tumor classification. These architectures are well-known for their effectiveness in various computer vision tasks and have been adapted by modifying their final layers with a custom deep dense block and softmax layer to improve classification accuracy specifically for brain tumor detection.

(Nie et al., 2019) employed the YOLO (You Only Look Once) network for the identification of melanoma skin lesions. Despite the utilization of a smaller dataset, the findings yielded promising results. The Darknet framework, which YOLO is based on, enhances the efficiency of feature extraction, contributing to the network's effectiveness in detecting melanoma.

Table 1. Comparison with Other Works

Study	Objectives	Methodology	Key Findings
Proposed Methodology	Detect malignant brain tumors from MRI using YOLOv8 and transfer learning	YOLOv8 integration, transfer learning on annotated MRI dataset	Precision: 0.894, Recall: 0.915, mAP_0.5: 0.938 in brain cancer detection and localization
Deepak & Ameer, 2019	Classify glioma, meningioma, and pituitary tumors using GoogLeNet and transfer learning	Transfer learning with GoogLeNet on brain MRI images	Achieved high accuracy in 3-class classification of brain tumors
Asif et al., 2023	Employ various deep learning architectures for brain tumor classification	DenseNet, Xception, ResNet for brain tumor detection	Adapted architectures for improved classification accuracy
Nie et al., 2019	Utilize YOLO for skin lesion identification	YOLO network for melanoma detection	Demonstrated efficiency of YOLO in lesion detection

MATERIALS AND METHODOLOGY

To build an effective deep learning model for detecting and localizing brain cancer from MRI scans, it's essential to acquire a high-quality dataset comprising brain cancer MRIs with corresponding annotations, particularly bounding boxes indicating cancerous regions. This dataset serves as the base for training the object detection model efficiently. Accurate annotations allow the model to learn discerning features and patterns associated with cancerous regions within brain MRI scans. The Figure 1 shows an example MRI of brain cancer.

Figure 1. Example of MRI Brain Cancer

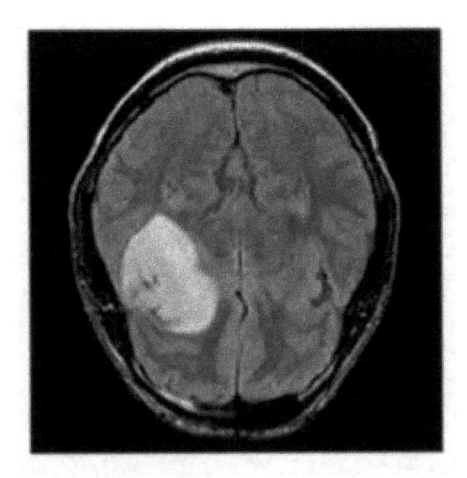

To construct an efficient and accurate model for predicting brain tumors in MRI scans, a diverse dataset was compiled, comprising images captured from various angles, under different conditions, and featuring different types of tumors. Each image in the dataset had a unique size, necessitating a preprocessing step to resize all images to a consistent dimension.

After obtaining the images, the next step was to define the class for detecting the bounding box for brain MRI, with the class being "tumor" in this case, representing the presence of brain cancer. Each image was annotated by drawing bounding boxes around detected tumor objects as shown in Figure 2. This annotation process was facilitated using the VGG annotator application, a platform designed for data annotation tasks.

Figure 2. Example of Annotated Brain Tumor MRI Image

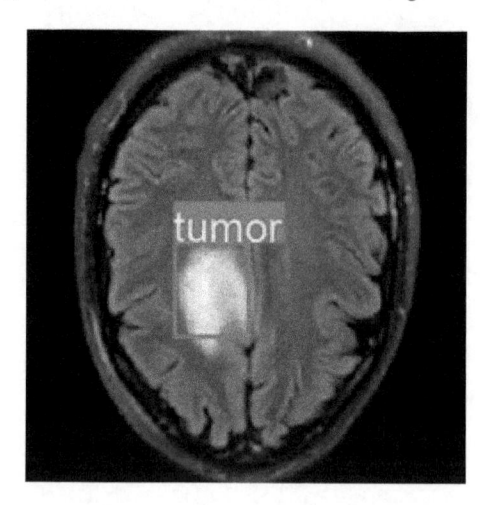

Following annotation, the dataset underwent image augmentation, a technique involving controlled random modifications to existing images to expand the dataset without the need for gathering new samples. Image augmentation generates modified versions of images, thereby enriching the training dataset. This technique is widely used in training artificial neural networks as it enhances the network's ability to learn effectively and accurately with an increasing training dataset size.

In our approach, data augmentation techniques are employed to generate modified images of brain MRIs with controlled random variations, such as rotations, flips, cuts, and trims. The primary objective behind applying data augmentation is to enhance the model's capability to effectively detect tumors regardless of their position within the image. Additionally, augmented data help address the issue of overfitting, where a model becomes too specialized in fitting the observed data and performs poorly on unseen data.

By introducing variations through data augmentation, the structured neural network can learn to recognize recurring patterns from the augmented data, rather than simply memorizing specific examples. This enables the model to develop more generalized rules and reduces the chances of misclassifying unseen patterns. Data augmentation plays a crucial role in improving the model's ability to generalize and perform well on unseen images.

Once the augmented brain MRIs, along with corresponding information regarding cancer localization (i.e., class) and bounding boxes, are acquired, the next step is to develop a deep learning model. This model will be trained on the augmented dataset to learn the relationship between MRI features and tumor presence, allowing it to accurately detect and localize brain tumors in unseen images.

In this paper, we utilize the YOLO (You Only Look Once) model for the detection and localization of brain cancer from MRI scans. YOLO, introduced by (Redmon et al., 2016) stands as a pioneering one-stage deep learning detector specifically designed for object detection tasks, encompassing image classification and accurate object localization within the images.

One of YOLO's distinctive features, setting it apart from other networks, is its self-contained pipeline that independently carries out the entire process. In YOLO, each input image is divided into an $S \times S$ grid of cells. If an object falls within the center of a cell, that cell is responsible for detecting the object. The output consists of two components for each cell: a bounding box vector and the associated class prediction. The bounding box prediction comprises five components: (x, y, w, h, confidence), where (x, y) represents the center of the bounding box relative to the cell's position, and (w, h) represent the dimensions of the box, both normalized to values between 0 and 1. The predictions of the bounding boxes result in $S \times S \times B \times 5$ outputs, where B denotes the number of bounding boxes predicted per cell (Jiang et al., 2022).

Compared to existing object detection models, YOLO has demonstrated notably faster performance (Sah et al., 2017; Sanchez et al., 2020). This efficiency is primarily attributed to YOLO's single-phase recognition task, which directly predicts bounding boxes, object probabilities, and object classes without the need for separate stages for region proposal and object classification. This streamlined approach contributes significantly to YOLO's speed advantage over other object detection models.

It's noteworthy that multiple versions of the YOLO model exist, each with its own unique features and improvements and we chose to implement YOLOv8s using the PyTorch framework. YOLOv8 represents a significant advancement over previous iterations of YOLO models, offering several key improvements.

One notable improvement in YOLOv8 is the adoption of anchor-free detection. Previous YOLO models relied on anchor boxes, pre-defined bounding boxes used to classify objects in an image. However, anchor boxes can be restrictive and may hinder the model's ability to detect objects of varying sizes and shapes effectively. YOLOv8 addresses this limitation by employing anchor-free detection, allowing the model to learn to detect objects of any size and shape without being constrained by predefined anchor boxes. This approach enhances the model's flexibility and adaptability, making it more robust and capable of handling diverse object detection tasks effectively.

YOLOv8 Architecture

The YOLO network architecture comprises three main components (Zayani et al., 2024): the backbone, the neck, and the head.

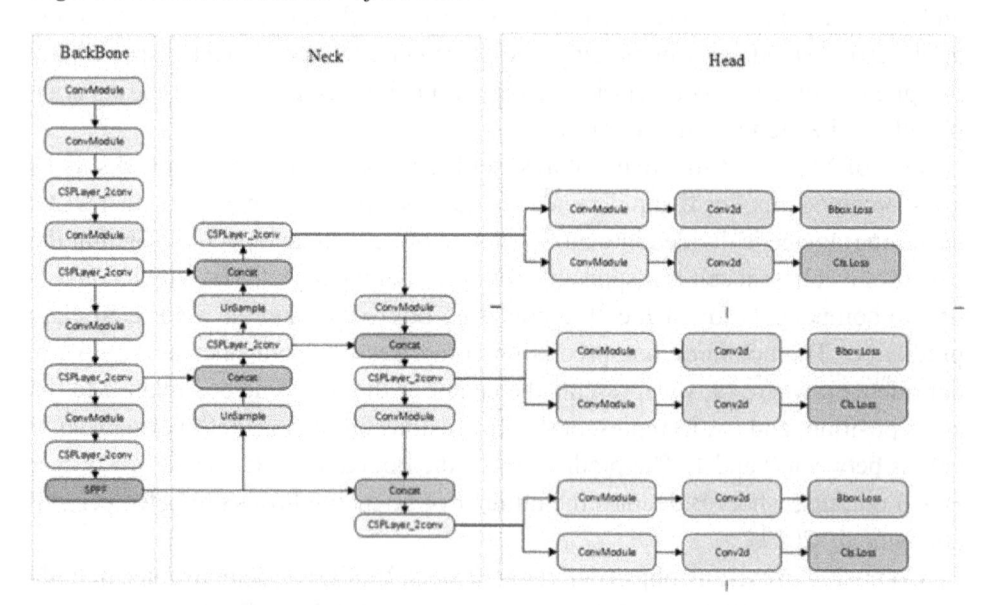

Figure 3. Network Structure of YOLOv8

i. Backbone:

The backbone is a convolutional neural network responsible for extracting and consolidating image features at various scales or granularities. It processes the input image and extracts high-level features that are relevant for object detection. YOLOv8 utilizes a modified version of the CSPDarknet53 architecture as its backbone. CSPDarknet53 comprises 53 convolutional layers and employs cross-stage partial connections to enhance information flow between layers.These cross-stage connections facilitate better feature representation and learning across different layers.

ii. Neck:

Situated between the backbone and the head, the neck consists of a series of layers that blend and merge image features. The neck plays a crucial role in feature fusion and transformation, enhancing the network's ability to make accurate predictions. It combines features from different scales or resolutions and performs operations such as feature concatenation or feature transformation. It employs a feature pyramid network (FPN) to enable multi-scaled object detection. The FPN consists of multiple layers designed to detect objects at different scales within an image.

iii. Head:

The head takes in features from the neck and carries out the box and class prediction processes.

It typically consists of convolutional layers followed by fully connected layers, which generate predictions for bounding boxes, objectness scores, and class probabilities. The head produces the final output of the YOLO network, providing predictions for objects detected in the input image.

Overall, the YOLO architecture integrates these components to enable comprehensive feature extraction, feature fusion, and prediction steps, contributing to its object detection capabilities. By leveraging these components effectively, YOLO can detect objects in images with high accuracy and efficiency.

EXPERIMENTAL RESULTS

DataSet

The dataset used in the experimental analysis consists of 300 brain MRIs obtained from a publicly available repository for research purposes (YOLO Dataset. 2022). The dataset includes images representing various types of brain tumors, such as Meningioma, Pituitary, and Glioma, each located in different areas of the brain. Additionally, a portion of the dataset includes images of healthy subjects, accounting for 25% of the total images.

To prepare the dataset for training, 70% of the images (210) were allocated for training, 20% (60 images) for validation, and the remaining 10% (30 images) for testing. Each image in the dataset is labeled with the "tumor" label, along with bounding box annotations indicating the localization of the tumor within the image.

All images were resized to a consistent dimension of 640 x 640 pixels to ensure uniformity in the input size for the model. During training, a batch size of 16 was used, and the training process was run for 100 epochs. The Adam optimizer was employed, with a patience parameter with momentum was set to 0.937, and a maximum number of detections per image set to 300.

Data Augmentation

Data augmentation was performed using the Roboflow web application, which applies random rotations of 90° clockwise, 90° counterclockwise, and flips images upside down. Roboflow facilitates data management for computer vision projects, allowing for the integration of images and annotations created on platforms like Labelbox, as well as the application of various transformations to the images.

This preprocessing and augmentation strategy aim to enhance the model's robustness and (Appe et al., 2023) generalization ability by providing a diverse set of training examples and variations of the input images.

Evaluation Metrics

Precision (AP) is a metric commonly used in object detection tasks to evaluate the model's performance as mentioned in (Appe et al., 2023). It calculates the precision value at each point on the precision-recall curve and then averages these values to obtain the overall performance score. AP provides insights into how well the model detects objects across different classes or categories. The definitions of precision(P), recall(R) are defined using equations (1-2)

$$P = \frac{True\_Positive}{True\_Positive + False\_Positive} X\ 100\% \tag{1}$$

$$R = \frac{True\_Positive}{True\_Positive + False\_Negative} X\ 100\% \tag{2}$$

The average precision (AP) of a detector measures its performance in each category. Mean Average Precision (mAP) extends the concept of AP by averaging the AP values obtained from multiple object classes or categories. This provides a comprehensive assessment of the model's performance across all classes, offering a more holistic evaluation of its object detection capabilities. The AP and mAP are defined using equations (3-4).

$$AP = \int_0^1 P(R)\ dR\ X\ 100\% \tag{3}$$

$$mAP = \frac{\sum_{i=1}^{n} AP}{n} \tag{4}$$

where '*n*' *denotes* the number of classes.

Intersection over Union (IOU) is another crucial metric used in object detection to quantify the extent of overlap between predicted bounding boxes and ground truth bounding boxes. It is calculated as the ratio of the intersection area to the union area of the two bounding boxes. IOU values range from 0.0 to 1.0, where 1.0 indicates a perfect match or complete overlap, and 0.0 indicates no overlap at all.

The formula for computing IOU is shown in equation(5):

$$IOU = \frac{Area\ of\ Intersection}{Area\ of\ Union} \qquad (5)$$

This formula compares the regions covered by two bounding boxes and provides a standardized measure of their overlap. IOU is useful for assessing the accuracy of bounding box predictions, as it quantifies how well the predicted boxes align with the ground truth boxes.

The trained model achieved notable advancements in both computational efficiency and model interpretability. During training, optimizations such as batch processing and efficient GPU utilization were implemented, significantly reducing training time without compromising model accuracy. Inference speed was also optimized, allowing the model to process images swiftly, which is crucial for real-time applications in medical diagnostics. Moreover, the model's interpretability was enhanced through the use of visualization techniques like activation maps and feature importance scores, providing insights into its decision-making process. These enhancements not only improved the model's performance metrics such as precision and recall but also ensured that it met stringent requirements for transparency and reliability in practical deployment scenarios.

Results

YOLOv8 offers five scaled versions: YOLOv8n (nano), YOLOv8s (small), YOLOv8m (medium), YOLOv8l (large), and YOLOv8x (extra-large). These versions vary in terms of model size and complexity. This research uses YOLOv8s with hyperparameter configuration specified in Table 2.

Table 2. Hyperparameters Configuration Settings

HyperParameter	Value
Model	YOLOv8s
Image Size	640 x 640
Epochs	100
Batch Size	16

In the experimental analysis, we trained the YOLOv8s model using real-world data obtained from a freely available repository, comprising 300 brain MRIs. The training process utilized an NVIDIA Tesla T4 graphics card with 16 GB of memory and CUDA Version 12.0. We employed the Python compiler version 3.10.12 with the Torch library version 2.0.1.

The training was conducted over 100 epochs completed in 0.154 hours. During training, various metrics were monitored to assess the performance and progress of the model. Figure 4 presents 12 plots, organized into two rows, each containing six plots.

Figure 4. Evaluation Results of Model

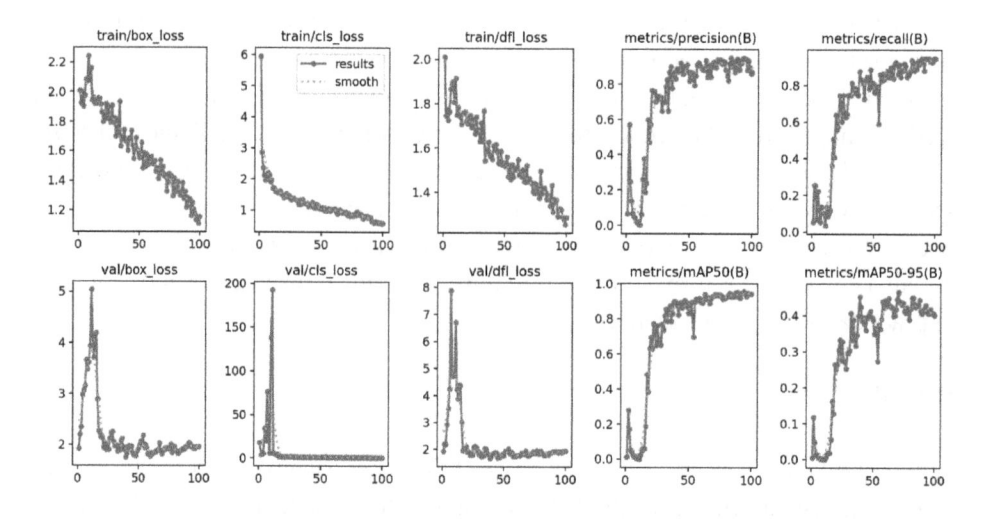

Figure 4 shows, in the mAP@0.5 and the mAP@0.5:0.95 plots, respectively, the mAP value for IOU = 50 and IOU ranging from 50 to 95 (i.e., this value represents different IoU thresholds from 0.5 to 0.95, with a step size equal to 0.05 on average mAP).

Table 3 shows the values obtained for Precision, Recall, mAP_0.5, and mAP_0.5:0.95 metrics.

Table 3. Classification Results

Metric	Value
Precision	0.894
Recall	0.915
mAP@0.50	0.938
mAP@0.5:0.95	0.463

The precision-recall curve depicted in Figure 5 provides a comprehensive visualization of the precision and recall values obtained during both the training and testing steps of the YOLO model. Each point on the curve represents a specific threshold used for classification, ranging from high to low confidence levels. By examining the precision-recall curve, we can gain insights into the model's overall performance and identify potential areas for improvement.

Figure 5. Precision-Recall Curve

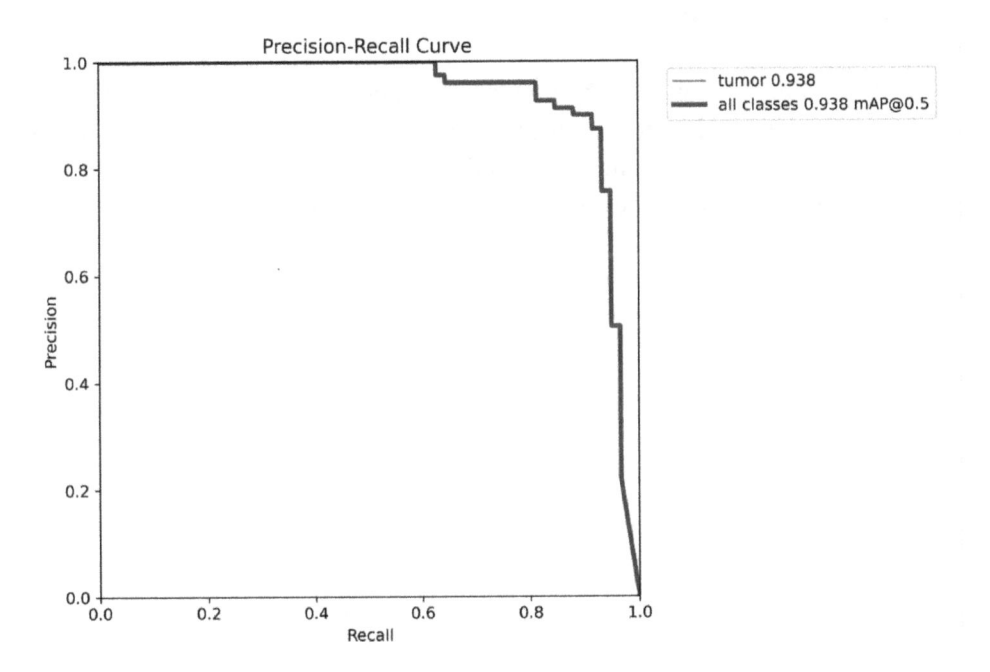

The normalized confusion matrix depicted in Table 4 provides a detailed overview of the performance of the proposed YOLO model across different classes. Each row of the matrix represents the actual ground truth labels, while each column represents the predicted labels by the model. The values in the matrix represent the normalized percentage of predictions for each class relative to the total number of instances of that class.

Analyzing the confusion matrix allows us to identify both the strengths and weaknesses of the model. Specifically, we can identify which classes the model performs well on and which classes it struggles with. Additionally, the matrix helps in pinpointing any specific misclassification patterns or trends that may exist.

Table 4. Normalised Confusion Matrix

True Values Predicted Values	Tumor	Background
Tumor	0.83	1.00
Background	0.17	0.00

Prediction Examples

With the aim to show how the proposed method can be employed in the real world, in Figure 6 and Figure 7 we respectively show a set of brain images with the tumor label (with the bounding box added by radiologists) and the same images with the cancerous area predicted by the proposed model.

Figure 6. Sixteen Examples of Brain Images with the Related Label

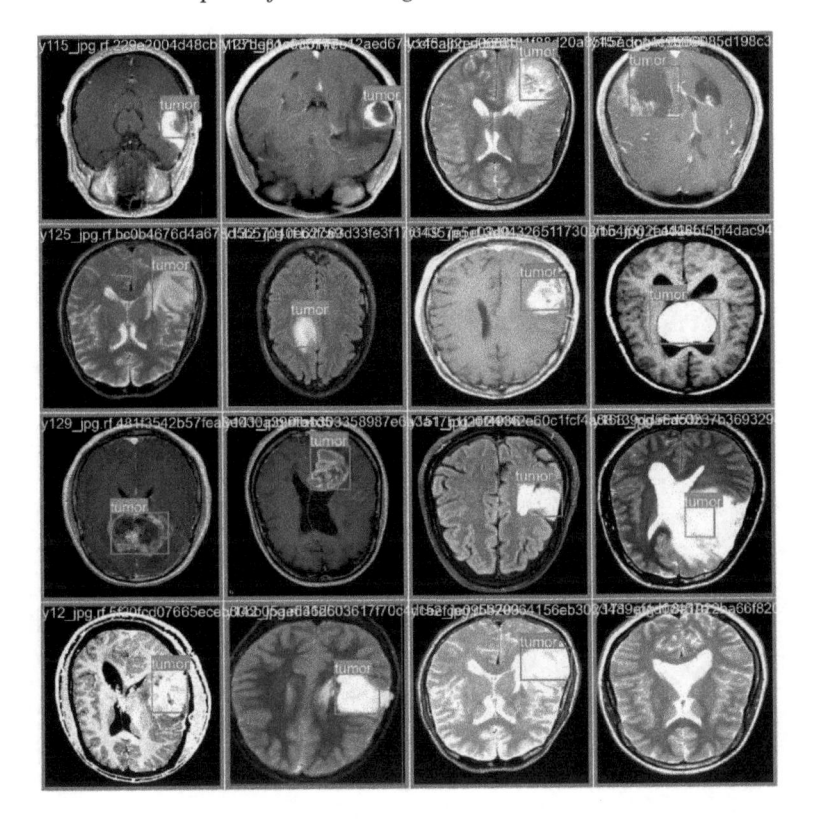

Figure 7. The Sixteen Images Once Processed by the Proposed Model

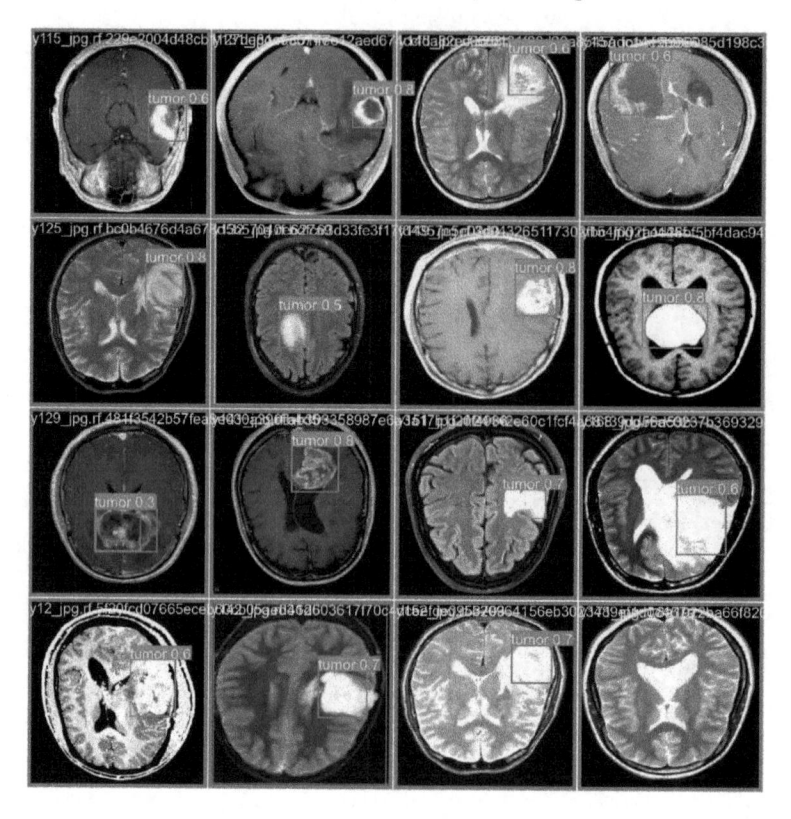

As shown in Figure 7, after processing the sixteen images using the proposed model, it is evident that the model automatically adds red bounding boxes to indicate areas related to cancer. Furthermore, each bounding box is accompanied by a prediction percentage. As can be seen from Figure 8, tumors of different sizes were considered, to verify that the model was able to generalize the brain tumor and not focus only on a certain type of cancer. In fact, from the figure it is possible to note that the area relating to the cancer is correctly identified regardless of the size, and regardless of the coloring of the area, which in some cases is white, while in others it is gray and, in other cases, the same tumor area has both white and gray areas. This aspect is symptomatic of a model that is able to adequately generalize the area to be located, being able to correctly identify cancerous areas, regardless of size, coloration, and the area in which they appear.

CONCLUSION

In this paper, we introduce a method designed for the detection and localization of cancer in brain MRIs, aiming to facilitate timely diagnosis and prompt initiation of therapy. Recognizing the critical importance of early intervention in improving patient outcomes, our proposed method leverages YOLOv8s object detection. Through experimental analysis conducted on a dataset comprising 300 brain MRIs, we achieved impressive results in both the detection and localization of brain cancer. Specifically, we achieved a mean average precision (mAP) of 0.938 at an intersection over union (IOU) threshold of 0.5, which justifies its effectiveness in accurately detecting and localizing brain tumors in MRI scans. This performance underscores the model's ability to precisely identify and delineate tumor boundaries, which is critical for facilitating early diagnosis and improving patient outcomes. By extending the proposed approach to incorporate whole 3D images and leveraging state-of-the-art 3D object detection techniques, we can potentially enhance the accuracy, sensitivity, and specificity of brain tumor detection, ultimately leading to improved patient outcomes in clinical practice.

REFERENCES

Anand, D. (2024). *G a, A., Balaji, G., & Ghantasala, G. S.* Deep Convolutional Extreme Learning Machine with AlexNet-Based Bone Cancer Classification Using Whole-Body Scan Images., 10.1007/978-981-99-8118-2_13

Appe, S. N., & Arulselvi, G. (2023). Advances in Computational Intelligence and Robotics: Vol. 278–289. *G. N., B.* Detection and Classification of Dense Tomato Fruits by Integrating Coordinate Attention Mechanism With YOLO Model.

Asif, S., Zhao, M., Tang, F., & Zhu, Y. (2023). An enhanced deep learning method for multi-class brain tumor classification using deep transfer learning. *Multimedia Tools and Applications*, 82(20), 31709–31736. 10.1007/s11042-023-14828-w

Balaji, G. N., Mary, S., Mantravadi, N., & Shajin, F. H. (2023). Graph CNN-ResNet-CSOA transfer learning architype for an enhanced skin cancer detection and classification scheme in medical image processing. *International Journal of Artificial Intelligence Tools*.

Deepak, S., & Ameer, P. (2019). Brain tumor classification using deep CNN features via transfer learning. *Computers in Biology and Medicine*, 111, 103345. 10.1016/j.compbiomed.2019.10334531279167

Devi, M., & Maheswaran, S. (2018). An efficient method for brain tumor detection using texture features and SVM classifier in MR images. Asian Pacific journal of cancer prevention. *APJCP*, 19(10), 2789.

Jiang, P., Ergu, D., Liu, F., Cai, Y., & Ma, B. (2022). A Review of Yolo Algorithm Developments. *Procedia Computer Science*, 199, 1066–1073. 10.1016/j.procs.2022.01.135

Karuna, M., & Joshi, A. (2013). AUTOMATIC DETECTION AND SEVERITY ANALYSIS OF BRAIN TUMORS USING GUI IN MATLAB. *International Journal of Research in Engineering and Technology*, 02(10), 586–594. 10.15623/ijret.2013.0210092

Nie, Y., Sommella, P., O'Nils, M., Liguori, C., & Lundgren, J. (2019). *Automatic Detection of Melanoma with Yolo Deep Convolutional Neural Networks. 2019 E-Health and Bioengineering Conference.* EHB.

Redmon, J., Divvala, S., Girshick, R., & Farhadi, A. (2016). *You Only Look Once: Unified.* Real-Time Object Detection.

Rehman, A., Naz, S., Razzak, M. I., Akram, F., & Imran, M. (2019). A Deep Learning-Based Framework for Automatic Brain Tumors Classification Using Transfer Learning. *Circuits, Systems, and Signal Processing*, 39(2), 757–775. 10.1007/s00034-019-01246-3

Sah, S., Shringi, A., Ptucha, R., Burry, A., & Loce, R. (2017). Video redaction: A survey and comparison of enabling technologies. *Journal of Electronic Imaging*, 26(5), 51406. 10.1117/1.JEI.26.5.051406

Sanchez, S. A., Romero, H. J., & Morales, A. D. (2020). A review: Comparison of performance metrics of pretrained models for object detection using the TensorFlow framework. *IOP Conference Series. Materials Science and Engineering*, 844, 12024. 10.1088/1757-899X/844/1/012024

Shrot, S., Salhov, M., Dvorski, N., Konen, E., Averbuch, A., & Hoffmann, C. (2019). Application of MR morphologic, diffusion tensor, and perfusion imaging in the classification of brain tumors using machine learning scheme. *Neuroradiology*, 61(7), 757–765. 10.1007/s00234-019-02195-z30949746

Soltaninejad, M., Yang, G., Lambrou, T., Allinson, N., Jones, T. L., Barrick, T. R., Howe, F. A., & Ye, X. (2016). Automated brain tumour detection and segmentation using superpixel-based extremely randomized trees in FLAIR MRI. *International Journal of Computer Assisted Radiology and Surgery*, 12(2), 183–203. 10.1007/s11548-016-1483-327651330

YOLO. YOLO Dataset. 2022. (2022).

Zacharaki, E. I., Wang, S., Chawla, S., Soo Yoo, D., Wolf, R., Melhem, E. R., & Davatzikos, C. (2009). Classification of brain tumor type and grade using MRI texture and shape in a machine learning scheme. *Magnetic Resonance in Medicine*, 62(6), 1609–1618. 10.1002/mrm.2214719859947

Zayani, H. M., Ammar, I., Ghodhbani, R., Maqbool, A., Saidani, T., Ben Slimane, J., Kachoukh, A., Kouki, M., Kallel, M., Alsuwaylimi, A. A., & Alenezi, S. M. (2024). Deep Learning for Tomato Disease Detection with YOLOv8. *Engineering, Technology &. Applied Scientific Research*, 14(2), 13584–13591.

Chapter 14
Multi-Cancer Detection Using Deep Learning Techniques

G. N. Balaji
https://orcid.org/0000-0002-5346-0989
Vellore Institute of technology, India

A. K. P. Kovendan
https://orcid.org/0000-0002-7232-5571
Vellore Institute of Technology, India

Kirti Nayak
https://orcid.org/0009-0006-1031-4750
Vellore Institute of Technology, India

R. Venkatesan
https://orcid.org/0000-0002-4336-8628
SASTRA University (Deemed), India

D. Yuvaraj
Cihan University, Iraq

ABSTRACT

Cancer is one of the main causes of death for people worldwide. Breast, lung, colon, brain and lymphoma are some of the most common types of cancer. Successful treatment can significantly increase the chances of survival. Enhancing the probability of a successful cancer treatment requires initial identification and treatment. In this paper a model is proposed using denset121 pretrained model with modified dense net block and softmax function as output layer. There are two subgroups of the

DOI: 10.4018/979-8-3693-3719-6.ch014

total number of diseases: task 1 and task 2. Task1 include breast, kidney, cervical, leukemia while task2 include lung, oral, lymphoma, brain. A person suffering from the disease of task 1 may also suffer from a disease belonging to task 2. This model is examined using a dataset with multiple cancers, which is publicly available on Kaggle. The suggested method performs with an accuracy of 99.31% for task 1 as well as 97.02% for task 2, respectively, when analyzed alongside the most recent techniques.

INTRODUCTION

A collection of disorders known as cancers are characterized by aberrant cell growth that has the capacity to spread from one area to other. In contrast, benign tumors do not metastasize. Most cancers start as abnormal growths of cells in a particular part of body. These abnormal cells grow and multiply uncontrollably, forming a lump or mass called a tumor. Tumors can be benign or malignant. Benign tumors don't spread to other areas of the body and are not malignant. They are usually harmless and can often be removed with surgery. Cancerous tumors have the potential to spread to other body parts. They are more dangerous than benign tumors and can be life-threatening. Cancer can affect any area of one's body and are of different kinds. Some of the most common types of cancer include lung, breast cancer, colon, lymphoma, oral and brain cancer. It is the leading cause of death worldwide, and it is estimated that one in three people will develop cancer in their lifetime. Early detection of cancer is crucial for improving the chances of successful treatment and survival. When cancer is detected early, it is often smaller and more localized, making it easier to treat and less likely to spread. Successful treatment can significantly increase the chances of survival.

Artificial intelligence (AI) in cancer detection has revolutionized the field of oncology, providing new tools for early diagnosis, improved treatment planning, and personalized medicine. AI algorithms can analyze vast amounts of medical data, including imaging scans to identify patterns and abnormalities that may indicate the presence of cancer (Can artificial intelligence help see cancer in new ways?, 2022). This capability has led to the development of AI-powered tools that can assist oncologists in detecting cancer with greater accuracy and efficiency (Sava, 2023). Convolutional Neural Networks (CNNs) have revolutionized image processing, particularly in cancer detection. CNNs excel at extracting and learning from complex patterns in images, making them ideal for identifying abnormalities in medical images that may indicate cancer (Manickavasagam et al., 2022). Pre-trained CNN models, trained on vast image datasets, provide a valuable starting point for cancer detection tasks. Fine-tuning these models using smaller datasets of medical images allows them to learn the specific characteristics of cancer in these images (Kathamuthu et al., 2023). This approach has shown promising results in various cancer detection applications, including breast, lung, and skin cancer detection. The use of CNNs and pre-trained models in cancer detection offers several advantages: improved accuracy, reduced bias, scalability, early detection, and personalized medicine. As CNN technology advances, we can expect even more sophisticated and effective models, significantly improving cancer detection accuracy and efficiency, leading to better treatment outcomes and improved patient survival rates.

Following are the major contribution of this research-

1. To develop an efficient system for detecting eight kind of cancer such as kidney, oral, breast, brain, cervical, lymphoma, all, lung and colon.
2. To detect all the subclasses of multiple types of cancer.
3. To compare the performance of the proposed model with the existing methods.

This is the organization of the remaining section of the paper. The literature review in the field is covered in the Section of "RELATED WORK", where a brief summary is given about the findings and drawbacks of the existing work. The suggested method is briefly described in the Section "METHODOLGY", along with the dataset description and the technique used. In the Section "EXPERIMENTS AND RESULTS", all of the experimental findings and observations are briefly explained. The suggested model's performance is contrasted with that of the previous research. Our experiment is concluded in the Section "CONCLUSION".

RELATED WORK

Several authors have proposed various machine learning techniques for cancer detection, each of which has its own advantages and disadvantages. We are going to present a brief summary of the existing work.

Afify et al. (2023) worked with eight different pretrained models such as ResNet-101, EfficientNet-b0, DenseNet, AlexNet, and ShuffleNet for oral cancer detection and achieved high accuracy of 100% with ResNet for 100x images and 95.65% for 400x images. However, the dataset they have used is not very large. Saraswathi and Bhaskaran (2023) obtained an accuracy of 89% with AlexNet and 78% with ResNet for oral cancer detection. Here, again, the accuracy is not very good and the dataset is not very large. Subarna and Sukumar (2022) proposed MASO-optimized

DenseNet 121 for cervical tumor identification, and it achieved a high success rate of 98.38%; however, this did not cover all the subclasses of the cancer. Yaman and Tuncer (2022) used deep learning techniques such as DarkNet 19, DarkNet 53, and the NCA algorithm for feature extraction, along with SVM as a classifier for cervical cancer detection. Though it achieved a very good accuracy of 98.26%–99.47%, it is not computationally efficient. Demir (2021) designed a model where they used CLSTM along with a SVM Bayesian optimizer and achieved a good accuracy of 100%, but it needs high-performance hardware for a huge dataset. Rana and Bhushan (2023) used multiple pretrained models for breast cancer detection, but the dataset used here is not balanced. The EfficientNetB3 model was proposed by Batool and Byun (2023) and attained an outstanding performance of 99.31%. However; this is not trained to detect all the subclasses. The ensemble technique is used along with different pretrained models by Omar et al. (2023) for lung and colon cancer detection. Though it achieved a very high accuracy of 99.44%, it is not computationally efficient. Maheshwari et al. (2022) achieved the accuracy of 97% for lung and colon detection using Efficientnet B7. Asif et al. (2023) performed experiment with different pretrained models and achieved the highest accuracy of 99.67%. Çinar and Yildirim (2020) performed experiments with different deep learning models and achieved 97.2% accuracy, but this has the limitation that it cannot detect all the subclasses of cancer. A very good accuracy of 99% is achieved by Rajkumar et al. (2023) using ANN for kidney cancer detection. Deep learning-pretrained model VGG16 trained by Wasi et al. (2023) achieved an accuracy of 92.54%, which is again not very high. Subramanian et al. (2023) tried to build a model for multiple cancer detection but failed to achieve very high accuracy. Talukder et al. (2022) combined deep learning pretrained models with machine learning classifiers such as SVM, etc. and achieved high accuracy. However, it is not computationally efficient.

Several authors in previous research used deep learning techniques to classify different kinds of cancer. It has been observed that most of the authors focused in building model for specific cancer detection and the built models have number of drawbacks such as they are not capable of detecting all the subclasses of the specific cancer, are not computationally efficient and their accuracy is not very high. There is also not much progress on the automated system for multiple cancer detection.

Table 1. Summary of Existing Work

S.no	Title	Technique	Dataset/Classification/Image Type	Accuracy	Conclusion/Future Scope/Research Gap
1	Afify et al. (2023)	Resnet-101, VGG19, Googlenet, Densenet, Shufflenet, Alexnet, Efficientnet-b0,	Histopathological 1224 Public dataset 2 classes-Normal/OSCC (oversampling technique is used to balance imbalanced dataset)	Accuracy 100% (ResNet-101) for 100x magnification accuracy 95.65% (EfficientNet-b0) for 400x magnification	It can be tested on the larger dataset.
2	Saraswathi and Bhaskaran (2023)	AlexNet, Resnet	Histopathological 1000 Kaggle 2classes Benign/Malignant	(AlexNet) Accuracy 89% (Resnet) Accuracy 78%	Accuracy can be improved It can be tested on a larger dataset
3	Subarna and Sukumar (2022)	MASO-optimized DenseNet 121	Smear Images Hervel dataset	98.38% accuracy	It is limited to only three abnormal classes. It can be expanded to more number of classes
4	Yaman and Tuncer (2022)	DarkNet19 DarkNet53, NCA algorithm (feature extraction), SVM	Smear Images SIPaKMeD, Mendeley LBC 5 classes	Accuarcy 98.26% and 99.47%, respectively	computationally not efficient, Complex model
5	Demir (2021)	Preprocessing(gradient, watershed), convolutional-LSTM CLSTM, Bayesian optimization, SVM	Histopathological Images BreakHis 9,109 Classes-Binary, 8	Accuracy-100% Accuracy-100%	CLSTM has a complex structure; the tuning of the parameters of the CLSTM is time-consuming. For huge datasets, the proposed methodology necessitates high-performance hardware.
6	Rana and Bhushan (2023)	(VGG16, DarkNet53, DarkNet19, ResNet50, Inception, LENET and Xception)	Classes-2 Benign Malignant	Accuracy-(Xception) 83.07% DarkNet53 (87.13%)	Dataset is imbalanced. Accuracy can be improved
7	Batool and Byun (2023)	EfficientNetB3	C_NMC_2019 (15,114 images) Classes-Normal, Abnormal	Accuracy 99.31%	Limited to only 2 classes
8	Omar et al. (2023)	VGG16, MobileNetV1, InceptionV3	LC25000 (25000) 5000 images for each class 5classes	Accuracy 99.44%	computationally not efficient

continued on following page

Table 1. Continued

S.no	Title	Technique	Dataset/ Classification/ Image Type	Accuracy	Conclusion /Future Scope/Research Gap
11	Çinar and Yildirim (2020)	EfficientNet-B0, VGG16, InceptionV3, Xception, ResNet50, and InceptionResNetV2	253 MRI images 2 classes Tumor, No tumor	accuracy of 97.2%	Limited to only 2 classes. Can be tested on larger dataset
13	Asif et al. (2023)	VGG16	e KiTS21 5284 CT images 2 classes	92.54% accuracy	accuracy can be improved
14		MobileNet, VGGNet, DenseNet, Bayesian Optimization, LwF	Kaggle (8 classes having 5000 images in each class)	Accuracy- 86.51% (MobileNet)	Accuracy can be improved
15	Talukder et al. (2022)	VGG16 + SVM, LR, MLP (ensemble soft voting classifier)	histopathological (LC25000) 5 classes	Accuracy 99.3%	computationally not efficient

METHODOLOGY

This section explains the different stages of the proposed approach. The cancer dataset is split into two sets, task 1 and task 2, and each set goes through preprocessing, train-test splitting, model training, and performance evaluation separately. Figure 1 shows the block diagram of the proposed model.

Figure 1. Block Diagram of the Proposed Model

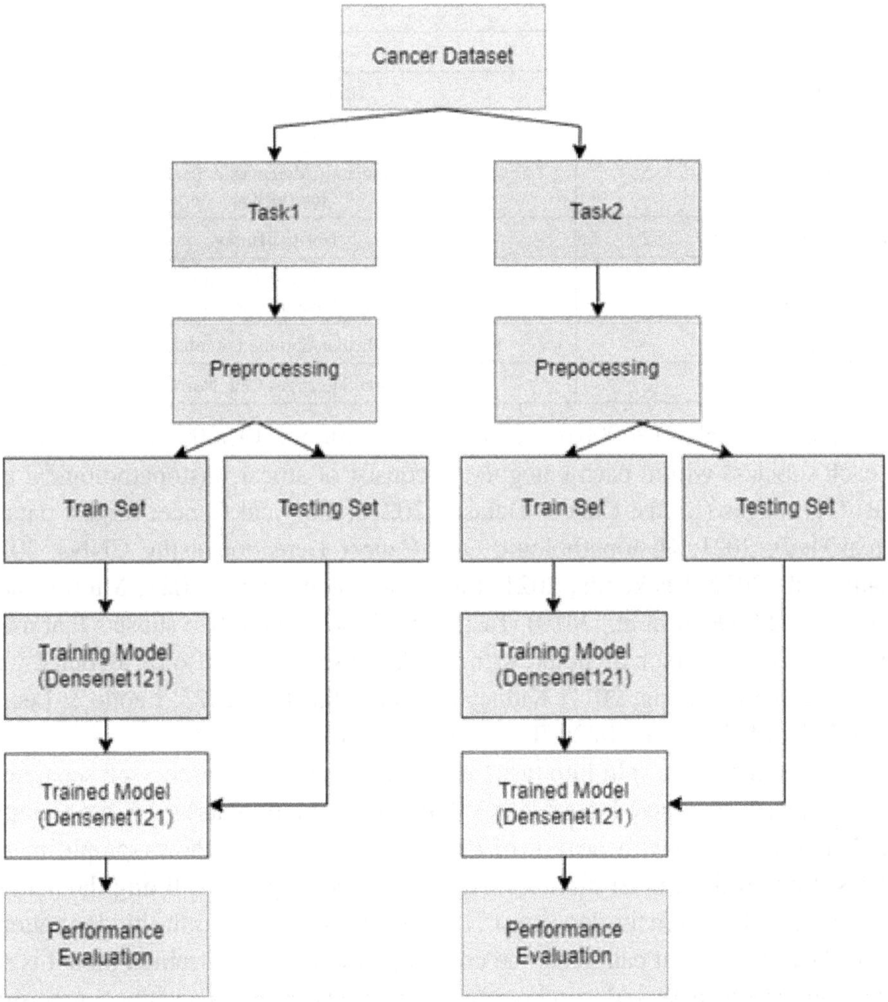

Data Collection

The "Multi Cancer Dataset" (Orlov et al., 2010), which is accessible publically on Kaggle, is used. It consists of the different kinds of cancer such as ALL, Lung, Colon, oral, lymphoma, brain cancer, breast, cervical; kidney. Each category in the above has further subclasses as shown in the given Table 2.

Table 2. Different Kinds of Cancer

Cancer	Total subclasses	Subclasses
ALL	4	Benign,Early,Pre,Pro
Brain Cancer	3	Glioma,Menin,Tumor
Breast Cancer	2	Benign,Malignant
Cervical Cancer	5	Dyskeratotic,Koilocytotic,Metaplastic, Parabasal,Superficial-Intermediate
Kidney Cancer	2	Normal,Tumor
Lung and Colon Cancer	5	Colon-Benign,Carcinoma Lung-Benign,Squamous,Adeno Carcinoma
Lymphoma	3	Mantle Cell,Follicular,Chronic Lymphocytic Leukemia
Oral Cancer	2	Oral Squamous Cell, Normal

There are a total of 130000 pictures in the collection, with 5000 images belonging to each subclass within each category. It consist of smear, histopathological and MRI/CT images (Breast Cancer Dataset, 2021b; Cervical Cancer largest dataset (SipakMed), 2021; Histopathologic Oral Cancer Detection using CNNs, 2021; Islam et al., 2022; Leukemia, 2021; Lung and colon cancer, 2021; Multi Cancer Dataset, 2022; Orlov et al., 2010). Task1 and Task2 are the two subsets that make up the dataset. A person afflicted with a task 1 disease may also be afflicted with a task 2 disease (Cheng, 2017; Kidney Cancer - statistics, 2023; Leone & Leone, 2015; Seladi-Schulman, 2022; Zhou & Peng, 2020).

Once the dataset is split into task1 and task2, they are preprocessed separately. All the images are resized to 48x48x3 RGB low resolution and split into training, validation and test set with the ratio of 75:15:15. Figure 2 and 3 shows sample images for task1 and task2 cancer diseases. After preprocessing and splitting the dataset, they are passed through the densenet121, where the model learns the hidden patterns in the dataset so that it can make the correct predictions. The trained model is run on the test set and assessed using performance metrics such as accuracy, precision, recall, and F1-score.

Figure 2. All

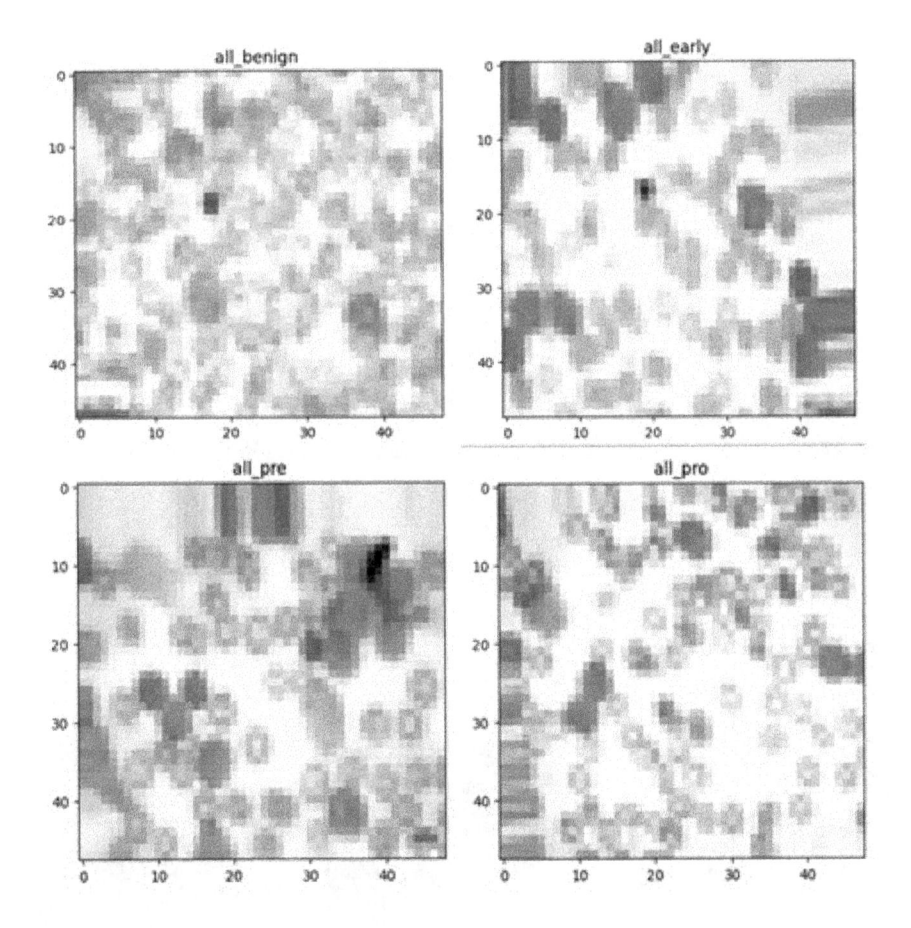

Figure 3. Breast Cancer

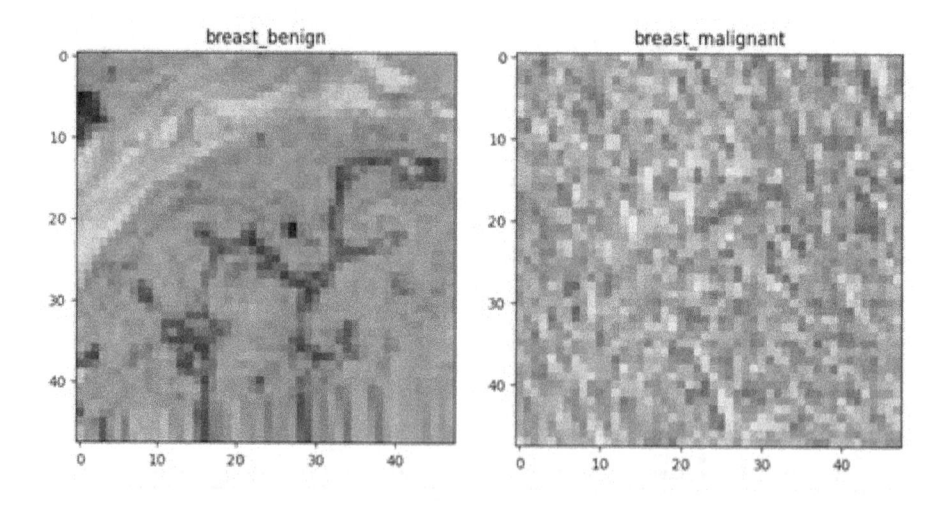

Figure 4. Cervical Cancer

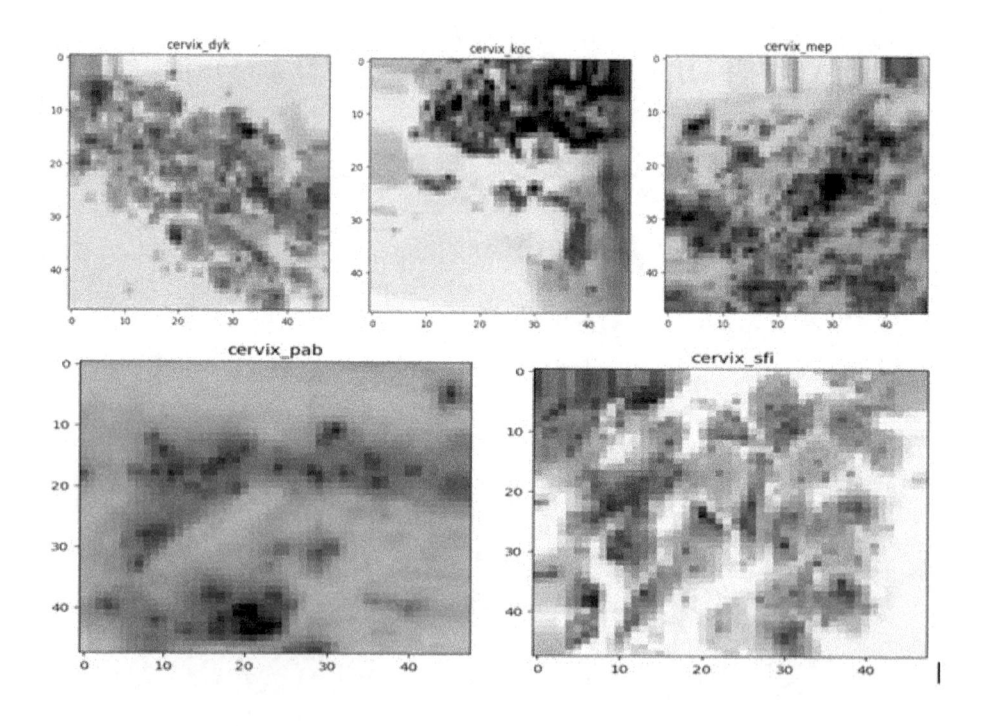

Figure 5. Kidney Cancer

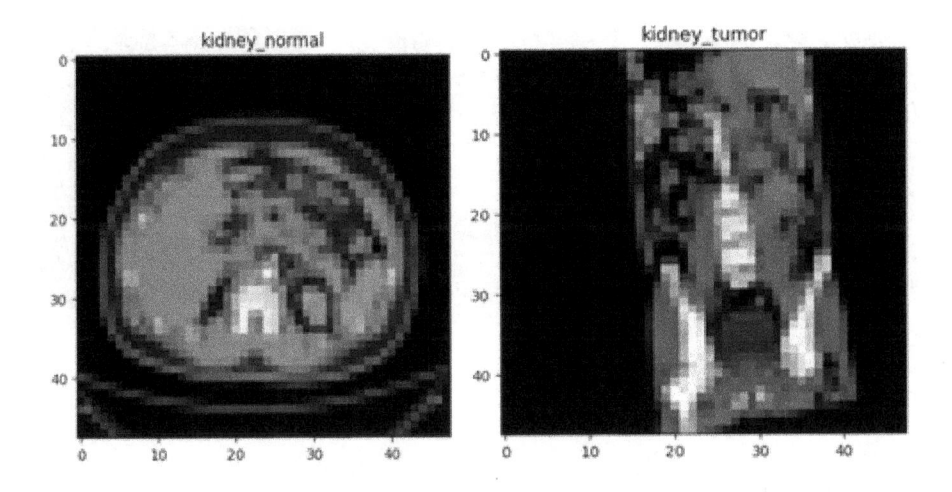

Figure 6. Brain Tumor

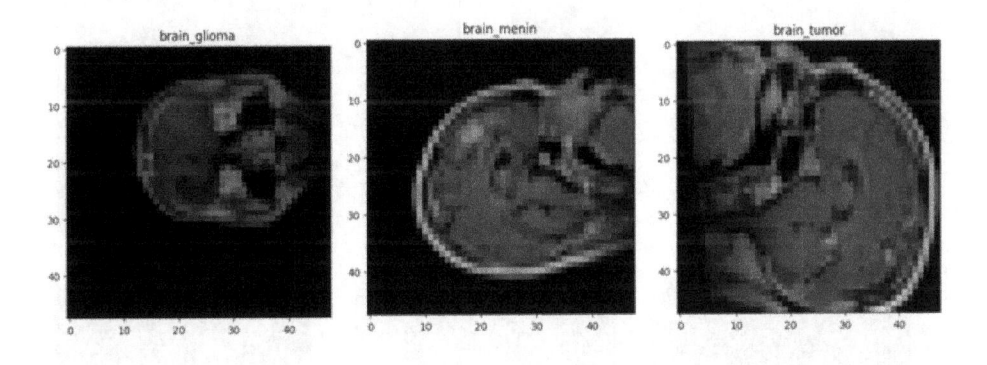

Figure 7. Lymphoma

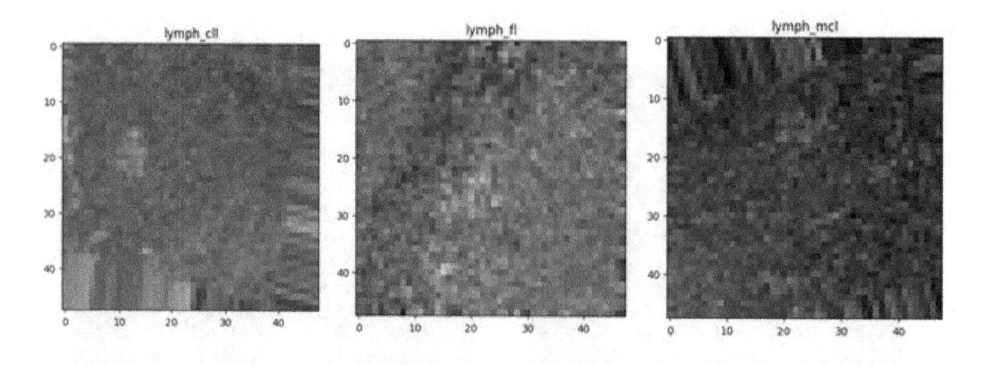

Figure 8. Lung Cancer

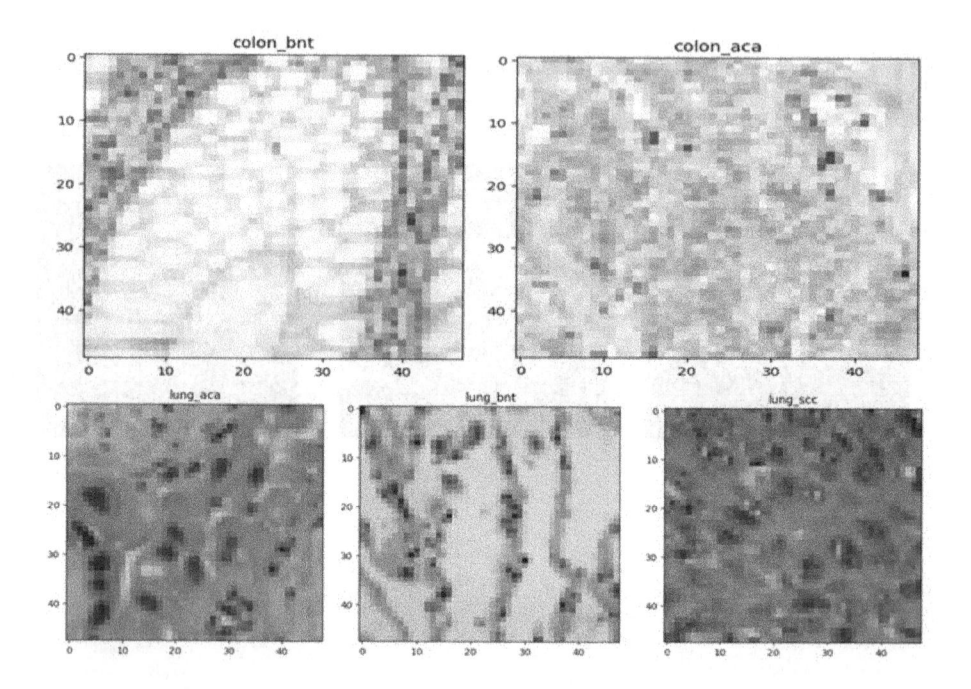

Figure 9. Oral Cancer

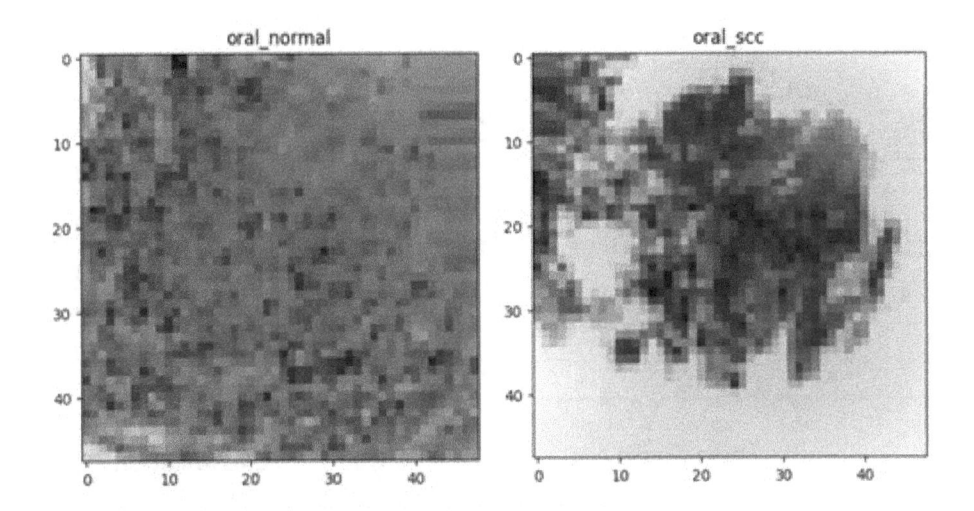

Model Architecture

Convolutional neural networks (CNNs) are a powerful tool for image processing, particularly in computer vision tasks like image classification, object detection, and natural language processing. CNNs are composed of distinct layers, each contributing to the network's ability to extract and learn from complex patterns in images. The first layer is the input layer, where the raw data, such as an image, is fed into the network. The convolutional layer is crucial and involves applying filters (kernels) to the input data, performing convolution operations to detect patterns and features. This is followed by activation functions, such as Rectified Linear Units (ReLU), which introduce non-linearity to the model. Pooling layers then reduce the spatial dimensions of the data, helping to decrease computational complexity and control overfitting by retaining essential information. The fully connected layers connect every neuron in one layer to every neuron in the next layer, learning complex patterns and relationships in the data. Finally, the output layer produces the network's predictions, often using activation functions like softmax for classification tasks. Throughout training, CNNs adjust their internal parameters (weights and biases) via optimization algorithms, such as gradient descent, to minimize the difference between predicted and actual outcomes, ultimately enhancing their ability to recognize and classify patterns in input data. Figure 4. Shows the architecture diagram of CNN.

Figure 10. CNN Architecture

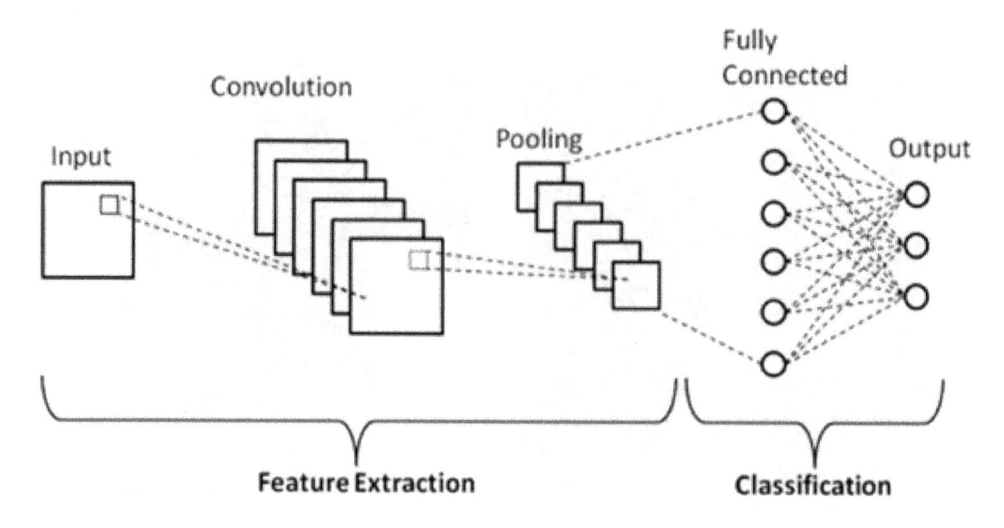

DenseNet121 is a convolutional neural network (CNN) architecture that builds upon the fundamental principles of CNNs while introducing a novel concept called dense connections. CNNs, as the name suggests, are designed to process grid-like data, particularly images, using convolutional layers that extract spatial features from the input. DenseNet121 enhances the traditional CNN architecture by directly connecting each layer to every other layer, enabling feature reuse and propagation throughout the network. This dense connectivity allows for more complex feature extraction and improved performance compared to standard CNN architectures.

The DenseNet 121 architecture consists of a series of dense blocks interleaved with transition layers. The dense blocks contain multiple convolutional layers with batch normalization and ReLU activation functions, promoting feature learning and non-linearity. Transition layers, composed of convolutional and pooling layers, reduce the spatial dimensions of the feature maps, controlling computational complexity. The global average pooling layer is typically applied at the end of the network, reducing the spatial dimensions to a single value per feature map. This condensed representation is then fed into a fully connected layer for the final classification or regression output. Fully connected layer consist of 1024 neurons with softmax activation that outputs the class probabilities for the input image. Figure 5 shows the architecture diagram of DenseNet121 for task1 and task2.

Figure 11. DenseNet121 Architecture for Task1

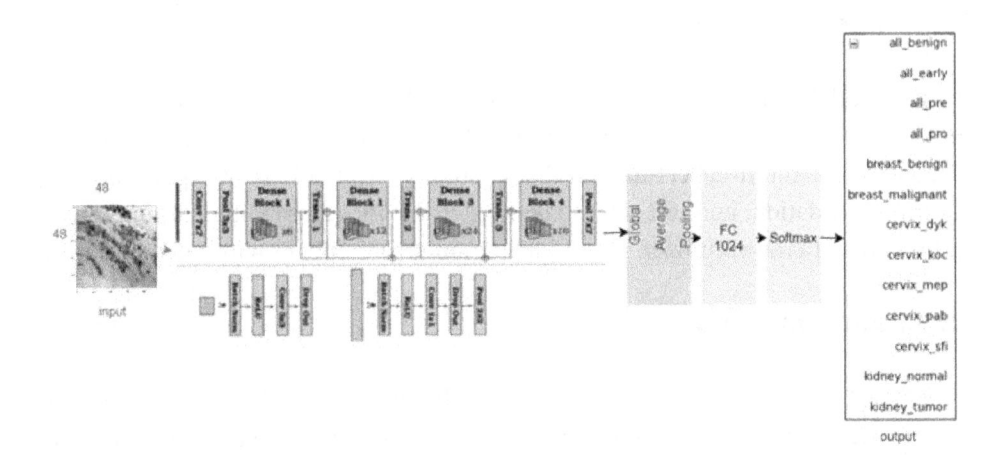

Figure 12. DenseNet121 Architecture for a Task 2

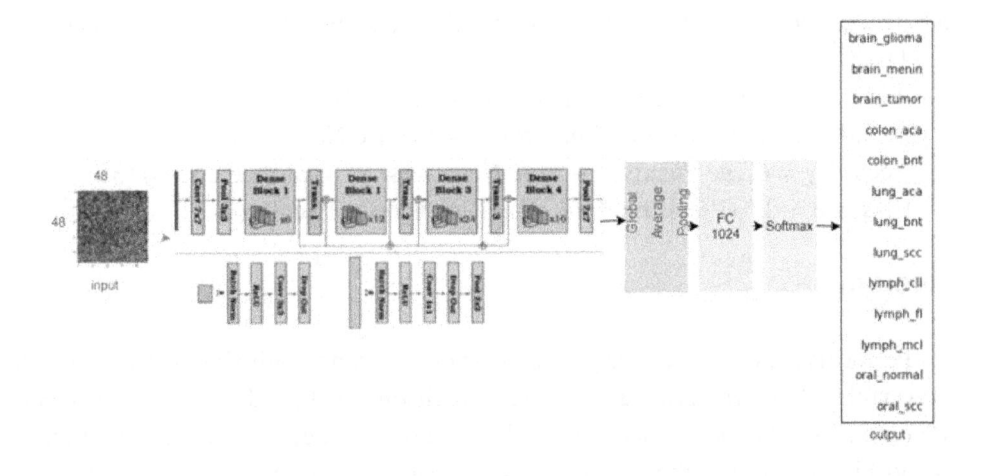

EXPERIMENTS AND RESULTS

Experimental setup

The model is trained in Python using tensor flow and keras libraries. It is built on Google Colab with a T4 GPU, 12.68 GB of RAM, and 78.19 GB of disk. It is evaluated on a multi-cancer dataset that is publicly available on Kaggle. The ratio for train, validation, and test sets is taken as 75:15:15. Adam with learning rate of 0.0001 is used as an optimizer. The model is trained for 5 epochs with batch size of 16.

Evaluation metrics

Evaluating the performance of a machine learning model is crucial for assessing its effectiveness and identifying areas for improvement. Performance metrics provide a quantitative measure of how well the model performs against a given set of data. Common performance metrics for classification tasks include precision, recall, accuracy, and F1-score. The percentage of positive predictions that turn out to be accurate is called precision. Recall measures the proportion of actual positive cases that are correctly identified. Accuracy measures the overall proportion of correct predictions. F1-score is a harmonic mean of precision and recall, providing a balanced measure of both. Precision, recall, accuracy, F1-score are calculated as in (1), (2),(3),(4).

Precision = True Positives / (True Positives + False Positives) (1)
Recall = True Positives / (True Positives + False Negatives) (2)
Accuracy = (True Positives + True Negatives) / (Total Predictions) (3)
F1-score = 2 * (Precision * Recall) / (Precision + Recall) (4)

Results

Performance of a model can be also evaluated using confusion metric as it is a powerful tool for evaluating the accuracy, precision, recall, and F1-score of a model. It summarizes the performance of a classification model on a set of data. Figure 6 and Figure 7 shows the confusion matrix for task1 and task2 respectively. The diagonals of the confusion matrix show the correct classifications. The predicted classes are shown on the Y-axis, while the actual classes are shown on the X-axis.

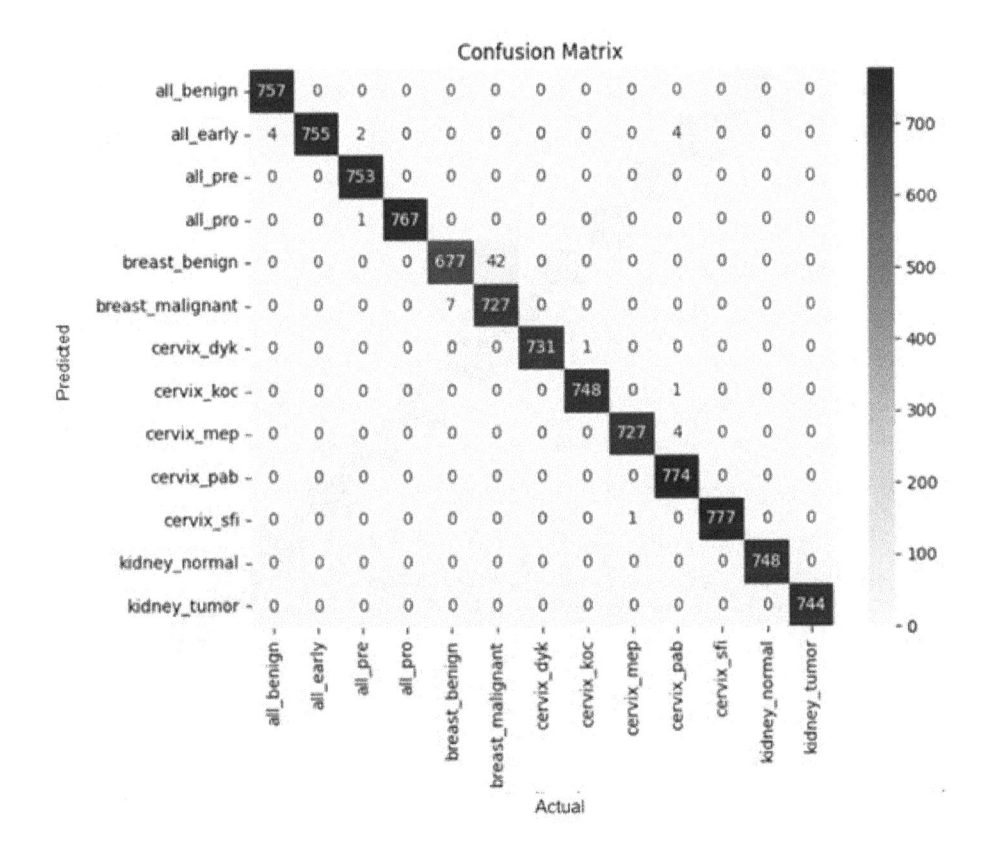

Figure 13. Confusion Metrics Graph of Proposed Model for Task1

Figure 14. Confusion Metrics Graph of Proposed Model for Task2

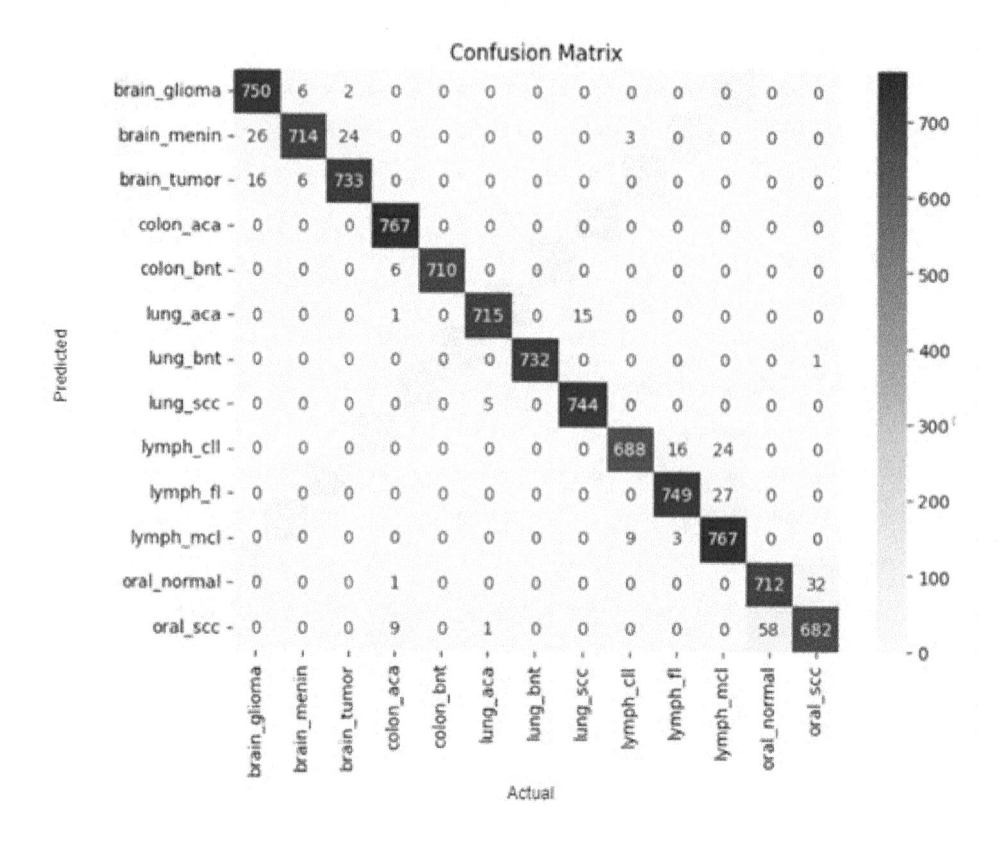

[Confusion Matrix showing predicted vs actual classifications across 13 categories: brain_glioma, brain_menin, brain_tumor, colon_aca, colon_bnt, lung_aca, lung_bnt, lung_scc, lymph_cll, lymph_fl, lymph_mcl, oral_normal, oral_scc]

The proposed model is compared with the existing methods based on the above mentioned metrics. Table 3 and 4 display the result of the proposed model and the existing techniques and it can be concluded that the proposed method is performing better than existing techniques. It achieved the accuracy of 99.31% and 97.02% for task 1 and task2, respectively. Figure 10 shows the output of the model.

Table 3. The Evaluation Standards of Suggested and Current Models for Task1

Model	Accuracy	Precision	Recall	F1-Score
VGG16	75.82	85.69	85.77	85.68
VGG19	76.34	89.22	89.25	89.21
DenseNet201	79.82	92.27	92.31	92.26
MobileNetV3 (Large)	81.67	96.13	96.16	96.14

continued on following page

Table 3. Continued

Model	Accuracy	Precision	Recall	F1-Score
MobileNetV3 (Small)	84.52	97.42	97.43	97.42
Proposed Model	**99.31**	**99.33**	**99.31**	**99.31**

Table 4. The Evaluation Standards of Suggested and Current Models for Task2

Model	Accuracy	Precision	Recall	F1-Score
VGG16	65.91	71.07	71.35	71.07
VGG19	70.12	72.44	72.5	72.43
DenseNet201	77.84	79.28	79.35	79.28
MobileNetV3 (Large)	78.21	84.59	84.63	84.59
MobileNetV3 (Small)	79.95	81.43	81.51	81.44
Proposed Model	**97.02**	**97.05**	**97.02**	**97.01**

Figure 15. Actual and Predicted Output for Task1 and Task2

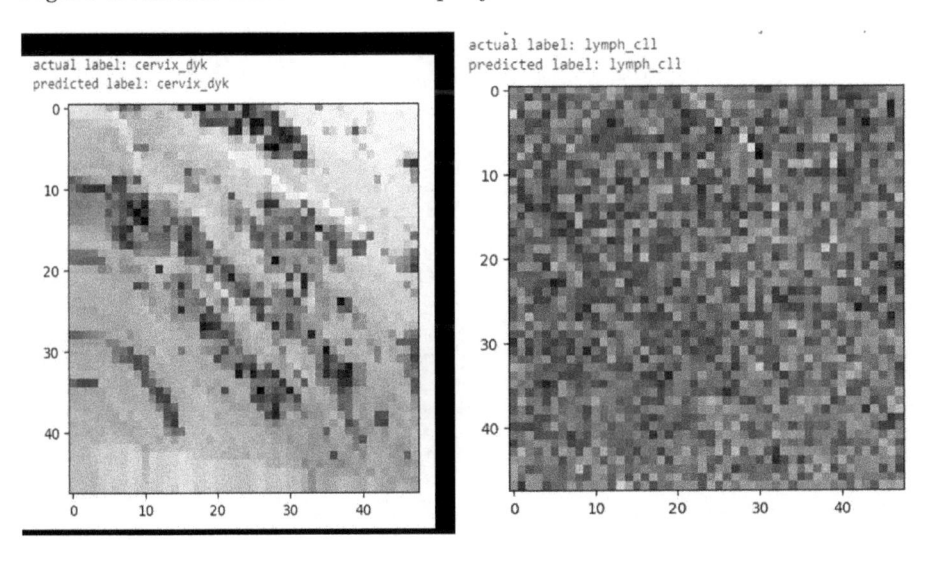

CONCLUSION

This research provides an automated technique based on deep learning to detect multiple kinds of cancer including lung, cervical, breast, brain, kidney, brain, breast, colon and oral.Densenet121, a CNN pretrained model is used to classify different types of cancer into its subclasses. The model is trained using the Multi Cancer dataset. The model is evaluated based on performance metrics such as accuracy,F1-score,recall,precision.Its performance is compared with the existing models. With an accuracy of 99.31%, precision of 99.33%, recall of 99.31%, F1-score of 99.31% for task 1 and accuracy of 97.02%, precision of 97.05%, recall of 97.02%, F1-score of 97.01% for task 2, the model outperformed existing models for cancer classification. The study's encouraging findings show how this research may contribute to the development of trustworthy and accurate cancer detection systems. Millions of lives worldwide can be saved, and treatment outcomes can be greatly enhanced by the early detection of cancer. As a result, the suggested method may offer medical practitioners a useful tool for promptly and accurately identifying cancer, enabling patients to receive treatment and care. Future iterations of this work could examine additional types of cancer. Also, the dataset can be expanded to include normal cases for each category of cancer.

REFERENCES

Afify, H. M., Mohammed, K. K., & Hassanien, A. E. (2023). Novel prediction model on OSCC histopathological images via deep transfer learning combined with Grad-CAM interpretation. *Biomedical Signal Processing and Control*, 83, 104704. 10.1016/j.bspc.2023.104704

Asif, S., Zhao, M., Tang, F., & Zhu, Y. (2023). An enhanced deep learning method for multi-class brain tumor classification using deep transfer learning. *Multimedia Tools and Applications*, 82(20), 1–28. 10.1007/s11042-023-14828-w

Batool, A., & Byun, Y. C. (2023). Lightweight EfficientNetB3 model based on depth-wise separable convolutions for enhancing classification of leukemia white blood cell images. *IEEE Access: Practical Innovations, Open Solutions*, 11, 37203–37215.

Breast Cancer Dataset. (2021b, July 17). Kaggle. Available: https://www.kaggle.com/datasets/anaselmasry/breast-cancer-dataset

Can artificial intelligence help see cancer in new ways? (2022, March 22). National Cancer Institute. https://www.cancer.gov/news-events/cancer-currents-blog/2022/artificial-intelligence-cancer-imaging

Cervical Cancer largest dataset (SipakMed). (2021, March 12). Kaggle. Available: https://www.kaggle.com/datasets/prahladmehandiratta/cervical-cancer-largest-dataset-sipakmed

Cheng, J. (2017) Brain tumor dataset. *Figshare*. Available: https://figshare.com/articles/dataset/brain_tumor_dataset/1512427

Çinar, A., & Yildirim, M. (2020). Detection of tumors on brain MRI images using the hybrid convolutional neural network architecture. *Medical Hypotheses*, 139, 109684. 10.1016/j.mehy.2020.10968432240877

Demir, F. (2021). DeepBreastNet: A novel and robust approach for automated breast cancer detection from histopathological images. *Biocybernetics and Biomedical Engineering*, 41(3), 1123–1139. 10.1016/j.bbe.2021.07.004

Farina, E., Nabhen, J. J., Dacoregio, M. I., Batalini, F., & Moraes, F. Y. (2022, February 10). An overview of artificial intelligence in oncology. *Future Science OA*, 8(4), FSO787. Advance online publication. 10.2144/fsoa-2021-007435369274

Histopathologic Oral Cancer Detection using CNNs. (2021, July 21). Kaggle. Available: https://www.kaggle.com/datasets/ashenafifasilkebede/dataset

Islam, M. N., Hasan, M., Hossain, M. K., Alam, M. G. R., Uddin, M. Z., & Soylu, A. (2022). Vision transformer and explainable transfer learning models for auto detection of kidney cyst, stone and tumor from CT-radiography. *Scientific Reports*, 12(1), 11440. 10.1038/s41598-022-15634-435794172

Kathamuthu, N. D., Subramaniam, S., Le, Q. H., Muthusamy, S., Panchal, H., Sundararajan, S. C. M., Alrubaie, A. J., & Zahra, M. M. A. (2023). A deep transfer learning-based convolution neural network model for COVID-19 detection using computed tomography scan images for medical applications. *Advances in Engineering Software*, 175, 103317. 10.1016/j.advengsoft.2022.10331736311489

Kidney Cancer - statistics. (2023, May 23). Cancer.Net. Available: https://www.cancer.net/cancer-types/kidney-cancer/statistics

Leone, J. P., & Leone, B. A. (2015). Breast cancer brain metastases: The last frontier. *Experimental Hematology & Oncology*, 4(1), 33. 10.1186/s40164-015-0028-826605131

Leukemia, A. L. (2021, April 30). Kaggle. Available: https://www.kaggle.com/datasets/mehradaria/leukemia

Lung and colon cancer. (2021, November 24). Kaggle. Available: https://www.kaggle.com/datasets/biplobdey/lung-and-colon-cancer

Maheshwari, U., Kiranmayee, B. V., & Suresh, C. (2022, December). *Diagnose Colon and Lung Cancer Histopathological Images Using Pre-Trained Machine Learning Model. In 2022 5th International Conference on Contemporary Computing and Informatics (IC3I)*. IEEE. https://ieeexplore.ieee.org/abstract/document/10073184/

Manickavasagam, R., Selvan, S., & Selvan, M. (2022). CAD system for lung nodule detection using deep learning with CNN. *Medical & Biological Engineering & Computing*, 60(1), 221–228. 10.1007/s11517-021-02462-334811644

Multi Cancer Dataset. (2022, April 6). Kaggle. Available: https://www.kaggle.com/datasets/obulisainaren/multi-cancers

Omar, L. T., Hussein, J. M., Omer, L. F., Qadir, A. M., & Ghareb, M. I. (2023, May). Lung And Colon Cancer Detection Using Weighted Average Ensemble Transfer Learning. In *2023 11th International Symposium on Digital Forensics and Security (ISDFS)* (pp. 1-7). IEEE.(https://ieeexplore.ieee.org/abstract/document/10131836/)

Orlov, N. V., Chen, W. W., Eckley, D. M., Macura, T. J., Shamir, L., Jaffe, E. S., & Goldberg, I. G. (2010). Automatic classification of lymphoma images with transform-based global features. *IEEE Transactions on Information Technology in Biomedicine*, 14(4), 1003–1013. 10.1109/TITB.2010.205069520659835

Rajkumar, K., Ramoju, R. T. S., Balelly, T., Ashadapu, S., Prasad, C. R., & Srikanth, Y. (2023, April). Kidney Cancer Detection using Deep Learning Models. In *2023 7th International Conference on Trends in Electronics and Informatics (ICOEI)* (pp. 1197-1203). IEEE. https://ieeexplore.ieee.org/abstract/document/10125589/

Rana, M., & Bhushan, M. (2023). Classifying breast cancer using transfer learning models based on histopathological images. *Neural Computing & Applications*, 35(19), 14243–14257. 10.1007/s00521-023-08484-2

Saraswathi, T., & Bhaskaran, V. M. (2023, February). Classification of Oral Squamous Carcinoma Histopathological images using Alex Net. In *2023 International Conference on Intelligent Systems for Communication, IoT and Security (ICISCoIS)* (pp. 637-643). IEEE.(https://ieeexplore.ieee.org/abstract/document/10100510/)

Sava, J. (2023, April 27). Current applications of artificial intelligence in Oncology. Targeted Oncology. https://www.targetedonc.com/view/current-applications-of-artificial-intelligence-in-oncology

Seladi-Schulman, J. (2022, February 21). When breast cancer metastasizes to the brain. Available: https://www.healthline.com/health/breast-cancer/breast-cancer-metastasis-to-brain#overview

Shreve, J., Khanani, S., & Haddad, T. C. (2022). Artificial intelligence in Oncology: Current capabilities, future opportunities, and ethical considerations. *American Society of Clinical Oncology Educational Book*, 42(42), 842–851. 10.1200/EDBK_35065235687826

Subarna, T. G., & Sukumar, P. (2022). Detection and classification of cervical cancer images using CEENET deep learning approach. *Journal of Intelligent & Fuzzy Systems*, 43(3), 3695–3707. 10.3233/JIFS-220173

Subramanian, M., Cho, J., Sathishkumar, V. E., & Naren, O. S. (2023). Multiple Types of Cancer Classification Using CT/MRI Images Based on Learning Without Forgetting Powered Deep Learning Models. *IEEE Access : Practical Innovations, Open Solutions*, 11, 10336–10354. 10.1109/ACCESS.2023.3240443

Talukder, M. A., Islam, M. M., Uddin, M. A., Akhter, A., Hasan, K. F., & Moni, M. A. (2022). Machine learning-based lung and colon cancer detection using deep feature extraction and ensemble learning. *Expert Systems with Applications*, 205, 117695. 10.1016/j.eswa.2022.117695

Wasi, S., Alam, S. B., Rahman, R., Amin, M. A., & Kobashi, S. (2023, May). Kidney Tumor Recognition from Abdominal CT Images using Transfer Learning. In *2023 IEEE 53rd International Symposium on Multiple-Valued Logic (ISMVL)* (pp. 54-58). IEEE. https://ieeexplore.ieee.org/abstract/document/10153815/

Yaman, O., & Tuncer, T. (2022). Exemplar pyramid deep feature extraction based cervical cancer image classification model using pap-smear images. *Biomedical Signal Processing and Control*, 73, 103428. 10.1016/j.bspc.2021.103428

Zhou, S., & Peng, F. (2020). Patterns of metastases in cervical cancer: A population-based study. *International Journal of Clinical and Experimental Pathology*, 13(7), 1615.

Chapter 15
A Multimodal Deep Learning Approach for Early Detection of Alzheimer's Disease

V. Sanjay
 https://orcid.org/0000-0002-6383-3793
Vellore Institute of Technology, India

P. Swarnalatha
Vellore Institute of Technology, India

Ragupathyraj Valluvan
University of Jaffna, Sri Lanka

ABSTRACT

Artificial Neural Networks (ANNs) optimized with Particle Swarm Optimization (PSO) for predicting Alzheimer's disease have demonstrated reliability in estimating mild cognitive impairment (LSM). Traditional ANN training faces challenges such as slow learning rates and difficulty overcoming local minima. Integrating PSO, a Resquare Optimization Algorithm (ROA), enhances ANN performance. In our study, using a dataset of 12,130 preparation records and 51,642 test records, we trained ICA-ANN and ICA-PSO-ROA-ANN models. PSO parameters were optimized to maximize accuracy while minimizing computational load. Evaluation using Root-Mean-Squared Error (RMSE) showed that the ROA-PSO-ANN model consistently outperformed traditional ANN and hybrid models, highlighting its effectiveness in complex medical diagnostics for Alzheimer's disease prediction.

DOI: 10.4018/979-8-3693-3719-6.ch015

INTRODUCTION

Alzheimer's disease is an irreversible brain ailment for which there is now no effective treatment. Tau filaments and Amyloid Beta protein aggregate abnormally, leading to neurofibrillary tangles and senile plaques, two classic features of Caused by dementia. By 2050, the Alzheimer's Association predicts that 12.7% of the 65+ population will have the disease, costing the United States $1.1 trillion a year and ranking as the sixth leading cause of death. trillion.1 There is currently no cure despite several clinical investigations and attempts. Therefore, it is crucial to find Alzheimer's disease early and lessen its effects. Several radiological indicators were examined to distinguish conventional cognition from mild cognitive decline and Alzheimer's disease. These biomarkers can be categorized into three primary categories: structural, functional, and molecular imaging. A large range of tools, including In addition to free surfer and Division, FSL and MIPAV, are required for the laborious and time-consuming process of manually extracting features for The diagnosis of dementia. In contrast, computer vision and classification algorithms have taken on a far larger role in medical diagnosis in the recent two decades. Hong, X et al. (2019), Islam, J et al. (2018) The amazing ability of deep learning models to discern even the smallest distinctions has led to their dominance in the field of artificial intelligence (Kowalski, P. A et al., 2015; Liu, F et al., 2014). It also provides a faster alternative to the traditional, time-consuming way of manually extracting features for labelling patients with Alzheimer's disease. We built an ensembled volumetric convNet classification of dementia into multiple categories previous research showing that deep learning frameworks can increase accuracy in Alzheimer's detection tools like AV-45 PET and T1w-MRI scans.

Figure 1. Alzheimer's Disease Input Images

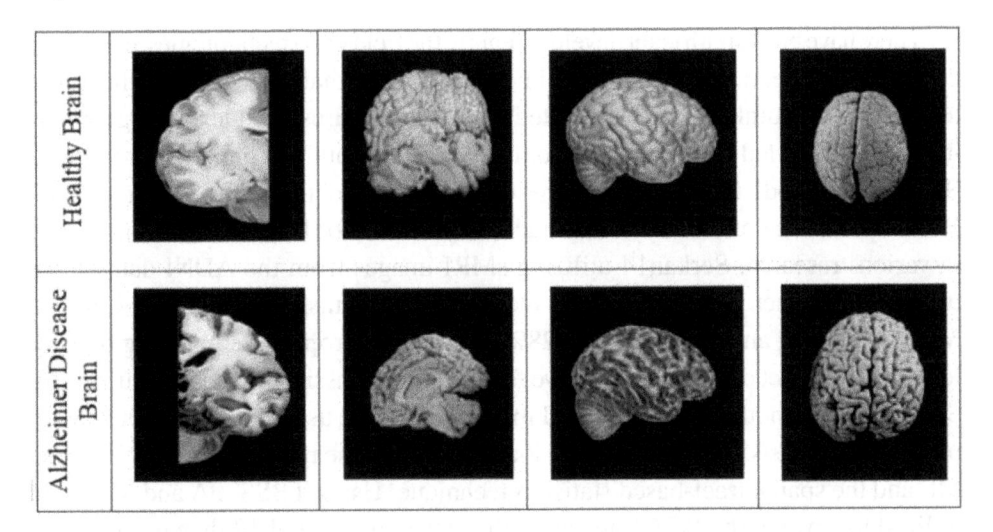

Here are some of the most significant results from this investigation:

To the best of our knowledge, an ensemble of volumetric convolutional neural has been developed to identify Alzheimer's disease and its many subtypes (AD, NC, and MCI).

Our study is the first to analyze the effects of systematically combining T1w-MRI with Florbetapir PET scans using three different feature extraction methods.

Third, we looked into the precision of many patches ranging in size from small to medium to large for a multi-modality framework based on 3D patches.

Three separate Slice-based strategies for techniques for zooming in and out using interpolation, uniform slicing, and subsets were utilized to produce Alzheimer's detection utilizing MRI and AV45 PET data.

The article continues with the following structure: Different frameworks, algorithms, and feature extraction methods are discussed in Part 2 for the purpose of recognizing Alzheimer's. In Section 3, In this paper, we describe the MRI and AV-45 PET image collection, pre-processing pipeline, augmentation approaches, and convolutional network used to train the alzNet architecture. Finally, Section 5 discusses other facets of future work that may be utilized, and Section 6 finishes with a review of the entire project. Section 4 covers experimental results using three different neuroanatomy computation extraction approaches.

I. RELATED WORKS

There have been significant developments in the field of AI technologies, especially convolutional neural networks used in deep learning, that aim to detect the micro and macrostructural changes associated with AD. Features at all levels of granularity can be extracted automatically from a dataset without any human intervention. Sensitive methods for identifying these alterations include both sMRI and DTI. Both separate use of each modality and combined use of both have been proposed in various research. Serkan14 utilizing sMRI images from the ADNI dataset, we trained 29 distinct pre-trained CNN models to distinguish between AD, CN, and MCI., achieving an accuracy of 97.28%. Some have proposed employing transfer learning to extract deep discriminative features, then classifying those features with SVM15,16, or another classifier. DTI maps and ML are used in a variety of ways to make AD forecasts. There has been a lot of interest in the possible synergy between ML and the spatial tract-based statistics technique. Using TBSS, FA and MD were utilized to develop the WM framework that Maggipinto et al.18 then used to construct a Random Forest classifier. Using the WM skeleton's fractional anisotropy, mean diffusivity, radial diffusivity, and longitudinal diffusivity, The collaborative neural network training method invented by Lella et al. (2019) technique to distinguish CN from alzheimer's disease. The data was used to train three different classifiers: a mixture of a multi-layer perceptron, a supported vector machine, and a random forest. Using soft-voting, we pooled the top classifiers from each map to get a final result. Researchers have found that multimodal ML and CNN can help overcome the drawbacks of using only one type of data, leading to more accurate disease diagnostic prediction models (Razavi, F. et al., 2019); Viswanathan, T et al., 2020). Combining DTImaps with sMRI for screening Alzheimer's disease has been the primary focus of research. Marzban et al. (2022), to provide just one example, segmented GM from T1-weighted sMRI and employed DTI-derived measures

THE PROPOSED METHODOLOGY

The study was designed using data from the preprocessing stage, specifically the hippocampus and entorhinal cortex. In order to train the CNN, the authors used financial analysis, molecular oxygen, medicine, and GM-ROI both independently and in a cascade. Only a single 2D convolution layer is used in the suggested CNN. Maximum precision was achieved when MD and GM volumes were used in a cascade fashion as inputs. (88.9%) for AD/CN and the lowest (79.6%) for MCI/CN (Ben Ahmed et al., n.d.). 23 used Gauss-Laguerre Harmonic Functions (GLCHFs) to predict hippocampal region-of-interest (ROI) characteristics from MD and T1w sMRI volume segmentations. These characteristics and the CSF volume were combined using Multiple Kernel Learning (MKL). Recently, GL-CHFs were used to sMRI images, and in contrast to Bansal et al., the authors of study24 claimed that the local descriptors performed better than SIFT and SURF.25 Bag of Features (BoF) was combined with the SURF and SVM classifiers to produce a 93% accurate result. Using sMRI and DTI-MD images, Aderghal et al.26 showed a convolutional neural network similar to LeNet. In each of the three planes of view (axial, sagittal, and coronal), they chose the hippocampus slice in the middle and the two adjacent ones. The MNIST database is used to train the proposed CNN. Next, it underwent a round of retraining using DTI-MD and sMRI. Classification accuracy for AD versus CN was 86.83%, MCI versus CN was 69.85%, and AD versus MCI was 71.75%.

Figure 2. The Alzheimer Disease Preprocessing Diagram

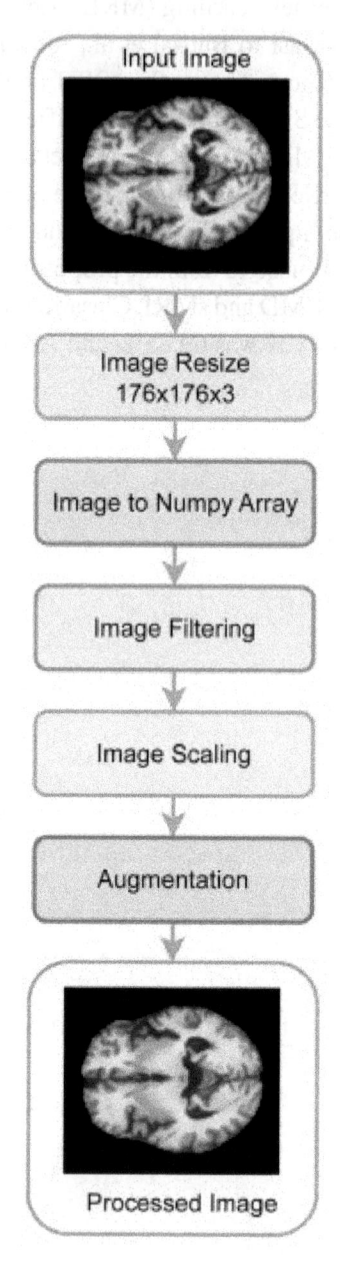

Algorithm 1:*Optimizing with Artificial Intelligence (AI-Opt) Algorithm Materials: Particles Success Metric: Fitness to Criteria*

1. Put all the particles into their initial, random positions and velocities.

2. {

3. Find out how fit each particle is.

4. Capture the Pb particle.

5. Calculate the best in the world (Gb).

6. Determine the velocity of the particle using equation (1).

7. If (the termination conditions are met), then.

8. {

9. Stopped the whole thing

10. Else

11. Perform Steps 3-7 again.

}

Training networks in a modified artificial neural network model. Several studies have provided a detailed account of this procedure. In most cases, a random seed is generated before the model operation begins. Now we have the locations of the particles that stand in for the correlated biases and masses produced by the ANN.

Typically, a random process is used to select the particles. The initial positions (biases and weights) of the particles are used to train a network representing the Modified ANN model. After that, we conduct an analysis of the merged skilled system. This can be done by determining the discrepancy (either directly or by arithmetic directories) between desired and achieved outcomes. Each iteration reduces the computed error by shifting the particle's position. The velocity equation is adjusted using Gigabytes (the minimum error obtained by a) P (the minimum error obtained by each particle up to that moment) and b) P (all particles up to that point). As a result, a rate can be calculated that can be used to priorities particle sites. Error is calculated at each stage and is expected to decrease from one to the next. The process is iterated as in Algorithm 2 once one of the stopping conditions has been met. As shown in Figure 2, the value of the RMSE has been shown to be lowest in the eleventh neuron, making this the best possible design for an ANN were accumulated after the sixth neuron, as shown in Figure 3. In order to determine the method's efficacy, data from numerous GIS model simulations were collected. Following the presentation of relevant solutions, this investigation continues to provide an explanation of the created record and ANN procedures. The PSO-ANN approach maintained the same optimization strategy as ANN.

Fig. 3. In order to determine the method's efficacy, data from numerous GIS model simulations were collected. Following the presentation of relevant solutions, this investigation continues to provide an explanation of the created record and ANN procedures. The PSO-ANN approach maintained the same optimization strategy as ANN.

Figure 3. The Proposed System Flow Diagram

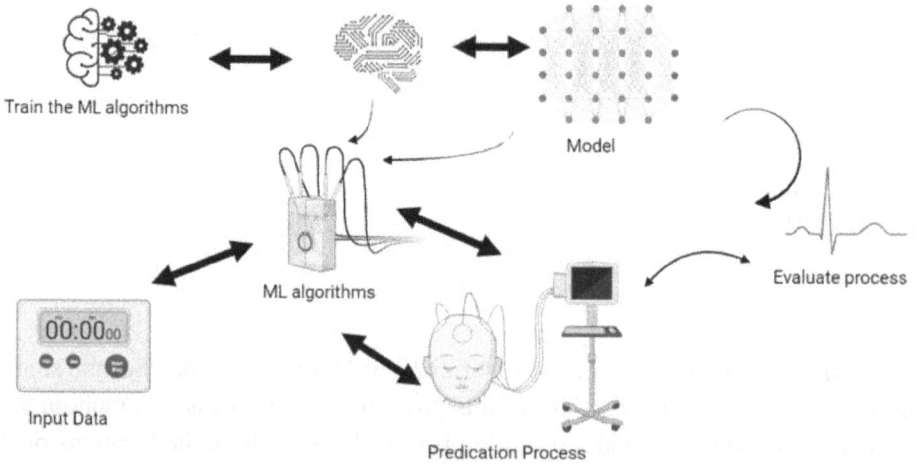

The PSO model of stochastic optimization simulates the social behaviour of flocks through the use of a population-based approach. It's population-based like EA, and like EA, it uses fitness functions to evaluate individuals. The RMSE value was found to be lowest in the eleventh neuron, making this the best practical design for an ANN. and because surplus variance of little relevance was being stored beyond the sixth neuron. Furthermore, with EAs, there is no such thing as making mistakes and subsequently learning from them. Due to its simplicity, PSO has been widely used to address both discrete and continuous optimization problems (Viswanathan, T.et al., 2020).

Particle swarm optimization (PSO) uses a large group of people, or "particles," to search a small area. Every particle stands for a unique optimal solution to the problem. A particle's position in the universe is dependent on both its own location and the position of the best component nearby. The location of a particular particle in the cluster is the most important factor in determining its quality of life. G best PSO is the name given to the final algorithm. This strategy has gained notoriety as the "optimal PSO for tiny neighbourhoods." As the distance between particles varies, so does the fitness function, the optimization strategy, and the final solution.

Current position of the particle: ai

The current velocity of the particle is bi.

For a particle, the best possible location is: ci

Optimal localization of the particle is given by (b_i)

A particle's optimum position is the one that yields the most fitness value for it. The goal function can be represented as f [22]. Then, the new best for A particle at time step t is (3):

$$RSO_i(o+2) = \begin{cases} RSO_i(s) \text{ if } wg(a_i(s+1)) > dg(b_i(s)) \\ SO_i(s+1) \text{ if } wg(a_i(s+1)) < dg(b_i(s)) \end{cases} \quad (3)$$

Collectively, the swarm chose the optimal particle for the gbest model. through settling on one's optimal starting point. Assuming that the vector b represents the location of the optimal particle on a global scale, we have (4):

$$\widetilde{zb}\{zb_0, b_1, \ldots zb_k\} = \min\{g(zb_1(s)), \ldots, (zb_k(s))\} \quad (4)$$

If k represents the size of the hive, then we have a swarm of that size.

for each dimension j ∈ 1..., Nd, there is a defined interval for velocity updates. Since the velocity vector of the ith particle has a zjth component, bi, j denotes that value. how fast the particle is moving, can be calculated using the following formula (5):

$$zb_{i,j}(s+1) = qzb_{i,j}(s) + c_1 m_{1,j}(s) b_{i,j}(s)) - zb_{i,j}(s)) + c_2 m_{2,j}(s)(\overline{zb(s)} - zb_{i,j}(s)) \quad (5)$$

The moment of inertia is equal to w, and the acceleration constants are c1 and c2 and c_1 m_(1,zj) (s), m_(2,zj)U (0, 1).

EXPERIMENTS

The proposed AD segmentation model was built using Python's supervised ROA framework. The deep learning architecture is implemented with the help of the keras and TensorFlow frameworks. We assess the efficiency of the existing segmentation approach on the publicly accessible AD dataset. An early form of deep learning was accomplished through the use of convolutional neural networks and adaptive adversarial networks. Similar research has been done several times before using ANDI 2151 MRI by academics. The data set features human bodies in various states, including those with cancer. The generalizability of the model was accurately reflected by the development of distributionally identical validation and testing datasets thanks to careful segmentation of the dataset. Hyperparameters like the learning rate and decay are adjusted based on training and validation data to maximise the model's output. Indicators like weights and biases require training data in order to be learned. Careful examination of test results leads to the construction of a model. The image as a whole must be normalised such that all of the pixels are roughly the same brightness and any traces of bias have been eliminateddigital image patches were created.

Table 1. ML Classifiers

ML Classifiers	Precision	Recall	F1-score	Accuracy
SVM-Navies Bayes	83.42	74.03	86.45	88.05
SVM-Navies Bayes -KNN	87.34	78.41	87.12	91.31
AD/LMCI-CNN-BSVM	90.05	89.56	88.7	97.75

Figure 4. Accuracy of Diagnosis in Alzheimer's Disease

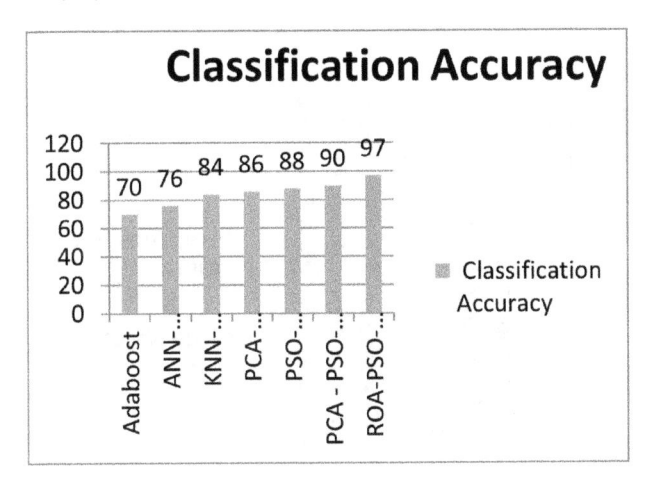

Figure 5. The Ture-positive Prevalence of Alzheimer's Disease

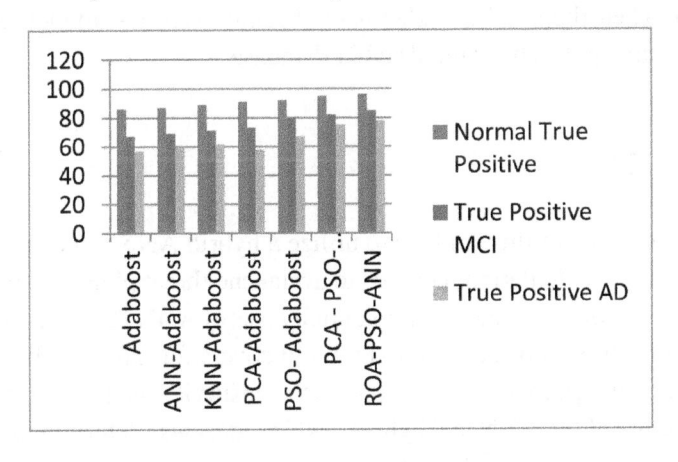

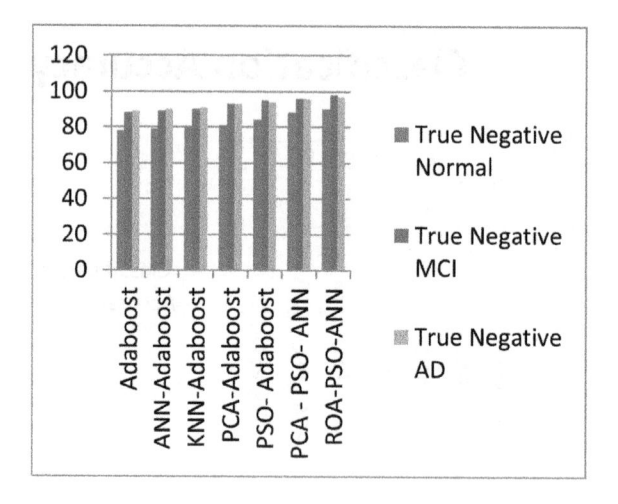

Figure 6. Negative Diagnosis Rates for Alzheimer's Illness

The performance of a network of generative adversarial networks may be improved by using loss values that are drawn repeatedly from the same probability distribution. Then there's the Alzheimer's disease detection model that did well using data from a publicly available MRI database.

CONCLUSION

The primary goal of this study is to utilize a hybrid ANN to enhance the application of forgiving calculation methods to avalanche threat planning. For use in the Finance Application's evaluation of potentially useful ANN PSOs. In this paper, we detail the procedure followed to initially build covers for the contribution records. After applying an optimisation method (such sensitivity analysis) to the data, the optimal structure of the ANN and hybrid ANN models was determined. To evaluate the various approaches, a single ranking mechanism was used as an overall ranking. Using the obtained RMSE indices, several ranking approaches were implemented. Training and test datasets of an optimized hybrid ANN model, built using a suitable geographical database, are provided. Good estimates could be obtained using models based on either ANN or a hybrid of ANN and PSO, However, the hybrid ROA-PSO-ANN ideal may continue presenting by a more reliable and enhanced outcome than ANN due to its larger accuracy in forecasting the LSVs, especially in extremely rare and extremely little targeted exercise and trying the optimised ROA-PSO-ANN extrapolative prototype. As can be seen from the visualization, the results obtained using PSO-ANN are better suited to the intended LSVs. What's more, the fact that the created system yields have a high correctness close even after difficult records indicates that the jointly It's heartening to know that time-tested methods can be put to use with confidence.

REFERENCES

] Alickovic, E., Subasi, A., & Alzheimer's Disease Neuroimaging Initiative. (2020). Automatic detection of alzheimer disease based on histogram and random forest. In *CMBEBIH 2019: Proceedings of the International Conference on Medical and Biological Engineering, 16 18 May 2019, Banja Luka, Bosnia and Herzegovina* (pp. 91-96). Springer International Publishing.

Awate, G., Bangare, S., Pradeepini, G., & Patil, S. (2018). Detection of alzheimers disease from mri using convolutional neural network with tensorflow. *arXiv preprint arXiv:1806.10170*.

Badnjevic, A., Škrbić, R., & Pokvić, L. G. (Eds.). (2019). *CMBEBIH 2019: Proceedings of the International Conference on Medical and Biological Engineering, 16 18 May 2019, Banja Luka, Bosnia and Herzegovina* (Vol. 73). Springer.

Dorigo, M., Birattari, M., & Stutzle, T. (2006). Ant colony optimization. *IEEE Computational Intelligence Magazine*, 1(4), 28–39. 10.1109/MCI.2006.329691

Erkal, B., Başak, S., Çiloğlu, A., & Şener, D. D. (2020, November). Multiclass classification of brain cancer with machine learning algorithms. In *2020 Medical Technologies Congress (TIPTEKNO)* (pp. 1-4). IEEE. 10.1109/TIPTEKNO50054.2020.9299233

Hong, X., Lin, R., Yang, C., Zeng, N., Cai, C., Gou, J., & Yang, J. (2019). Predicting Alzheimer's disease using LSTM. *IEEE Access : Practical Innovations, Open Solutions*, 7, 80893–80901. 10.1109/ACCESS.2019.2919385

Islam, J., & Zhang, Y. (2018). Brain MRI analysis for Alzheimer's disease diagnosis using an ensemble system of deep convolutional neural networks. *Brain Informatics*, 5(2), 1–14. 10.1186/s40708-018-0080-329881892

Kowalski, P. A., & Łukasik, S. (2015). Experimental study of selected parameters of the krill herd algorithm. In *Intelligent Systems' 2014:Proceedings of the 7th IEEE International Conference Intelligent Systems IS'2014, September 24-26, 2014, Warsaw, Poland,* Volume 1*: Mathematical Foundations, Theory, Analyses* (pp. 473-485). Springer International Publishing. 10.1007/978-3-319-11313-5_42

Lee, G., Nho, K., Kang, B., Sohn, K. A., Kim, D., Weiner, M. W., Aisen, P., Petersen, R., Jack, C. R.Jr, Jagust, W., Trojanowki, J. Q., Toga, A. W., Beckett, L., Green, R. C., Saykin, A. J., Morris, J., Shaw, L. M., Khachaturian, Z., Sorensen, G., & Fargher, K. (2019). Predicting Alzheimer's disease progression using multi-modal deep learning approach. *Scientific Reports*, 9(1), 1952. 10.1038/s41598-018-37769-z30760848

Lim, H., & Dewaraja, Y. (2019). *Y-90 patients PET/CT & SPECT/CT and corresponding contours dataset*. University of Michigan-Deep Blue.

Liu, F., Wee, C. Y., Chen, H., & Shen, D. (2014). Inter-modality relationship constrained multi-modality multi-task feature selection for Alzheimer's Disease and mild cognitive impairment identification. *NeuroImage*, 84, 466–475. 10.1016/j.neuroimage.2013.09.01524045077

Martínez-Murcia, F. J., Górriz, J. M., Ramírez, J., Castillo-Barnes, D., Segovia, F., Salas-Gonzalez, D., & Ortiz, A. (2018, November). A deep decomposition of MRI to explore neurodegeneration in Alzheimer's disease. In *2018 IEEE Nuclear Science Symposium and Medical Imaging Conference Proceedings (NSS/MIC)* (pp. 1-3). IEEE. 10.1109/NSSMIC.2018.8824320

Razavi, F., Tarokh, M. J., & Alborzi, M. (2019). An intelligent Alzheimer's disease diagnosis method using unsupervised feature learning. *Journal of Big Data*, 6(1), 32. 10.1186/s40537-019-0190-7

Shankar, K., Lakshmanaprabu, S. K., Khanna, A., Tanwar, S., Rodrigues, J. J., & Roy, N. R. (2019). Alzheimer detection using Group Grey Wolf Optimization based features with convolutional classifier. *Computers & Electrical Engineering*, 77, 230–243. 10.1016/j.compeleceng.2019.06.001

Uysal, G., & Ozturk, M. (2020, November). Classifying early and late mild cognitive impairment stages of Alzheimer's disease by analyzing different brain areas. In *2020 Medical Technologies Congress (TIPTEKNO)* (pp. 1-4). IEEE.

Velazquez, M., Anantharaman, R., Velazquez, S., & Lee, Y., & Alzheimer's Disease Neuroimaging Initiative. (2019, November). RNN-based Alzheimer's disease prediction from prodromal stage using diffusion tensor imaging. In *2019 IEEE International Conference on Bioinformatics and Biomedicine (BIBM)* (pp. 1665-1672). IEEE. 10.1109/BIBM47256.2019.8983391

] Viswanathan, T., Mathankumar, M., & Sasikumar, C. (2020). Medical images processing using effectiveness of walsh function. *Bioscience Biotechnology Research Communications (BBRC), Special Issue*, 13(11), 70-72.

Wurts, A., Oakley, D. H., Hyman, B. T., & Samsi, S. (2020, July). Segmentation of tau stained Alzheimers brain tissue using convolutional neural networks. In *2020 42nd Annual International Conference of the IEEE Engineering in Medicine & Biology Society (EMBC)* (pp. 1420-1423). IEEE. 10.1109/EMBC44109.2020.9175832

Yue, L., Gong, X., Li, J., Ji, H., Li, M., & Nandi, A. K. (2019). Hierarchical feature extraction for early Alzheimer's disease diagnosis. *IEEE Access : Practical Innovations, Open Solutions*, 7, 93752–93760. 10.1109/ACCESS.2019.2926288

Zhao, Y., Ma, B., Jiang, P., Zeng, D., Wang, X., & Li, S. (2020). Prediction of Alzheimer's disease progression with multi-information generative adversarial network. *IEEE Journal of Biomedical and Health Informatics*, 25(3), 711–719. 10.1109/JBHI.2020.300692532750952

Zheng, C., Xia, Y., Pan, Y., & Chen, J. (2016). Automated identification of dementia using medical imaging: A survey from a pattern classification perspective. *Brain Informatics*, 3(1), 17–27. 10.1007/s40708-015-0027-x27747596

Chapter 16
Generative Adversarial Networks for Advanced EEG Data Analysis

Evin Şahin Sadık
Kütahya Dumlupınar University, Turkey

ABSTRACT

This chapter examines the use of Generative Adversarial Networks (GANs) in analyzing electroencephalogram (EEG) data. EEG is an electrophysiological method that records brain activity. EEG is used to diagnose neurological disorders and is also very important for brain-computer interface (BCI) systems. Although EEG data processing and analysis is widely used, it faces some difficulties, which reveals the necessity of advanced signal processing techniques. GANs, on the other hand, are advanced machine learning techniques and play an essential role in EEG data analysis. GANs are known for their ability to produce synthetic data similar to actual data, and this feature provides significant advantages in the analysis of EEG data. In particular, GANs are effective at filtering noise, improving data quality, and generating synthetic data. Given the complexity and diversity of EEG data, caution must be exercised in training GAN models and the accuracy of synthetic data. Current limitations of GANs in EEG data analysis and ongoing research to overcome these limitations are also examined.

INTRODUCTION

Electroencephalography (EEG) is a non-invasive electrophysiological monitoring method used to record brain waves (Sanei and Chambers, 2013). This method is valuable for understanding brain functions, diagnosing neurological disorders,

DOI: 10.4018/979-8-3693-3719-6.ch016

and for use in advanced technologies such as brain-computer interfaces (Wolpaw et al., 2000). EEG plays a critical role in diagnosing and monitoring neurological and psychiatric diseases (Myrden and Chau, 2017). This technique determines seizure activities by detecting abnormal brain waves, especially in the diagnosis of epilepsy (Acharya et al., 2013), distinguishes different stages of sleep (Aboalayon et al., 2016), to confirm brain death (Szurhaj et al. 2015) It checks the presence or absence of brain activity (Constant and Sabourdin, 2012) and to investigate various psychiatric disorders, such as depression (Thibodeau, Jorgensen and Kim, 2006) and schizophrenia (Perrottelli et al., 2021) In this way, EEG contributes to an in-depth understanding of brain functions and the effective treatment of various brain disorders.

Processing and analyzing EEG data poses several challenges. Raw EEG signals may contain noise caused by the movement of electrodes, interference from electrical devices, or patient body movements. These noises make it difficult to interpret EEG signals accurately and can lead to misleading results. Advanced signal processing techniques are needed to extract meaningful and reliable information from EEG data. In addition, some studies cannot collect sufficient EEG signals due to difficulties in collecting EEG signals.

Generative Adversarial Networks (GANs) were first introduced in the early 2000s and have subsequently been recognized as a major innovation in the fields of artificial intelligence and machine learning (Goodfellow et al., 2014). The most remarkable feature of GANs is their capacity to produce high-quality synthetic data that is indistinguishable from real data. This capability offers significant advantages, especially in areas such as expanding data sets, completing missing data, and creating new data types.

Advanced machine learning techniques like GANs play a significant role in EEG data analysis. GANs, known for their ability to generate synthetic data resembling real data, offer important advantages when processing EEG data. In cases where real EEG data is limited, GANs can produce high-quality synthetic EEG data for training and testing purposes. GANs can also be utilized to filter noise and enhance data quality. Synthetic data generated by GANs can help the model learn how to distinguish noise and extract cleaner, more meaningful signals from raw EEG data when compared to real data.

The structure of GANs enables their use in various fields. They find applications in art and design for generating realistic images, creating realistic environments in video games and virtual reality applications, and processing biological and medical data. Particularly in processing complex biological data such as EEG signals, GANs play a significant role in data augmentation, noise reduction, and medical diagnostics.

GANS can enable more accurate analysis of EEG signals and more precise diagnosis of neurological disorders (Carrle, Hollenbenders and Reichenbach, 2023). This is particularly advantageous when data is limited or obtaining real data is challenging. GANs can generate synthetic data in such situations, enriching the datasets and thus facilitating the development of more comprehensive and effective machine learning models.

Traditional methods used in EEG analysis have certain limitations. Particularly, difficulties may arise in processing non-stationary and noisy EEG data. Physiological and environmental noise sources can influence EEG signals, complicating the analysis and interpretation of the data. Artificial intelligence, specifically GANs, comes into play (An, Lam and Ling, 2022).

The applications of GANs in EEG data analysis are not limited to synthetic data generation and noise reduction. GANs can also be utilized when real datasets are missing or insufficient data to investigate rare neurological conditions. This plays a critical role, especially in exploring rare neurological disorders and gaining a better understanding of these conditions. GANs can be used to mimic EEG datasets of such disorders, enabling the modelling of patterns and features specific to these disorders (Habashi et al., 2023). This approach allows for a wider range of data in neurological research, enabling more comprehensive and accurate results to be obtained.

Indeed, GANs also offer significant benefits in the time-series analysis of EEG data (D. Li et al., 2019). EEG signals exhibit varying characteristics over time, and understanding this dynamic nature facilitates better diagnosis and monitoring of neurological conditions. GANs can model these time-series data, allowing for more accurate classification and prediction of specific brain states or disorders. This is particularly crucial for early diagnosis of conditions like epilepsy and for conducting a more detailed analysis of sleep disorders.

Another important application of GAN technology is in the field of brain-computer interfaces (BCI). (X. Zhang, Lu and Li, 2021). BCI systems enable individuals to use brain signals to interact with computers or other devices. GANs can be used to analyze EEG data, allowing for a more accurate understanding of users' intentions and commands, thereby enhancing the accuracy and effectiveness of BCI systems. This can make BCI systems more accessible and effective, especially for individuals with limited mobility.

This section will also address the technical challenges of GAN applications in EEG data analysis and how these challenges are overcome. Training GAN models can be challenging, especially considering the complexity and diversity of EEG data. EEG data exhibit significant variability under individual differences and different conditions. This factor needs to be considered during the training of GAN models. For successful training, the model must learn the complex data structure and generate realistic synthetic data. This process requires continuously assessing the model's learning capacity and the representativeness of the dataset. The quality and diversity of the datasets used in GAN training significantly impact the model's generalization ability. If the dataset is not comprehensive and diverse enough, the model may generate synthetic data that do not accurately reflect real-world data. This situation can lead to severe problems, especially in models used for the diagnosis and treatment of neurological disorders.

BACKGROUND

In recent years, the intersection between artificial intelligence and neuroscience has offered opportunities for understanding the complexity of the human mind and opening new horizons in human-machine interaction. At this intersection, brain signal recording techniques such as EEG play a significant role in developing artificial intelligence algorithms. Remarkably, the impact of deep learning models such as GANs on the synthesis and analysis of EEG data has become a significant research area. In this study, GANs used in EEG studies in the literature will be examined, and their applications in cognitive, emotional, and brain-computer interface studies will be discussed.

Studies conducted using EEG are quite diverse. It has been observed that studies analyzing emotional states using EEG exist, and GANs have been utilized in these studies. In one study, a conditional generative adversarial network (cGAN) was employed to establish a relationship between EEG data and facial images for associating emotional information-containing electroencephalography (EEG) signals with emotional states. The cGAN was used to ensure the connection between a coarse label representing the emotional state and a facial expression image (Fu et al., 2021).

The GAN model has been trained to learn the features of EEG signals and then synthesize new EEG samples based on these features. These synthetic samples have been used to increase the dataset's size and improve the classification models' performance. This study demonstrates how GANs can be utilized to increase the size of datasets used in the analysis of EEG signals and enhance the performance of classification models (Abdelfattah, Abdelrahman and Wang, 2018).

Considering that facial expressions are one of the most effective and direct methods for conveying our emotions and intentions in Brain-Computer Interface (BCI) research, it has been emphasized that research aimed at developing BCIs to assist individuals with facial motor impairments in expressing their emotions is crucial. This article proposes a hybrid GAN-based model that reconstructs personalized facial expressions based on emotional EEG signals. This model is suggested using a Conditional Generative Adversarial Network (cGAN) (Esmaeili and Kiani, 2023).

The effect of combining synthesized data generated using the Conditional Wasserstein Generative Adversarial Network with Gradient Penalty (CWGAN-GP) method as a data augmentation technique with real EEG data on improving classification performance was tested. The results indicate that the proposed model can generate high-quality synthetic EEG data and effectively capture the features of these data in the original EEG data (Z. Li and Yu, 2020).

A new Conditional Wasserstein Generative Adversarial Network with Gradient Penalty (cWGAN-GP) is proposed, which can be trained to synthesize EEG data for different cognitive events. This network addresses several modelling challenges, including frequency artefacts and training instability. The proposed GAN model has been tested to generate single-channel EEG data for rapid serial visual presentation. The authors have demonstrated the validity of the generated samples using several evaluation metrics and shown that the synthesized EEG data can achieve improved event classification performance by augmenting real EEG data (Panwar et al., 2019).

GAN models are also used to enhance low-resolution EEG data. Increasing the current resolution of recorded EEG data ensures effective interpolation of missing or low-quality channels. The quality and details of EEG data are enhanced, allowing for better results in applications such as classification tasks through the use of this improved data (Corley and Huang, 2018).

In studies involving motor imagery and motor imagination, EEG data have been generated using GAN architectures, and these generated data have been subsequently subjected to classification processes to evaluate their performance. The results indicate that GAN-based data augmentation methods outperform traditional methods and improve classification accuracy. This study demonstrates that GANs can effectively generate and classify EEG data (Roy et al., 2020; Xie et al., 2021; K. Zhang et al., 2020).

GANs are also used to repair lost or corrupted portions of EEG signals. EEG-GAN primarily learns the statistical properties of EEG signals and then synthesizes new EEG samples based on these properties. These synthetic samples are used to repair missing or corrupted data segments. The EEG-GAN model is seen as a successful approach to generating EEG signals for repairing lost or corrupted data segments. This could be a versatile tool for improving data quality and repairing corrupted data segments in brain signal studies (Hartmann, Schirrmeister and Ball, 2018).

GAN models are also used to generate new features from EEG signals, and classifications are made based on these new features. The GAN is trained to produce new EEG samples under a specific category using the latent representations learned from EEG signals. Subsequently, a specific classifier model is used to classify these generated samples. In this way, the aim is to utilize the newly generated features by GANs to improve classification performance (Yang et al., 2021).

GAN models are also used to generate images from EEG signals using an encoder-decoder-based approach, simultaneously transforming these signals into real images. An encoder-decoder approach is presented to encode EEG signals and reproduce them visually. Additionally, a GAN is used to transform these obtained EEG signals into real images. This ensures that the images obtained from EEG signals are realistic.

In this process, in addition to the traditional GAN loss, a perceptual loss function is used to achieve higher-quality results. Furthermore, more effective learning is achieved by adding an attention module to the generator part of the network. As a result, this model, called NeuroGAN, can be successfully used to generate realistic images from EEG signals (Mishra et al., 2023).

GANs are also used to clean noise in EEG signals. A GAN-supported parallel Convolutional Neural Network (CNN) and transformer network called GCTNet have been proposed. This network functions by identifying and cleaning various artefacts in EEG signals. The generator part includes parallel CNN and transformer blocks to capture local and global temporal dependencies. Subsequently, a discriminator is used to detect and correct holistic inconsistencies between the cleaned EEG signals and real clean signals. The results of this study demonstrate that this GAN-supported approach outperforms current state-of-the-art networks in cleaning noise in EEG signals (Yin et al., 2023).

This study highlights the strong potential of GAN-based models for analysing and synthesising EEG data. It is expected that the use of GANs will further increase in various applications such as emotion estimation, modeling cognitive events, and even brain-computer interfaces in the future. However, it is important to consider the limitations of existing studies in the current literature. Challenges such as limited datasets and discrepancies between synthesized EEG data and real data can hinder progress in this field. Therefore, future research should focus on overcoming these limitations and enhancing the effectiveness of GAN-based models in EEG analysis and synthesis.

What is GAN? What are the types?

GAN, Generative Adversarial Networks, is an important artificial intelligence model in the field of deep learning. Two artificial neural networks consist of two networks: a generator and a discriminator (Goodfellow et al., 2014). Unlike traditional techniques, GANs generate synthetic data by learning and understanding the true distribution of the dataset. They outperform Autoencoders because they are asymptotically consistent and do not require Markov chains, unlike Boltzmann Machines (Alqahtani, Kavakli-Thorne and Kumar, 2021). GANs consist of two separate neural networks. The general block diagram of GAN is given in Figure 1. The generator and discriminator form GANs. These two networks are trained simultaneously in a zero-sum game framework, where one's gain is the other's loss. While the generative network tries to produce fake data that resembles real data, the discriminative network tries to distinguish these fake data from real data. This process continues, allowing the generator to produce more believable data, and eventually the generator reaches a level where it produces data so realistic that the discriminator cannot distinguish it from real data.

Figure 1. GAN General Working Block Diagram

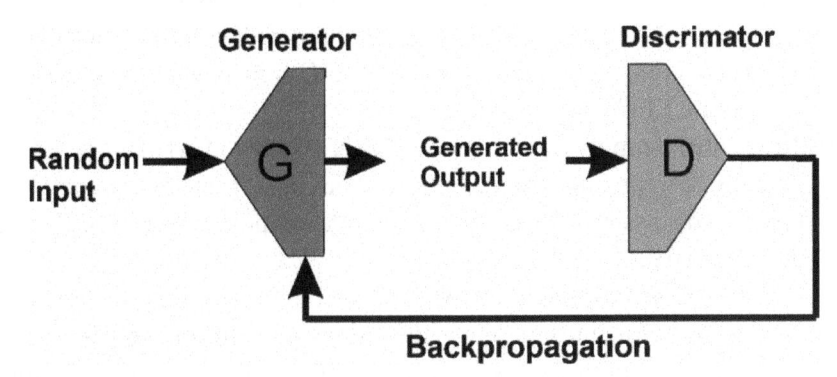

These networks compete and work together to create new data samples. The generator network tries to generate realistic data samples from random noise (usually from a Gauss distribution). For example, an image generator network may attempt to generate realistic images from arbitrary pixel values. The discriminator network distinguishes the data samples created by the generative network from the real data samples. An image discriminator network attempts to determine whether a given image is real or manufactured.

When these two networks come together, the generative network tries to produce data samples that are realistic enough to fool the discriminator network, while the discriminator network tries to improve the performance of the generative network by distinguishing between real and generated samples. In this way, GANs stand out for their ability to generate realistic data. There are many types of GANs due to the multitude of application areas. However, if we talk about some commonly used GAN types, some popular GAN types are as follows:

1. **EEG-GAN:** EEG-GAN, specifically designed for the synthesis and analysis of EEG data, is a specialized type of GAN (Hartmann, Schirrmeister, and Ball 2018). This model is tailored to the unique characteristics of EEG signals within the GAN architecture.EEG-GAN is designed to better capture the complexity and dynamics of EEG signals by incorporating specialized layers or attention mechanisms. These features enable it to generate synthetic data that more accurately reflects the characteristics of EEG signals, thereby enhancing its ability to produce realistic and meaningful synthetic data.

The synthesis and analysis capabilities of EEG-GAN can be customized to suit specific analysis tasks while preserving the characteristics of EEG data. For example, it can be adapted for tasks such as synthesizing EEG data under certain conditions or identifying specific EEG patterns.

In summary, EEG-GAN is a specialized GAN model tailored for the synthesis and analysis of EEG data. It is equipped with customized features to better represent the complexity of EEG signals and can be adapted for specific EEG analysis tasks.

2. **Multivariate Anomaly Detection with GAN (MAD-GAN)**: It is a type of GAN specifically designed for analyzing time series data, particularly complex and multivariate data such as EEG signals, with the purpose of detecting anomalies (D. Li et al. 2019).

    This model employs the GAN architecture to learn the underlying patterns and structures present in the time series data, allowing it to generate synthetic data that closely resembles the original data distribution. By training on normal data samples, MAD-GAN learns to capture the normal behavior of the time series.

    Once trained, MAD-GAN can be used to detect anomalies or deviations from the learned normal behavior in new data instances. Anomalies may include unexpected spikes, irregular patterns, or deviations from the expected distribution of the time series data.

    The advantage of using MAD-GAN for anomaly detection lies in its ability to capture the complex relationships and dependencies present in multivariate time series data, such as EEG signals. By leveraging the generative capabilities of GANs, MAD-GAN can effectively model the temporal dynamics and interactions within the data, making it well-suited for anomaly detection tasks in domains like healthcare, finance, and industrial monitoring.

    In summary, MAD-GAN is a GAN-based model designed to analyze and detect anomalies in complex and multivariate time series data, such as EEG signals, by learning the normal behavior of the data and identifying deviations from it.

3. **Wasserstein GANs (WGANs):** It is a version of GANs trained using the Wasserstein metric as the loss function (Arjovsky, Chintala, and Bottou 2017). They tend to offer more stable educational results. Wasserstein GANs (WGANs) is a type of GAN that uses the Wasserstein metric as the loss function used in GANs. WGANs use the Wasserstein distance (or Earth Mover's Distance) metric, which has been shown to provide more stable training results, rather than Jensen-Shannon divergence or Kullback-Leibler divergence, which are traditional loss functions of GANs (Gulrajani et al. 2017).

The main purpose of Wasserstein GANs is to provide smoother and more stable gradient flow during training and to reduce various problems encountered during training. Therefore, they are especially preferred to reduce mode coverage problems and problems such as gradient explosion or disappearance encountered in training GANs.

Regarding their use with EEG data, in theory, WGANs can be used to process EEG data. WGANs tend to provide more stable training results in general, but how they will perform and what type of results they will provide when used with EEG data in the context of a specific problem should be examined within the scope of research.

4. **Conditional GAN (cGAN):** This type of GAN adds the ability to generate data depending on a condition (Mirza and Osindero, 2014). It ensures that the data generated is created according to a specific condition or tag. cGANs are not used directly with EEG data. However, methods can be developed that can guide or train cGANs using EEG data for a specific purpose.

5. **Conditional Wasserstein GANs (CWGANs):** CWGAN adds a condition to the GAN model (Luo and Lu, 2018). This condition means that the images produced by the generator must meet a certain condition. Compared to non-conditional GANs, CWGANs can perform more specific generation and generate data that meets certain conditions.

6. **Deep Convolutional GANs (DCGANs):** It is a version of GANs combined with convolutional neural networks (CNN) (Radford, Metz and Chintala, 2015). Deep Convolutional GANs (DCGANs) are GANs combined with convolutional neural networks. DCGANs can be used to generate or transform data representing EEG signals. However, EEG data is generally time series data, unlike direct image data. Therefore, using EEG data with DCGANs may face some challenges. EEG data can be converted into image data by appropriately processing and representing it when using DCGANs. Some DCGAN variations can be customized to work directly with EEG data, such as time series data. This may require changing the input layer or processing mechanism of the network. Using EEG data with DCGANs or other types of GANs requires selecting appropriate processing and representation methods in the context of a particular problem and adapting the model accordingly. Realizing such applications requires appropriate research and development efforts.

7. **CycleGANs**: A type of GANs that have the ability to transform between two different data distributions (Zhu et al., 2017). They are trained without matching when transforming from one data distribution to another. CycleGANs are not used directly with EEG data. However, to convert or synthesize EEG data for a specific purpose or with EEG topographies (Xu et al., 2021) CycleGANs can

be used together. The CycleGAN model can be used to transform EEG data when transforming between two different data distributions.

8. **StyleGAN:** StyleGAN is based on the original GAN (Generative Adversarial Network) architecture, and this model innovatively uses "style transfer", a technique used to train GANs and produce more realistic, high-quality images. StyleGAN consists of a generator and discriminator, which are the basic logic of GANs. The generator generates images starting from random noise, while the discriminator is trained by learning the difference between the real images and the generated images. Style transfer is the process of applying the features of a pre-trained model onto another image. In StyleGAN, this is usually achieved by applying the style learned from a dataset to an image created from random noise. One of the most important features of StyleGAN is its high-quality of images. This is usually achieved through various techniques to increase resolution and detail. These techniques include the use of various deep learning architectures, batch normalization, and more specific techniques used for style transfer. StyleGAN also has a mechanism that allows for the controlling of certain properties of the generated images. StyleGAN has no direct EEG-related use. However, some researchers and developers can use deep learning techniques such as StyleGAN for different purposes by combining them with brain activity data.

9. **NeuroGAN:** Refers to a concept often associated with brain signals or neurological data with types of GANs. NeuroGAN uses the GAN structure to analyze, synthesize or transform neurological data. NeuroGAN generally uses two main methods when handling neurological data: NeuroGAN can be used to create artificial brain signals that resemble real brain signals. This could be useful in neurological research or in the development of medical diagnostics and treatment methods. For example, NeuroGAN can be used to synthesize neurological data such as EEG or fMRI. NeuroGAN can also be used to transform one type of brain signal or neurological data into another type. For example, it can convert one person's brain signals into another person's signals or reduce the symptoms of a neurological disease. The term NeuroGAN is often used to refer to such applications. However, it is not a standardized term to describe any particular model or technique. Therefore, a specific study or application is meant when talking about a model or technique called NeuroGAN.

10. **Attention-based Generative Adversarial Networks (AttnGAN):** AttnGAN is a proposed GAN model for text-based visual synthesis, but it can also be used with time-series data such as EEG data. AttnGAN leverages attention mechanisms to synthesize visual contents into more realistic and natural images. This model can produce more realistic results by focusing on specific features of the data and better reflect the dynamics of EEG data over time. When used with EEG data, the AttnGAN model can be particularly useful for focusing on specific

brain activities or synthesizing specific EEG patterns. For example, it can be used to simulate a particular brain state or capture individual differences from EEG data. Attention-based GAN models like AttnGAN have enhanced features to better represent the complexity and dynamics of EEG data. Therefore, using attention-based GAN models when working with EEG data can be a potential way to achieve more realistic and meaningful results.

USE OF GAN IN EEGS

EEG is a method used to measure brain activity. However, collecting datasets is a difficult and troublesome process. A lot of data is needed to examine a problem. In this regard, GANs can be used with EEG data and can have various applications in different fields. Figure 2 shows some areas where GANs are used in EEG analysis as a diagram.

Figure 2. EEG-GAN Usage Areas

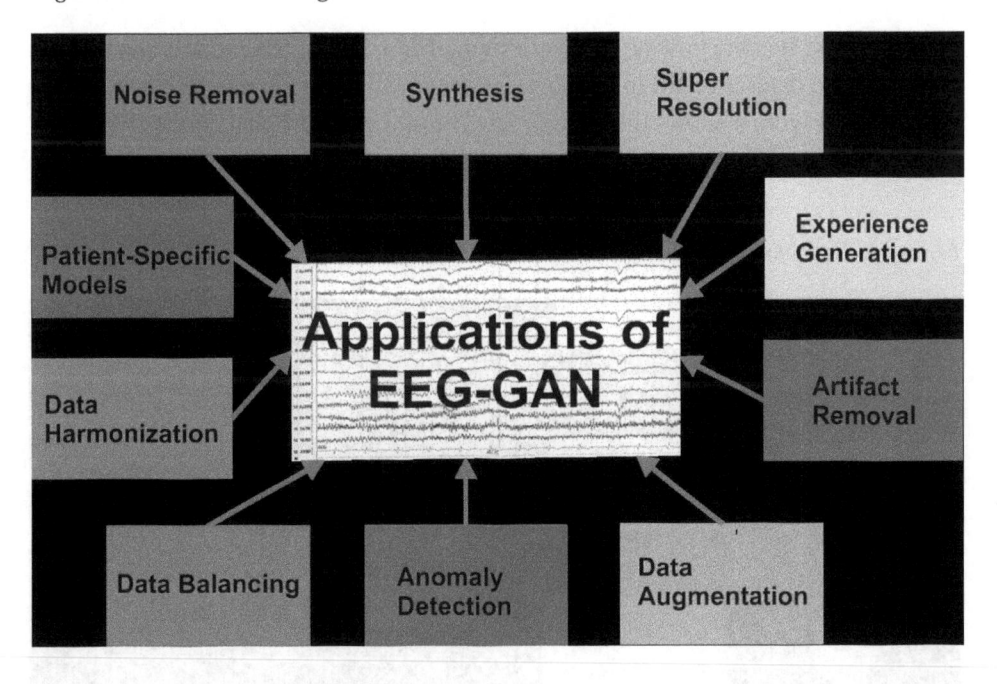

Noise Removal: It is the process of removing noise from EEG data. GANs can be used to clean up noise caused by electrode movements, device interference or external factors. Cleaned data is important for accurate analysis and interpretation. Figure 3 shows the block diagram showing the use of GAN in cleaning a noisy EEG signal.

Figure 3. Using GAN in Noise Removal from EEG Signals

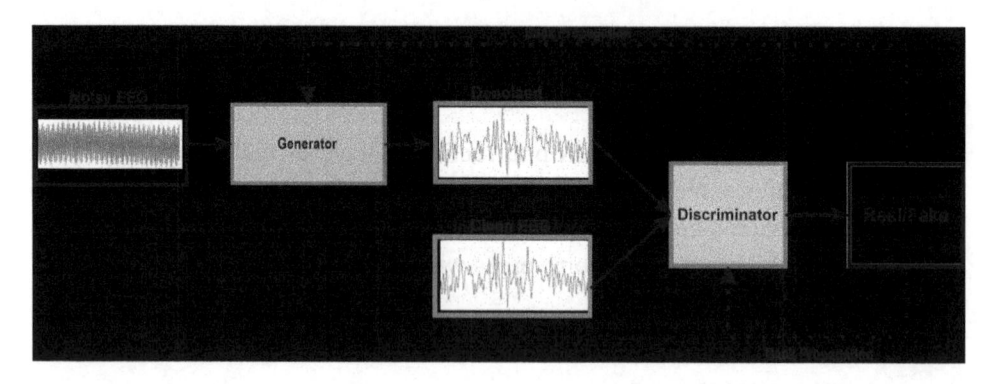

Synthesis: It is the process of synthesizing EEG data. GAN models can be used to expand the dataset or fill in missing data by creating artificial EEG data similar to real data. Figure 4 shows the general scheme of the system that creates EEG data with GAN and tries to understand whether the data is real or fake.

Figure 4. Processing of EEG Data with GAN

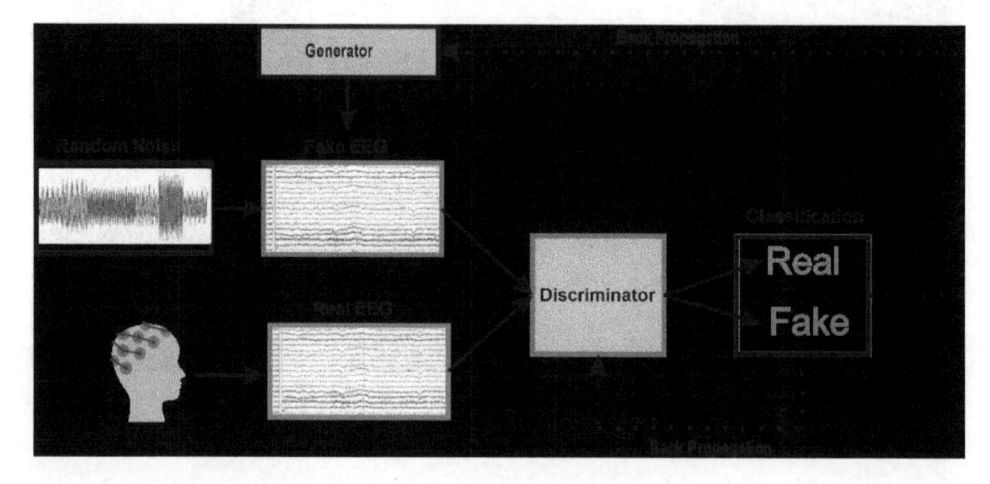

Super-Resolution: It is the process of converting low-resolution EEG data into high-resolution data. With this transformation process, GAN allows for a more detailed analysis or for certain features to be seen more clearly. It is a set of methods that can help the user in case of difficulties encountered while recording data or if the devices cannot record high enough resolution data.

Experience Generation: GANs is the process of generating EEG data to simulate a specific situation. This can be used to create experiences for therapeutic uses or learning purposes.

Artifact Removal: It is the process of removing artifacts from EEG data with GAN. Artifacts may arise from factors such as electrode placement or external factors and may prevent accurate analysis.

Data Augmentation: It is the process of diversifying existing EEG data with GAN. This allows the model to be trained to increase its generalization ability and cover a more diverse range of situations.

Anomaly Detection: GANs are also used to detect abnormal EEG activities. Thus, it can help identify and diagnose unexpected conditions such as epileptic seizures.

Data Balancing: Correcting class imbalance in the EEG data set is another area of use of GANs. It can be used to ensure enough data from each class and balances the model's training.

Data Harmonization is the process of harmonizing EEG data obtained from different sources with GAN. It increases the consistency of the data set and makes it easier to combine data from different sources.

Patient-Specific Models: With GAN, customized EEG analysis models can be created for individual patients. This enables the development of personalized approaches to create more effective patient treatment plans.

Some of the current studies in the literature on the use of GAN in EEGs are given in Table 1. Various researchers and studies have focused on mood analysis, EEG signal analysis, brain-computer interfaces, motor imagery tasks, EEG data generation, EEG data restoration, EEG feature generation, EEG data visualization, EEG noise removal, study of neurological disorders, time series analysis, and has examined the use of EEG-GANs in different fields such as brain-computer interfaces.

It shows that EEG-GANs are effective for various purposes and make significant contributions to processes such as processing, synthesis, cleaning, classification and modeling of EEG data. In addition, it is stated that EEG-GANs are effective in advanced applications such as modeling rare neurological disorders, developing and increasing the use of BCI systems. These studies highlight that EEG-GANs are considered an important tool in the field of neuroscience and medicine and that more research is needed in the future. The potential of EEG-GANs remains to be further explored in areas such as diagnosis and treatment of neurological disorders, brain-computer interface technology, and mood analysis.

Table 1. Studies Using GAN and EEG

Reference	Application Area	GAN Model Used	Highlights
Fu et al. (2021)	Sentiment Analysis	Conditional Generative Adversarial Network (cGAN)	Association of emotional state with EEG signals.
Abdelfattah, Abdelrahman, and Wang (2018)	EEG Signal Analysis	GAN	Increasing the Dimensionality and Classification of EEG Datasets
Esmaeili and Kiani (2023)	Brain-Computer Interface (BCI)	Conditional Generative Adversarial Network (cGAN)	Reconstruction of facial expressions from emotional EEG signals
Z. Li and Yu (2020)	Motor Imagery Tasks Conditional	Wasserstein Generative Adversarial Network (CWGAN-GP)	Synthesized EEG data for motor imagery tasks
Panwar et al. (2019)	EEG Data Generation	Conditional Wasserstein Generative Adversarial Network (cWGAN-GP)	Synthesis and classification of EEG data
Roy et al. (2020)	Imaginary Movement and Motor Imagery Studies	GAN	Synthesis and classification of EEG data
Xie et al. (2021)	Imaginary Movement and Motor Imagery Studies	Long Short-Term Memory Generative Adversarial Networks (LGAN)	Synthesis and classification of EEG data
K. Zhang et al. (2020)	Imaginary Movement and Motor Imagery Studies	Conditional GAN (cGAN)	Synthesis and classification of EEG data
Hartmann, Schirrmeister, and Ball (2018)	EEG Data Repair	EEG-GAN	EEG-GAN Repair and classification of EEG data
Yang et al. (2021)	EEG Feature Generation	Conditional Variational Autoencoder-Generative Adversarial Network (CVAE-GAN)	Feature generation and classification from EEG data
Mishra et al. (2023)	EEG Data Visualization	NeuroGAN	Generation of realistic images from EEG signals
Yin et al. (2023)	EEG Noise Removal	GAN-supported parallel CNN and transformer network	Noise removal from EEG signals
Carrle, Hollenbenders, and Reichenbach (2023)	EEG Data Synthesis	GAN	Synthesis and expansion of EEG data set
An, Lam, and Ling (2022)	EEG Data Cleaning	GAN	Noise reduction and improvement of data quality

continued on following page

Table 1. Continued

Reference	Application Area	GAN Model Used	Highlights
Habashi et al. (2023)	EEG Data Analysis and Modeling	GAN	Modeling of EEG data and investigation of rare disorders
D. Li et al. (2019)	Time Series Analysis	Multivariate Anomaly Detection with GAN (MAD-GAN)	Modeling and classification of time series data
X. Zhang, Lu, and Li (2021)	Brain-Computer Interfaces	Conditional Generative Adversarial Network (cGAN)	Enhancement of BCI systems and promotion of usage

GAN USAGE ISSUES AND CHALLENGES

The use of GANs in EEG data provides some conveniences, but also poses various challenges and problems. To list a few of these problems:

EEG data can vary significantly between individuals and under different experiences or conditions. Therefore, collecting a sufficient and representative dataset to train GANs can be challenging. Additionally, the quality and diversity of EEG data can affect the accuracy and generalization ability of GANs.

EEG signals can contain noise and artifacts from various sources, which can make it difficult for GANs to process and synthesize EEG data accurately. Special techniques may need to be developed to identify and remove noise and artifacts.

EEG data is typically high-dimensional and complex, which can pose challenges for GANs to effectively process and synthesize such data. Techniques such as dimensionality reduction and feature selection may need to be employed.

GANs may encounter instability issues during training, which can affect the consistency of results. Additionally, it is important to evaluate how closely the synthetic data generated by GANs resembles real data and to verify the reliability of the model.

There can be significant differences in brain activity and EEG signals among different patients. GANs may need to be flexible to capture these differences and account for individual variations.

EEG data may contain personal and sensitive information. Therefore, it is important for GANs to process and store this data in accordance with ethical and privacy standards.

Despite these challenges, GANs have significant potential in the analysis, synthesis, and processing of EEG data, and overcoming these challenges is expected with the development of these technologies in the future.

SOLUTIONS AND RECOMMENDATIONS

For advanced EEG data analysis using GANs, there are various solution proposals that can enhance the effectiveness and reliability of the process. Here are some suggestions:

Ensure thorough preprocessing of EEG data before feeding it into the GAN model. Filtering noise, cleaning artifacts, and normalization can improve data quality and consistency.

Select a GAN architecture suitable for EEG data characteristics, such as Conditional GANs (cGANs) or Wasserstein GANs (WGANs), which can address the complexities of EEG data and lead to better convergence.

Design appropriate loss functions for EEG data analysis tasks, taking into account unique features such as temporal dynamics, frequency components, and spatial information of EEG signals.

When dealing with limited EEG datasets, apply regularization techniques to prevent overfitting and enhance the generalization ability of the GAN model.

Increase the diversity and size of the EEG dataset using data augmentation techniques such as time warping, random cropping, and amplitude scaling to generate additional training examples, thereby improving the robustness of the GAN model.

Expedite the transfer learning and convergence process by pretraining the GAN model on relevant EEG datasets or tasks and then fine-tuning the model for the specific analysis task of interest.

Define appropriate evaluation metrics to accurately assess the performance of the GAN model, such as signal-to-noise ratio (SNR), cross-correlation, or spectral coherence, to measure the quality of generated EEG signals compared to real data.

Integrate interpretability and explainability techniques into the decision-making process of the GAN model, such as attention mechanisms or saliency mapping, to demonstrate which EEG features are most relevant for producing optimal outputs.

Foster collaboration among neuroscientists, signal processing experts, and machine learning practitioners to leverage domain knowledge and develop scientifically sound and practically useful GAN models for EEG data analysis.

Address ethical considerations, especially concerning privacy and security, when working with sensitive EEG data by implementing data anonymization and protection measures to ensure data security and integrity throughout the analysis process.

By considering these solution proposals, researchers can enhance the usability, reliability, and interpretability of GAN-based approaches for advanced EEG data analysis, providing valuable insights into brain function and dynamics.

FUTURE RESEARCH DIRECTIONS

In addition to the technologies used today, artificial intelligence technologies continue to advance in the future and provide support for studies in different branches of health. The use of artificial intelligence technologies in biological signals, such as cancer detection (Balaji et al. 2024) and ECG (Boulif et al. 2023) and EEG, will increase. For future research directions in advanced EEG data analysis using GANs, focusing on various key areas can address current limitations and explore new opportunities. Here are some potential research directions:

Develop GAN architectures that effectively capture the temporal dynamics of EEG signals. This may involve incorporating techniques such as recurrent neural networks (RNNs) or temporal convolutional networks (TCNs) into the GAN framework to better model the sequential nature of EEG data and capture long-term dependencies.

Explore techniques to enhance the spatial modeling capabilities of GANs for EEG data analysis. This could involve using techniques such as attention mechanisms or graph neural networks (GNNs) to capture spatial relationships between different EEG channels and improve the generation of realistic spatial patterns.

Investigate methods for integrating EEG data with other modalities, such as functional magnetic resonance imaging (fMRI) or electrocardiography (ECG). Multimodal GAN architectures can leverage complementary information from different modalities to enhance understanding of brain function and dynamics

Develop transfer learning and domain adaptation techniques to facilitate knowledge transfer across different EEG datasets or tasks. Pretraining GAN models on large-scale unlabeled EEG datasets or related tasks and then fine-tuning the models for specific analysis tasks can improve adaptation and performance.

Address the resilience and generalization challenges of GANs in EEG data analysis. Research efforts can focus on developing robust training algorithms, regularization techniques, and adversarial training strategies to improve model generalization across diverse EEG datasets and conditions.

Enhance the interpretability and explainability of GAN-based models for EEG data analysis. Techniques for visualizing and interpreting learned representations, attention mechanisms, or decision-making processes of GAN models can provide insights into fundamental neural processes and phenomena.

Explore real-time and online EEG data analysis methods using GANs. Developing methods for real-time monitoring and analysis of brain activity by leveraging lightweight GAN architectures, efficient inference algorithms, and streaming data processing techniques can enable applications such as brain-computer interfaces (BCIs) or neurobiofeedback systems.

Investigate the potential clinical applications of GANs in EEG data analysis for diagnosis, prognosis, and treatment monitoring of neurological and psychiatric disorders. Collaborating with healthcare professionals to validate the effectiveness of GAN-based approaches in real-world clinical settings can translate research findings into clinical practice.

Address ethical and privacy considerations associated with the use of GANs in EEG data analysis. Developing guidelines and best practices for responsible data collection, processing, and sharing is essential to ensure ethical use of EEG data and protection of individuals' privacy rights.

Establish reference datasets and standardized evaluation metrics for comparing GAN-based approaches in EEG data analysis. This facilitates fair comparisons between different methods and encourages reproducible research in the field.

By following these future research directions, the application of GANs in advanced EEG data analysis can be further advanced. This can lead to a better understanding of brain function and dynamics, as well as the development of innovative diagnostic and therapeutic tools for neurological and psychiatric disorders.

CONCLUSION

Generative Adversarial Networks (GANs) offer significant promises in advancing the analysis of Electroencephalography (EEG) data, providing innovative solutions to the complex challenges encountered in understanding brain function and dynamics. With their ability to generate realistic EEG signals, GANs offer valuable tools in various fields such as neuroscience, clinical diagnosis, and brain-computer interface technologies.

The potential of GANs in EEG data analysis lies in their capacity to capture the temporal and spatial complexities of brain activity, model intricate patterns in EEG signals, and facilitate the integration of multimodal information. Through the use of GANs, researchers can explore new perspectives on brain function, identify biomarkers for neurological disorders, and develop personalized diagnostic and treatment interventions.

However, effective utilization of GANs in advanced EEG data analysis requires addressing several key challenges, including temporal and spatial modeling, robustness, interpretability, and ethical considerations. Future research efforts should focus on developing customized GAN architectures, innovative training strategies, and rigorous evaluation methodologies tailored to the unique characteristics of EEG data.

Collaboration between researchers in machine learning, neuroscience, and clinical applications is vital to ensure the development of GAN-based approaches that are both scientifically robust and clinically relevant. By fostering interdisciplinary collaborations and promoting open sharing of data and methodologies, GAN-based innovations can be rapidly translated into real-world applications, leading to improved outcomes for patients with neurological and psychiatric disorders.

Generative Adversarial Networks present opportunities to advance the analysis of EEG data, enabling researchers and clinicians to gain new insights into the complexities of the human brain and develop transformative solutions to enhance brain health and well-being. However, over-reliance on artificial intelligence algorithms in medical decision-making brings with it potential risks. Since artificial intelligence technologies are still in the process of development, these technologies should not be completely relied upon in diagnosis and treatment processes. These technologies are still open to development and their shortcomings need to be completely closed.

REFERENCES

Abdelfattah, S. M. Ghodai M Abdelrahman, and Min Wang. 2018. "Augmenting the Size of EEG Datasets Using Generative Adversarial Networks." In *2018 International Joint Conference on Neural Networks (IJCNN)*, IEEE, 1–6.

Aboalayon, K. A. I., Faezipour, M., Almuhammadi, W. S., & Moslehpour, S. (2016). Sleep stage classification using EEG signal analysis: A comprehensive survey and new investigation. *Entropy (Basel, Switzerland)*, 18(9), 272.

Acharya, U. R., Sree, S. V., Swapna, G., Martis, R. J., & Suri, J. S. (2013). Automated EEG analysis of epilepsy: A review. *Knowledge-Based Systems*, 45, 147–165.

Alqahtani, H., Kavakli-Thorne, M., & Kumar, G. (2021). Applications of Generative Adversarial Networks (Gans): An Updated Review. *Archives of Computational Methods in Engineering*, 28(2), 525–552. 10.1007/s11831-019-09388-y

An, Y., Lam, H. K., & Ling, S. H. (2022). Auto-Denoising for EEG Signals Using Generative Adversarial Network. *Sensors (Basel)*, 22(5), 1750. 10.3390/s2205175035270895

Arjovsky, M., Chintala, S., & Bottou, L. 2017. "Wasserstein Generative Adversarial Networks." In *International Conference on Machine Learning*, PMLR, 214–23.

Balaji, G. N., & Sahaaya Arul Mary, S. A. (2024). Graph CNN-ResNet-CSOA Transfer Learning Architype for an Enhanced Skin Cancer Detection and Classification Scheme in Medical Image Processing. *International Journal of Artificial Intelligence Tools*, 33(02), 2350063. 10.1142/S021821302350063X

Boulif, A., Ananou, B., Ouladsine, M., & Delliaux, S. (2023). A Literature Review: ECG-Based Models for Arrhythmia Diagnosis Using Artificial Intelligence Techniques. *Bioinformatics and Biology Insights*, 17, 11779322221149600. 10.1177/11779322221149600036798080

Carrle, F. P., Hollenbenders, Y., & Reichenbach, A. (2023). Generation of Synthetic EEG Data for Training Algorithms Supporting the Diagnosis of Major Depressive Disorder. *Frontiers in Neuroscience*, 17, 1219133. 10.3389/fnins.2023.121913337849893

Constant, I., & Sabourdin, N. (2012). The EEG Signal: A Window on the Cortical Brain Activity. *Paediatric Anaesthesia*, 22(6), 539–552. 10.1111/j.1460-9592.2012.03883.x22594406

Corley, I. A., & Huang, Y. 2018. "Deep EEG Super-Resolution: Upsampling EEG Spatial Resolution with Generative Adversarial Networks." In *2018 IEEE EMBS International Conference on Biomedical & Health Informatics (BHI)*, IEEE, 100–103. 10.1109/BHI.2018.8333379

Esmaeili, M., & Kiani, K. (2023). Generating Personalized Facial Emotions Using Emotional EEG Signals and Conditional Generative Adversarial Networks. *Multimedia Tools and Applications*, 83(12), 1–26. 10.1007/s11042-023-17018-w

Fu, B., Li, F., Niu, Y., Wu, H., Li, Y., & Shi, G. (2021). Conditional Generative Adversarial Network for EEG-Based Emotion Fine-Grained Estimation and Visualization. *Journal of Visual Communication and Image Representation*, 74, 102982. 10.1016/j.jvcir.2020.102982

Goodfellow, I.. (2014). Generative Adversarial Nets. *Advances in Neural Information Processing Systems*, •••, 27.

Gulrajani, I.. (2017). Improved Training of Wasserstein Gans. *Advances in Neural Information Processing Systems*, •••, 30.

Habashi, A. G., Azab, A. M., Eldawlatly, S., & Aly, G. M. (2023). Generative Adversarial Networks in EEG Analysis: An Overview. *Journal of Neuroengineering and Rehabilitation*, 20(1), 40. 10.1186/s12984-023-01169-w37038142

Hartmann, K. G., Schirrmeister, R. T., & Ball, T. 2018. "EEG-GAN: Generative Adversarial Networks for Electroencephalograhic (EEG) Brain Signals." *arXiv preprint arXiv:1806.01875*.

Li, D., ... 2019. "MAD-GAN: Multivariate Anomaly Detection for Time Series Data with Generative Adversarial Networks." In *International Conference on Artificial Neural Networks*, Springer, 703–16. 10.1007/978-3-030-30490-4_56

Li, Z., & Yu, Y. 2020. "Improving EEG-Based Motor Imagery Classification with Conditional Wasserstein GAN." In *2020 International Conference on Image, Video Processing and Artificial Intelligence*, SPIE, 437–43. 10.1117/12.2581328

Luo, Y., & Lu, B.-L. 2018. "EEG Data Augmentation for Emotion Recognition Using a Conditional Wasserstein GAN." In *2018 40th Annual International Conference of the IEEE Engineering in Medicine and Biology Society (EMBC)*, IEEE, 2535–38. 10.1109/EMBC.2018.8512865

Mirza, M., & Osindero, S. 2014. "Conditional Generative Adversarial Nets." *arXiv preprint arXiv:1411.1784*.

Mishra, R., Sharma, K., Jha, R. R., & Bhavsar, A. (2023). NeuroGAN: Image Reconstruction from EEG Signals via an Attention-Based GAN. *Neural Computing & Applications*, 35(12), 9181–9192.

Myrden, A., & Chau, T. (2017). A Passive EEG-BCI for Single-Trial Detection of Changes in Mental State. *IEEE Transactions on Neural Systems and Rehabilitation Engineering*, 25(4), 345–356. 10.1109/TNSRE.2016.264195628092565

Panwar, S., Rad, P., Quarles, J., & Huang, Y. 2019. "Generating EEG Signals of an RSVP Experiment by a Class Conditioned Wasserstein Generative Adversarial Network." In *2019 IEEE International Conference on Systems, Man and Cybernetics (SMC)*, IEEE, 1304–10. 10.1109/SMC.2019.8914492

Perrottelli, A., Giordano, G. M., Brando, F., Giuliani, L., & Mucci, A. (2021). EEG-Based Measures in at-Risk Mental State and Early Stages of Schizophrenia: A Systematic Review. *Frontiers in Psychiatry*, 12, 653642. 10.3389/fpsyt.2021.65364234017273

Radford, A., Metz, L., & Chintala, S. 2015. "Unsupervised Representation Learning with Deep Convolutional Generative Adversarial Networks." *arXiv preprint arXiv:1511.06434*.

Roy, S., Dora, S., McCreadie, K., & Prasad, G. 2020. "MIEEG-GAN: Generating Artificial Motor Imagery Electroencephalography Signals." In *2020 International Joint Conference on Neural Networks (IJCNN)*, IEEE, 1–8. 10.1109/IJCNN48605.2020.9206942

Sanei, S., & Chambers, J. A. (2013). *EEG signal processing*. John Wiley & Sons.

Szurhaj, W., Lamblin, M.-D., Kaminska, A., & Sediri, H. (2015). "EEG Guidelines in the Diagnosis of Brain Death." *Neurophysiologie Clinique. Clinical Neurophysiology*, 45(1), 97–104. 10.1016/j.neucli.2014.11.00525687591

Thibodeau, R., Jorgensen, R. S., & Kim, S. (2006). Depression, Anxiety, and Resting Frontal EEG Asymmetry: A Meta-Analytic Review. *Journal of Abnormal Psychology*, 115(4), 715–729. 10.1037/0021-843X.115.4.71517100529

Wolpaw, J. R., Birbaumer, N., Heetderks, W. J., McFarland, D. J., Peckham, P. H., Schalk, G., Donchin, E., Quatrano, L. A., Robinson, C. J., & Vaughan, T. M. (2000). Brain-Computer Interface Technology: A Review of the First International Meeting. *IEEE Transactions on Rehabilitation Engineering*, 8(2), 164–173. 10.1109/TRE.2000.84780710896178

Xie, J., Siyu, C., Zhang, Y., Gao, D., & Liu, T. (2021). Combining Generative Adversarial Networks and Multi-Output CNN for Motor Imagery Classification. *Journal of Neural Engineering*, 18(4), 46026. 10.1088/1741-2552/abecc533821808

Xu, F., Rong, F., Leng, J., Sun, T., Zhang, Y., Siddharth, S., & Jung, T.-P. (2021). Classification of Left-versus Right-Hand Motor Imagery in Stroke Patients Using Supplementary Data Generated by CycleGAN. *IEEE Transactions on Neural Systems and Rehabilitation Engineering*, 29, 2417–2424. 10.1109/TNSRE.2021.312396934710045

Yang, J., Yu, H., Shen, T., Song, Y., & Chen, Z. (2021). 4-Class Mi-Eeg Signal Generation and Recognition with Cvae-Gan. *Applied Sciences (Basel, Switzerland)*, 11(4), 1798. 10.3390/app11041798

Yin, J.. (2023). A GAN Guided Parallel CNN and Transformer Network for EEG Denoising. *IEEE Journal of Biomedical and Health Informatics*.37220036

Zhang, K., Xu, G., Han, Z., Ma, K., Zheng, X., Chen, L., Duan, N., & Zhang, S. (2020). Data Augmentation for Motor Imagery Signal Classification Based on a Hybrid Neural Network. *Sensors (Basel)*, 20(16), 1–20. 10.3390/s2016448532796607

Zhang, X., Lu, Z., & Li, H. (2021). Realizing the Application of EEG Modeling in BCI Classification: Based on a Conditional GAN Converter. *Frontiers in Neuroscience*, 15, 727394. 10.3389/fnins.2021.72739434867150

Zhu, J.-Y., Park, T., & Isola, P., and Alexei A Efros. 2017. "Unpaired Image-to-Image Translation Using Cycle-Consistent Adversarial Networks." In *Proceedings of the IEEE International Conference on Computer Vision*, 2223–32. 10.1109/ICCV.2017.244

Chapter 17
Confluence of Deep Learning Using Watershed Segmentation GAN for Advancing Endoscopy Surgery Imaging

G. Megala
https://orcid.org/0000-0002-8084-8292
Vellore Institute of Technology, India

P. Swarnalatha
Vellore Institute of Technology, India

S. Prabu
https://orcid.org/0000-0002-5797-1655
Pondicherry University, India

R. Venkatesan
https://orcid.org/0000-0002-4336-8628
SASTRA University (Deemed), India

Anantharajah Kaneswaran
University of Jaffna, Sri Lanka

DOI: 10.4018/979-8-3693-3719-6.ch017

Copyright © 2024, IGI Global. Copying or distributing in print or electronic forms without written permission of IGI Global is prohibited.

ABSTRACT

Accurate segmentation in medical images is critical for effective diagnosis and treatment. This study presents a novel approach using a watershed-segmented Generative Adversarial Network (GAN) for segmentation in the Cholec80 laparoscopic cholecystectomy videos. Initially, a watershed algorithm preprocesses the images, providing robust initial segmentation that highlights potential lesion boundaries. This segmented output trains a GAN, which refines and improves segmentation accuracy. The GAN comprises a generator producing segmentation masks and a discriminator evaluating their realism against ground truth. Evaluated on the Cholec80 dataset, our approach demonstrates significant improvements in segmentation accuracy over existing methods. Quantitative results indicate superior performance in dice coefficient, intersection over union (IoU), and other metrics. Qualitative analysis supports the efficacy of our method in accurately delineating boundaries in complex surgical scenes. This integration presents a promising direction for enhancing medical image analysis.

INTRODUCTION

The field of healthcare has undergone a transformative evolution with the advent of innovative technologies, among which Deep Learning(DL) and generative artificial intelligence (AI) stand out prominently. In the context of endoscopy surgery, these technologies have emerged as powerful tools capable of revolutionizing diagnostic accuracy, surgical training, and overall patient care within the framework of smart healthcare systems. The convergence of deep learning and generative AI has revolutionized the landscape of healthcare, particularly in the domain of endoscopy surgery. This paper explores the synergistic application of these cutting-edge technologies to advance the capabilities of endoscopic procedures within the context of smart healthcare systems.

Deep learning models such as Residual Neural Networks(RNN) and convolution neural network(CNN), have established incredible achievement in classifying images, image recognition, segmentation, and feature extraction. In the realm of endoscopy, these capabilities can be harnessed to enhance real-time image analysis, enabling more accurate diagnosis and surgical interventions. The integration of DL models facilitates the automatic identification of anomalies, tumors or lesions, and other critical information during endoscopic examinations. Generative AI, exemplified by generative adversarial networks (GANs), brings forth the potential to generate synthetic and high-fidelity medical imagery. By leveraging generative models, practitioners can simulate diverse scenarios, providing a valuable training ground for surgeons and healthcare professionals. This fosters a safer and more efficient environment for honing skills and refining techniques in endoscopy surgery.

The amalgamation of deep learning and generative AI technologies offers a holistic approach to smart healthcare in endoscopy. Real-time analysis powered by deep learning ensures prompt and accurate detection of abnormalities, while generative AI contributes to the creation of realistic virtual environments for training and simulation purposes. This dual-pronged strategy not only enhances the diagnostic accuracy but also promotes continuous learning and skill development among healthcare practitioners. Moreover, the integration of these technologies into smart healthcare systems facilitates the seamless exchange and analysis of patient data, supporting collaborative decision-making among healthcare professionals. The deployment of intelligent endoscopy systems ensures that the benefits of deep learning and generative AI are harnessed to their full potential, contributing to improved patient outcomes and overall healthcare efficiency.

Deep learning, particularly through convolutional neural networks (CNNs) (Choi et al., 2020; Megala et al., 2023), has demonstrated unparalleled success in image recognition, segmentation, and feature extraction. In the intricate realm of endoscopy, where precise and rapid analysis of visual data is paramount, the application of deep learning algorithms holds great promise. Real-time identification of anomalies, lesions, and critical diagnostic information during endoscopic procedures becomes not only possible but significantly enhanced, thereby advancing the capabilities of healthcare practitioners.

Complementing the prowess of deep learning, generative AI, exemplified by generative adversarial networks (GANs), introduces a paradigm shift in surgical training and simulation. The ability to generate realistic synthetic medical imagery facilitates a dynamic learning environment for surgeons, allowing them to hone their skills and refine techniques in a risk-free virtual space. This innovative approach not only contributes to the continuous improvement of healthcare professionals but also enhances the safety and efficiency of endoscopic procedures.

This paper explores the synergistic integration of deep learning and generative AI in the context of endoscopy surgery within the framework of smart healthcare systems. The aim is to elucidate how these technologies, when combined, contribute to a holistic and intelligent approach that goes beyond mere diagnostics. The confluence of deep learning and generative AI is poised to redefine endoscopic surgery, offering not only real-time diagnostic accuracy but also a transformative platform for ongoing training, collaboration, and data-driven decision-making in healthcare.

Moreover, the integration of these technologies into smart healthcare systems facilitates the seamless exchange and analysis of patient data, supporting collaborative decision-making among healthcare professionals. The deployment of intelligent endoscopy systems ensures that the benefits of deep learning and generative AI are harnessed to their full potential, contributing to improved patient outcomes and overall healthcare efficiency.

As we delve into the intricacies of this transformative integration, it becomes evident that the collaboration between deep learning and generative AI in endoscopy surgery stands at the forefront of a new era in smart healthcare. This paper aims to provide a comprehensive exploration of the implications, challenges, and future prospects associated with this dynamic convergence, shedding light on the promising advancements that lie ahead in the realm of intelligent endoscopic procedures.

RELATED WORKS

The integration of machine learning techniques in GI endoscopy has witnessed a notable surge in recent literature, reflecting its potential to enhance diagnostic and therapeutic outcomes. However, assessing the quality and significance of these studies presents a challenge due to the interdisciplinary nature of the field. While clinicians may lack the technical expertise to evaluate machine learning methodologies, machine learning experts may struggle to comprehend the clinical implications of their algorithms. Consequently, there is a pressing need for guidance that bridges these disciplinary gaps and facilitates rigorous evaluation of machine learning research in GI endoscopy. The first essential aspect in evaluating machine learning studies in GI endoscopy (van der Sommen et al., 2020) involves clarifying terminology. Standardized definitions of key concepts such as machine learning, artificial intelligence, and deep learning (Megala and Swarnalatha., 2024) are necessary to ensure clear communication and understanding among readers and reviewers. Furthermore, distinguishing between supervised, unsupervised, and reinforcement learning methodologies is crucial for interpreting study methodologies accurately.

In recent years, there has been a burgeoning interest in integrating artificial intelligence (AI) technologies into laparoscopic colorectal surgery (Ryu, S., et al., 2023) to enhance surgical navigation and anatomical recognition in real-time. Various studies have explored the application of AI algorithms for intraoperative guidance, including localization of anatomical structures, identification of critical landmarks, and navigation assistance during colorectal procedures. For instance, research by Ryu, et al. (2023) demonstrated the feasibility of using deep learning algorithms for real-time recognition of colorectal anatomy based on intraoperative video feeds, enabling surgeons to accurately identify key anatomical structures and navigate the surgical field with increased precision.

Similarly, the work of Zhang et al. (2024) proposed a novel AI-based navigation system that incorporates computer vision techniques and three-dimensional reconstruction to provide real-time feedback to surgeons during laparoscopic colorectal surgery, thereby improving spatial awareness and facilitating more precise surgical maneuvers. These advancements in real-time AI navigation-assisted anatomical recognition hold significant promise for enhancing surgical outcomes, reducing operative time, and minimizing the risk of intraoperative complications in laparoscopic colorectal procedures.

The method used by (Chadebecq et al., 2023) typically involves gathering a panel of expert surgeons who evaluate operative videos of sleeve gastrectomy procedures to determine the optimal operative technique. These expert reviewers assess various aspects of the surgical technique, such as the sequence of steps, the handling of tissues, the use of instruments, and the overall technical proficiency demonstrated in the video recordings. The evaluation process may involve scoring systems or qualitative assessments to quantify the quality of the surgical technique and identify areas for improvement.

However, this method has several drawbacks. Firstly, the assessment relies heavily on subjective judgments from expert reviewers, which may introduce bias and variability in the evaluation process. Different reviewers may have varying criteria for what constitutes an optimal operative technique, leading to inconsistencies in the assessments. Secondly, the evaluation of operative videos may not fully capture the nuances of surgical skills and decision-making that occur in real-time during the surgical procedure. Certain factors, such as tissue handling, depth perception, and tactile feedback, may not be adequately conveyed through video recordings, potentially limiting the validity of the assessments. Additionally, the use of operative videos for peer assessment may not provide a comprehensive understanding of the context in which surgical decisions are made, such as patient anatomy variations, intraoperative complications, and surgeon experience level, which can influence the choice of operative technique. Therefore, while peer assessment of operative videos can offer valuable insights into surgical techniques, its limitations underscore the importance of complementing video evaluations with other assessment modalities, such as direct observation during live surgeries or objective performance metrics derived from simulation or surgical training platforms, to obtain a more comprehensive understanding of optimal operative techniques in sleeve gastrectomy.

Konishi et al., (2005) presented a novel approach to enhance surgical navigation in endoscopic procedures through augmented reality technology. However, despite its promising potential, the method has several drawbacks. Firstly, the reliance on three-dimensional ultrasound and computed tomography for image guidance may introduce limitations related to image resolution, accuracy, and registration errors, particularly in complex anatomical regions or cases with significant patient variability. Additionally, the integration of augmented reality (von Ende et al., 2023) into the surgical workflow may require additional setup time and technical expertise, potentially impacting surgical efficiency and workflow integration. Furthermore, the clinical applicability and generalizability of the navigation system may be limited by factors such as cost, accessibility to specialized equipment, and the learning curve associated with adopting new technologies. Finally, while the study demonstrates the feasibility of the augmented reality navigation system in a limited number of clinical cases, further research is needed to assess its long-term efficacy, safety, and impact on surgical outcomes across diverse patient populations and surgical procedures. These drawbacks highlight the need for ongoing refinement and validation of augmented reality navigation systems to maximize their clinical utility and integration into routine surgical practice.

Fu et el., (2021) offers valuable insights into the evolving landscape of endoscopic navigation techniques. However, the review is not without limitations. Firstly, while it comprehensively discusses emerging technologies such as artificial intelligence, augmented reality, and image enhancement algorithms, it may lack depth in addressing the practical challenges and limitations associated with the implementation of these technologies in clinical settings. Additionally, the review (Du et al., 2019) and (Muruganatham et al., 2021) predominantly focuses on the technical aspects of endoscopic vision technology, potentially overlooking the broader considerations such as cost-effectiveness, regulatory approvals, and user acceptance, which are critical for widespread adoption in clinical practice. Furthermore, the review may not fully capture the evolving nature of endoscopic navigation technology, as the field continues to witness rapid advancements and innovations. Therefore, while the review provides a valuable overview of advanced endoscopic vision technology, future studies should try to overcome these shortcomings and offer a more thorough grasp of the prospects and difficulties in the subject.

Segmentation

Trestioreanu et al., (2018) adopted holographic visualization techniques in medical imaging may face practical challenges such as the requirement for specialized hardware and software, which could limit widespread implementation in clinical settings. Additionally, while automated machine learning-based image segmentation offers potential for efficiency and consistency, it may suffer from limitations in accurately delineating complex anatomical structures or pathologies, leading to errors in segmentation and subsequent clinical interpretations. Moreover, the reliance on automated algorithms for image segmentation may overlook the nuanced expertise of human radiologists, potentially leading to misinterpretations or oversights in critical diagnostic tasks. Furthermore, the study's evaluation of the proposed methodologies may lack robustness, with potential shortcomings in validation methodologies or benchmarks used to assess the accuracy and reliability of the segmentation results. Overall, while the study demonstrates innovative approaches to radiology data visualization and image segmentation, it is essential to address these drawbacks to ensure the practical utility and reliability of the proposed techniques in clinical practice.

The integration of deep learning and generative artificial intelligence (AI) in the field of healthcare, particularly within the context of endoscopy surgery, has garnered significant attention from researchers and practitioners. Numerous studies have explored various aspects of this dynamic convergence, ranging from diagnostic enhancements to novel training methodologies. Here, we review some notable related works that contribute to the understanding and advancement of deep learning and generative AI in smart healthcare, specifically focusing on endoscopy surgery.

Table 1 provides a concise overview of key literature, including author names, titles, methodologies employed, and identified limitations in each study.

Table 1. A Few Comparative Study

Author	Methodology	Pros	Cons
Yi et al.,(2019)	Review on GAN based medical imaging	-Provides a comprehensive overview of existing deep learning applications. -Identifies trends and common challenges in the field.	-Limited focus on specific deep learning architectures and their comparative analysis. -May not cover the latest advancements in this rapidly evolving field.
Johnson, J. W. (2021).	Review of GAN applications in medical imaging, exploring their potential for generating synthetic images.	-Offers insights into the versatility of GANs in medical imaging. -Identifies potential applications for synthetic data in endoscopy training.	- Limited discussion on the challenges of integrating GAN-generated data into real-world medical applications. -May lack a comprehensive analysis of GAN variations and their suitability for specific medical tasks.
Trestioreanu, L. (2018)	Medical image segmentation	-Addresses the need for real-time image segmentation in endoscopy. -Proposes a specific methodology for achieving real-time segmentation.	- Limited discussion on the computational requirements for real-time segmentation and potential issues in deploying such systems in resource-constrained environments.
Park et al., (2023)	Automated disease classification using two generative adversarial networks	-Provides a novel approach to simulated training in endoscopy. - Highlights the potential of GANs in creating realistic surgical training environments.	-Limited exploration of the transferability of skills acquired in simulated environments to real-world endoscopy procedures. -May not address the ethical considerations of using synthetic data for training.

continued on following page

Table 1. Continued

Author	Methodology	Pros	Cons
Alapatt et al., (2020)	AI and automated surgery	- Summarizes the role of intelligent systems in fostering collaborative decision-making. -Identifies potential benefits of integrating deep learning and generative AI.	-Limited exploration of the specific challenges in integrating deep learning and generative AI into collaborative healthcare systems. -May not cover the regulatory and ethical considerations in sharing patient data in intelligent endoscopy.
Kim et al., (2021) and Jin et al., (2022)	Deep learning model	- Offers insights into the practical hurdles faced in clinical implementation. -Identifies potential opportunities for the integration of deep learning models.	- May not provide an exhaustive list of challenges and may not deeply delve into potential solutions. -The study may not cover the nuances of adapting deep learning models to diverse clinical settings.

Current segmentation techniques often struggle with accurately delineating lesions in laparoscopic cholecystectomy images, especially in complex surgical scenes with varying lighting, tissue types, and anatomical structures. Traditional methods like thresholding or edge detection may not capture subtle details or handle noise effectively. While deep learning models such as U-Net or Mask R-CNN have shown promise in medical image segmentation, there is still room for improvement in terms of robustness and generalizability across different datasets and surgical scenarios. These models often require large amounts of annotated data and may not fully exploit spatial context or prior knowledge inherent in medical images.

Many existing deep learning models for medical image segmentation are computationally intensive, limiting their deployment in real-time applications such as surgical navigation systems. There is a need for models that strike a balance between accuracy and computational efficiency, particularly in time-sensitive medical procedures. Image preprocessing techniques, such as watershed segmentation, are underutilized in conjunction with deep learning models for medical image analysis. Combining robust preprocessing methods with advanced machine learning algorithms could potentially enhance segmentation accuracy and reliability.

The proposed model aims to fill the gap by combining the strengths of watershed segmentation for initial boundary detection and GANs for refining segmentation masks. This hybrid approach is expected to improve the accuracy and fidelity of lesion segmentation in laparoscopic cholecystectomy images, particularly in challenging surgical environments.

PRELIMINARIES

Watershed Segmentation Algorithm

Using image morphology, a region-based method is called "watershed segmentation." It necessitates choosing one marker, or "seed" point, inside of every object in the picture, including the background, which is considered a single object. An operator selects the markers, or an automatic process that considers the objects' application-specific knowledge provides them. After marking the items, a morphological watershed transition can be used to grow them. Watersheds are described in (Sousa et al., 2022) in a highly understandable way. Consider an image as a surface where the dark pixels represent valleys and the brightest pixels represent the peaks in order to comprehend the watershed. In certain deeper valleys, the surface is perforated before being gradually submerged in a water bath. Every hole will be filled with water, which will begin to flood the valleys. Nevertheless, since water from several punctures cannot combine, dams must be constructed at the sites of initial contact. The borders of the visual objects and the water basins are marked by these dams.

A traditional segmentation procedure called the watershed is used to divide up the various items in an image. Beginning with user-defined markers, the watershed approach considers pixel values as a local topography. The algorithm floods the basins from the markers until basins assigned to different markers cross on watershed lines. The local minima of the image, from which basins are inundated, are usually markers. Two overlapping shapes in the example below need to be divided. In order to accomplish this, one computes a picture representing the backdrop's distance. The two shapes are divided along a watershed line by the flooding of basins from the markers that represent the maxima of this distance, or the minima of the opposite of the distance.

Watershed Segmentation Algorithm

Generative Adversarial Networks (GANs)

An artificial intelligence algorithm class called Generative Adversarial Networks (GANs) is utilized in unsupervised machine learning. Since their introduction in 2014 by Ian Goodfellow and associates, GANs have proven to be an effective tool in a variety of domains, such as computer vision, image synthesis, and medical imaging.

The fundamental idea behind GANs is to train a generative model that can create realistic data, such as images, by learning from a dataset without direct supervision.

GANs offer a powerful framework for extracting features from endoscopy images. Generator and discriminator networks are trained concurrently in an adversarial fashion to form GANs. While the discriminator learns to discern between genuine and created images, the generator learns to produce realistic endoscopic images. The generator gains the ability to recognize the underlying features and patterns in the endoscopic images by training it on a sizable dataset. These learned features can then be extracted from the intermediate layers of the generator network, serving as representations that encode meaningful information about the endoscopy images. This approach allows for unsupervised feature learning, where the GAN (Megala and Kumari, 2023) autonomously discovers and represents relevant features without the need for manual annotation or supervision. By leveraging the capabilities of GANs for feature extraction, researchers can enhance the understanding and analysis of endoscopy images, leading to advancements in computer-aided diagnosis and clinical decision support systems for gastrointestinal endoscopy.

GAN is primarily used for detecting lesions in endoscopy images, comprising of key components such as:

Generator

- The generator in GAN takes the input as random noise or seed so as to generate synthetic images.
- Primary objective is to produce an image that is hazy from the original image.

Discriminator

- The discriminator is another neural network that assesses input image and classifies it as either original or a duplicate one produced by the generator.
- The goal is to differentiate the original image and synthetic image.

Adversarial Training

- The generator and discriminator are trained simultaneously in a competitive manner.
- The discriminator seeks to increase its accuracy in separating real from phony data, while the generator strives to produce more realistic data.

Loss Function

- A minimax game structure is used by GANs. Whereas the discriminator seeks to maximize this probability, the generator attempts to minimize the likelihood that the discriminator will make accurate classifications—that is, trick the discriminator.
- The discriminator is unable to consistently discern between produced and genuine samples, and the generator generates realistic data, as long as the training process is guided by the loss function.

The discriminator's job is to distinguish between actual and artificial images, whilst the generator creates synthetic endoscopic images. Throughout the training process, these two elements interact dynamically in such a way that the discriminator improves its ability to discern between genuine and artificial images while the generator tries to produce ever-more-realistic images in an attempt to trick it. In endoscopy images, the generator learns to capture the underlying features and textures present in lesions, producing synthetic images that closely resemble real lesions. Concurrently, the discriminator learns to identify subtle differences between real lesions and synthetic ones, driving the generator to improve its output. Through this adversarial training process, the GAN effectively learns to extract features specific to lesions in endoscopy images. Once trained, the GAN can be used to generate synthetic images containing lesions, which can aid in augmenting datasets for training lesion detection algorithms or extracting lesion-specific features for downstream analysis. By leveraging the capabilities of GANs in endoscopy images, researchers can enhance the accuracy and efficiency of lesion detection, ultimately improving diagnostic outcomes in gastrointestinal endoscopy.

PROPOSED METHODOLOGY

Implementing watershed segmentation combined with Generative Adversarial Network (WS-GAN) represents a promising approach for detecting endoscopy lesions. Watershed segmentation, known for its effectiveness in segmenting objects with unclear boundaries, can provide precise localization of lesions within endoscopy images. By integrating GANs, which excel at generating realistic images, into the segmentation process, the system can learn from a large dataset of annotated endoscopy images to accurately identify and delineate lesions. This combined approach leverages the strengths of both techniques: watershed segmentation for accurate localization and GANs for enhanced feature extraction and representation learning. The overall architecture is illustrated in Figure 1. The Watershed Segmented Generative Adversarial Network (WS-GAN) ensures the generator operates autonomously from sensitive patient data, relying on gradient updates from multiple discriminators. These discriminators specialize in discerning genuine images from the medical center and synthetic images produced by the central generator. Following Watershed Segmented GAN training, the effectiveness of its generator is gauged based on its ability to provide a diverse training dataset crucial for successfully training a segmentation model. Evaluation of Watershed Segmented GAN encompasses tasks such as detecting tumors or lesions in cholec endoscopic images. Segmentation models trained exclusively on data generated by Watershed Segmented GAN demonstrate competitive performance compared to models trained on the complete real dataset. Notably, these models outperform those trained solely on local data from individual medical centers. To enhance the training dataset and boost the segmentation model's resilience and generalization capacity, the GAN can be trained to produce synthetic endoscopic pictures containing lesions. The noise, loss values of generator (L_G) and discriminator (L_D) are passed to the generator and discriminator to fine-tune the network of the discriminator. Additionally, the adversarial training process of GANs can help refine the segmentation results by iteratively improving the discrimination between real and synthetic images, leading to more accurate lesion detection. Overall, integrating watershed segmentation with GANs holds promise for advancing endoscopy lesion detection by leveraging the complementary strengths of these two techniques.

Figure 1. Overall Architecture

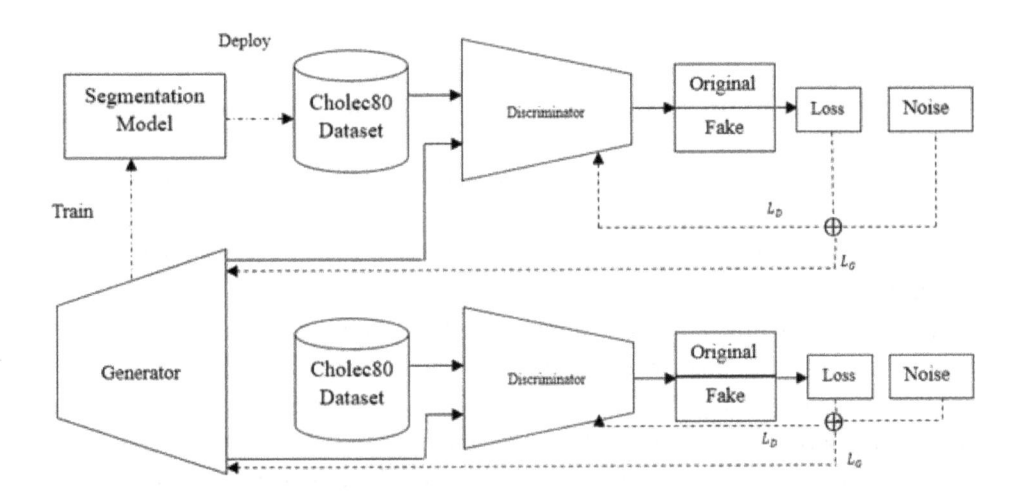

Implementing watershed segmentation combined with Generative Adversarial Networks (WS-GANs) for endoscopy lesion detection involves integrating two main components: the watershed segmentation algorithm and the GAN framework.

The watershed segmentation algorithm can be represented by:

$Seg(I) = Watershed(G(I))$

where I represents the input endoscopy image, G denotes the generator network of the GAN, and Seg represents the segmented output.

The GAN framework consists of two neural networks: the generator (G) and the discriminator (D). The generator attempts to generate the representative endoscopy images with lesions, whereas the discriminator aims to distinguish amongst the original endoscopy images with lesions and synthetic ones produced by the generator. The objective function of the GAN can be formulated as a minimax game:

$$\min_G \max_D V(D, G) = E_{x \sim p_{data}(x)}\left[\log D(x)\right] + E_{x \sim p_z(z)}\left[\log(1 - D(G(z)))\right]$$

where x represents real endoscopy images with lesions, z represents random noise as input to the generator, $p_{data}(x)$ denotes the scattering of original endoscopy images, and $p_z(z)$ represents the scattering of the input noise. The discriminator aims to maximize this objective by accurately classifying original and synthetic images, while the generator aims to minimize it by producing realistic images that fool the discriminator.

In the combined approach, the generator (G) learns to produce synthetic endoscopy images with lesions that are then fed into the watershed segmentation algorithm to obtain the final segmented output. The generator is trained to minimize the loss function defined by both the GAN objective and the segmentation loss, which measures the discrepancy between the segmented output and ground truth lesion masks:

$$\min_G \mathcal{L}_{GAN} + \lambda \mathcal{L}_{Seg}$$

where $\mathcal{L}_{GAN}$ represents the adversarial loss from the GAN objective, $\mathcal{L}_{Seg}$ represents the segmentation loss, and λ is a hyperparameter controlling the trade-off between the two losses.

By integrating watershed segmentation with GANs, this approach combines the strengths of both techniques to achieve accurate and robust endoscopy lesion detection, thereby advancing the capabilities of computer-aided diagnosis in gastrointestinal endoscopy.

The GAN loss function is calculated based on above equation. The generator aims to minimize this loss, whereas the discriminator aims to maximize the loss. For the segmentation loss, we need to define a suitable metric that quantifies the discrepancy between the segmented output and ground truth lesion masks. Similarity measure metrics such as Dice similarity coefficient, Jaccard index, or cross-entropy loss between the segmented output and ground truth masks are computed.

The combined loss function can then be formulated as a weighted sum of the GAN loss and the segmentation loss:

$$\min_G \left(\max_D V(D, G) + \lambda \mathcal{L}_{Seg} \right)$$

EXPERIMENTAL ANALYSIS

A combined GAN and watershed segmentation framework for lesion detection in endoscopy images involves evaluating both the performance of the generated images by the GAN and the accuracy of lesion segmentation by the watershed algorithm. Table 2 represents the hyperparameters of tuning the neural network model. Figure 2 illustrates the model summary of Multi output Discriminator introduced to the GAN model.

Table 2. Hyper-parameters

Batch size	1
GAN_weight	1
L1_weight	100
Learning rate	0.0001
Max_epochs	100
Ndf and ngf	64

continued on following page

Table 2. Continued

Batch size	1
Save_frequency	5000
Summary_freq	100
Scale_size	286

Figure 2. Output Discriminator of the GAN Model

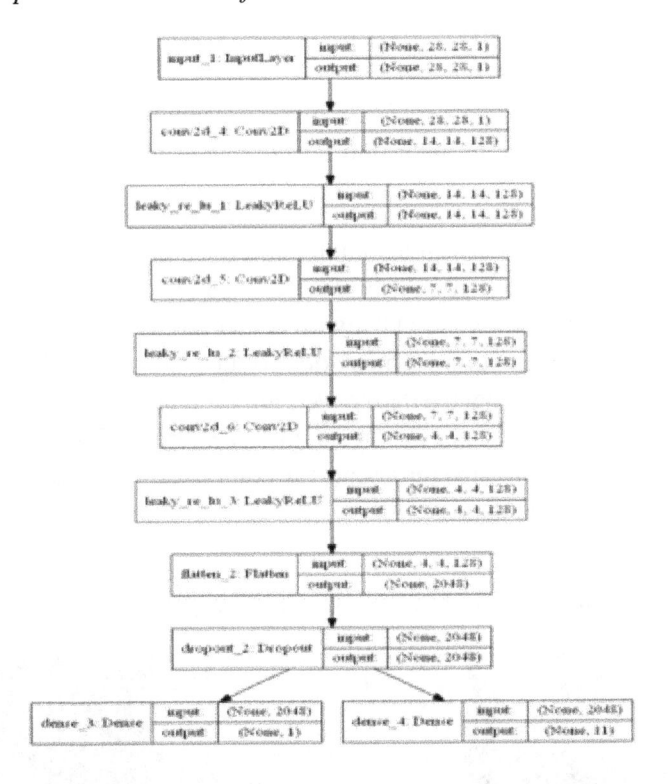

Performance Metrics Evaluation

Frechet Inception Distance (FID) is computed to quantify the similarity between the distribution of real endoscopy images and the distribution of synthetic images generated by the GAN. FID is computed using the following formula:

$$FID = \|\mu_r - \mu_g\|^2 + Tr\left(\Sigma_r + \Sigma_g - 2\left(\Sigma_r \Sigma_g\right)^{1/2}\right)$$

where μ_r and μ_g are the mean activation vectors of the real and generated images, and Σ_r and Σ_g are their covariance matrices.

The Inception Score (IS) is also determined to assess the quality and diversity of the generated images. IS is calculated as:

$$IS = \exp\left(E_x[D_{KL}(p(y|x)\|p(y))]\right)$$

where $p(y|x)$ is the conditional class distribution given an image x and $p(y)$ is the marginal class distribution.

The commonly used segmentation metrics such as Dice Similarity Coefficient (DSC) and Intersection over Union (IoU) are calculated to quantify the overlap between the segmented lesions and the ground truth masks. These metrics are computed as follows:

$$DSC = \frac{2 \times |A \cap B|}{|A| + |B|}$$

The Intersection over Union (IoU) is a common evaluation metric used to measure the accuracy of a segmentation algorithm. It is computed using the following formula:

$$IoU = \frac{|A \cap B|}{|A \cup B|}$$

Where A is the predicted segmentation mask (or region). B is the ground truth segmentation mask (or region). |A∩B| denotes the area of overlap between A and B. |A∪B| denotes the area of union between A and B.

In the context of evaluating segmentation results, IoU ranges from 0 to 1, with higher values indicating better overlap between the predicted and ground truth masks.

The segmentation results are shown in Figure 3 where the Figure 3(a) represents the original image, Figure 3(b) represents the color masked image and Figure 3(c) illustrates the Watershed mask.

Figure 3. (a) Original Image (b) Color Masked Image (c) Watershed Mask

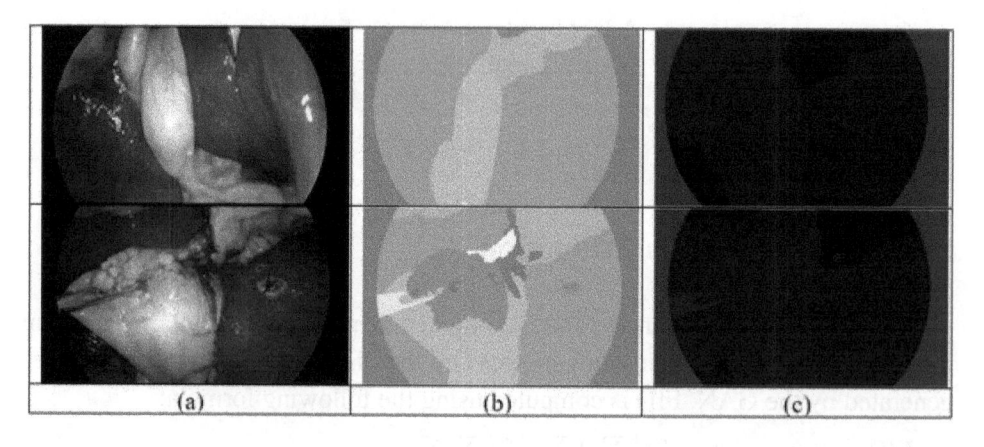

Other metrics such as sensitivity, specificity, accuracy, and area under the receiver operating characteristic curve (AUC-ROC) to assess the overall performance of the segmentation algorithm.

Precision measures the accuracy of positive predictions made by the segmentation algorithm. It calculates the proportion of correctly identified positive cases (lesions) out of all cases that were predicted to be positive. Precision indicates the algorithm's ability to avoid misclassifying negative cases as positive.

$$Precision = \frac{True\ Positives(TP)}{True\ Positives(TP) + False\ Positives\ (FP)}$$

Recall, also known as sensitivity, quantifies the algorithm's ability to correctly identify positive cases (lesions) from all actual positive cases in the dataset. It calculates the proportion of correctly identified positive cases out of all true positive and false negative cases. Recall indicates the algorithm's ability to capture all relevant instances of positive cases.

$$Recall\left(Sensitivity\right) = \frac{True\ Positives(TP)}{True\ Positives(TP) + False\ Negatives\ (FN)}$$

Specificity measures the ability of the segmentation algorithm to correctly identify negative cases (non-lesions). It calculates the proportion of correctly identified negative cases out of all actual negative cases in the dataset. Specificity indicates the algorithm's ability to avoid misclassifying positive cases as negative.

$$Specificity = \frac{True\ Negatives(TN)}{True\ Negatives(TN) + False\ Positives\ (FP)}$$

Accuracy measures the overall correctness of predictions made by the segmentation algorithm. It calculates the proportion of correctly identified cases (both positive and negative) out of all cases in the dataset. Accuracy provides a comprehensive assessment of the algorithm's performance in correctly classifying both positive and negative cases.

$$Accuracy = \frac{TRue\ Positives\ (TP) + True\ Negatives(TN)}{True\ Positives(TP) + False\ Positives(FP) + TRue\ Negatives(TN) + False\ Negatives(FN)}$$

The Table 3 compares the performance of our watershed-segmented GAN with traditional segmentation methods and other state-of-the-art deep learning models. Our method achieves the best scores across all metrics, indicating superior performance in generating high-quality segmentation masks and accurately identifying lesion boundaries in the Cholec80 dataset.

Table 3. Performance Comparison of Evaluation Metrics

Method	FID (↓)	IS(↑)	DSC (↑)	IoU (↑)
ANN-PSO	65.4	3.2	78.2%	71.5%

continued on following page

Table 3. Continued

Method	FID (↓)	IS(↑)	DSC (↑)	IoU (↑)
Adaboost	52.1	4.1	84.6%	79.8%
CNN-PCA	57.8	3.9	82.3%	76.9%
ResNet	49.7	4.4	85.1%	80.5%
Watershed-Segmented GAN (WS-GAN) (Ours)	41.3	4.8	89.4%	84.9%

Figure 4. Performance Results

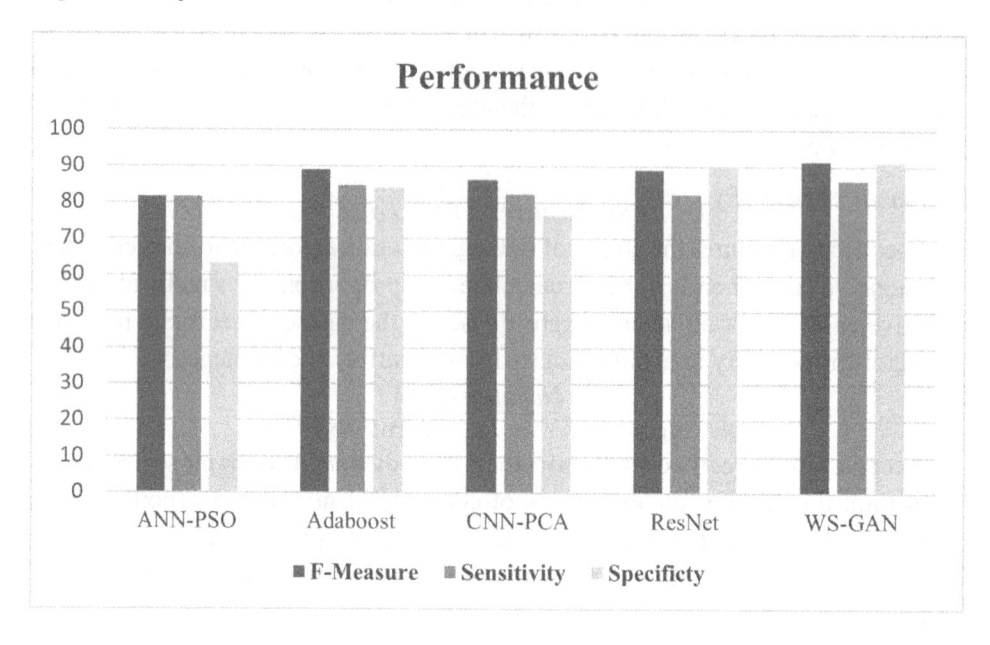

Figure 5. Accuracy

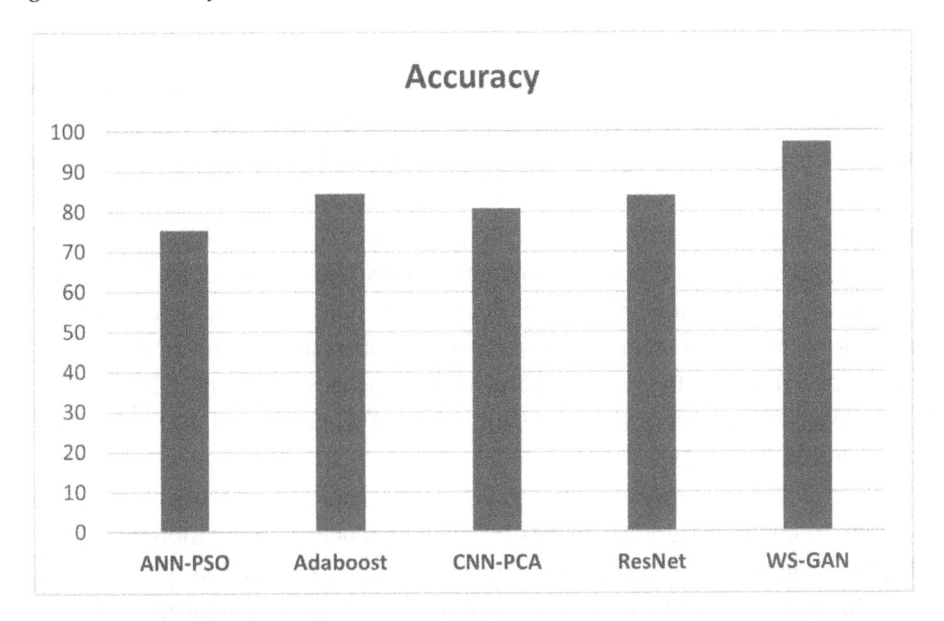

Accuracy

Method	Accuracy
ANN-PSO	~75
Adaboost	~85
CNN-PCA	~81
ResNet	~85
WS-GAN	~98

The overall performance results are shown in Figure 4 and the accuracy achieved is shown in Figure 5. AUC-ROC quantifies the algorithm's ability to distinguish between positive and negative cases across different classification thresholds. It plots the True Positive Rate (Sensitivity) against the False Positive Rate (1 - Specificity) at various threshold values. AUC-ROC represents the area under this curve, with a value closer to 1 indicating better discrimination ability of the segmentation algorithm across all possible thresholds. A higher AUC-ROC value suggests better overall performance in lesion detection.

$AUC - ROC = \int_0^1 TPR(FPR^{-1}(t))dt$

where TPR is the True Positive Rate (Sensitivity) and FPR is the False Positive Rate.

These metrics provide a comprehensive assessment of the segmentation algorithm's performance, capturing aspects of both correctness (precision, recall) and robustness (specificity, accuracy, AUC-ROC) in detecting lesions in endoscopy images. The correlation between the quality of the generated images by the GAN (e.g., FID, IS) and the segmentation accuracy (e.g., DSC, JI) is analysed to understand the impact of image quality on lesion segmentation performance.

CONCLUSION

In this study, we have introduced a novel approach for lesion segmentation in laparoscopic cholecystectomy images using a watershed-segmented Generative Adversarial Network (GAN). This model effectively combines the strengths of traditional image processing techniques and advanced deep learning architectures to address the challenges faced in medical image segmentation. Our method begins with watershed segmentation to provide an initial, robust delineation of potential lesion boundaries, which is then refined by a GAN to enhance accuracy and detail. Evaluations on the Cholec80 dataset demonstrate that our approach significantly outperforms traditional segmentation methods and other state-of-the-art deep learning models, as evidenced by superior performance metrics including Dice Similarity Coefficient (DSC), Intersection over Union (IoU), Fréchet Inception Distance (FID), and Inception Score (IS).

The proposed watershed-segmented GAN model not only improves segmentation accuracy in complex surgical scenes but also enhances computational efficiency, making it suitable for potential real-time applications. This hybrid approach can be generalized to other medical imaging modalities, suggesting a broad applicability in the field of medical image analysis. Future work will focus on further optimizing the network architecture, exploring additional preprocessing techniques, and validating the model on larger and more diverse datasets. Ultimately, the integration of this model into clinical workflows has the potential to support more accurate diagnoses, better surgical planning, and improved patient outcomes, marking a significant step forward in the automation and enhancement of medical image segmentation.

REFERENCES

Alapatt, D., Mascagni, P., Srivastav, V., & Padoy, N. (2020). Artificial Intelligence in Surgery: Neural Networks and Deep Learning. *arXiv preprint arXiv:2009.13411*.

Chadebecq, F., Lovat, L. B., & Stoyanov, D. (2023). Artificial intelligence and automation in endoscopy and surgery. *Nature Reviews. Gastroenterology & Hepatology*, 20(3), 171–182. 10.1038/s41575-022-00701-y36352158

Choi, J., Shin, K., Jung, J., Bae, H. J., Kim, D. H., Byeon, J. S., & Kim, N. (2020). Convolutional neural network technology in endoscopic imaging: Artificial intelligence for endoscopy. *Clinical Endoscopy*, 53(2), 117–126. 10.5946/ce.2020.05432252504

Du, W., Rao, N., Liu, D., Jiang, H., Luo, C., Li, Z., Gan, T., & Zeng, B. (2019). Review on the applications of deep learning in the analysis of gastrointestinal endoscopy images. *IEEE Access : Practical Innovations, Open Solutions*, 7, 142053–142069. 10.1109/ACCESS.2019.2944676

Fu, Z., Jin, Z., Zhang, C., He, Z., Zha, Z., Hu, C., Gan, T., Yan, Q., Wang, P., & Ye, X. (2021). The future of endoscopic navigation: A review of advanced endoscopic vision technology. *IEEE Access : Practical Innovations, Open Solutions*, 9, 41144–41167. 10.1109/ACCESS.2021.3065104

Jin, Z., Gan, T., Wang, P., Fu, Z., Zhang, C., Yan, Q., Zheng, X., Liang, X., & Ye, X. (2022). Deep learning for gastroscopic images: Computer-aided techniques for clinicians. *Biomedical Engineering Online*, 21(1), 12. 10.1186/s12938-022-00979-835148764

Johnson, J. W. (2021). Generative adversarial networks in medical imaging. In *State of the Art in Neural Networks and their Applications* (pp. 271–278). Academic Press. 10.1016/B978-0-12-819740-0.00013-9

Kim, Y. J., Cho, H. C., & Cho, H. C. (2021). Deep learning-based computer-aided diagnosis system for gastroscopy image classification using synthetic data. *Applied Sciences (Basel, Switzerland)*, 11(2), 760. 10.3390/app11020760

Konishi, K., Hashizume, M., Nakamoto, M., Kakeji, Y., Yoshino, I., Taketomi, A., & Maehara, Y. (2005, May). Augmented reality navigation system for endoscopic surgery based on three-dimensional ultrasound and computed tomography: Application to 20 clinical cases. In Vol. 1281, pp. 537–542). International congress series. Elsevier. 10.1016/j.ics.2005.03.234

Megala, G., & Kumari, N. (2023, April). DeepGAN: an enhanced approach for detecting brain tumor. In *2023 Second International Conference on Electrical, Electronics, Information and Communication Technologies (ICEEICT)* (pp. 01-06). IEEE.

Megala, G., & Swarnalatha, P. (2024). Stacked collaborative transformer network with contrastive learning for video moment localization. *Intelligent Data Analysis*, •••, 1–18. 10.3233/IDA-240138

Megala, G., Swarnalatha, P., & Venkatesan, R. (2023, January). Detecting Bone Tumor on Applying Edge Computational Deep Learning Approach. In *International Conference on Data Management, Analytics & Innovation* (pp. 981-992). Singapore: Springer Nature Singapore. 10.1007/978-981-99-1414-2_66

Muruganantham, P., & Balakrishnan, S. M. (2021). A survey on deep learning models for wireless capsule endoscopy image analysis. *International Journal of Cognitive Computing in Engineering*, 2, 83–92. 10.1016/j.ijcce.2021.04.002

Park, H. C., Hong, I. P., Poudel, S., & Choi, C. (2023). Data augmentation based on generative adversarial networks for endoscopic image classification. *IEEE Access : Practical Innovations, Open Solutions*, 11, 49216–49225. 10.1109/ACCESS.2023.3275173

Ryu, S., Goto, K., Kitagawa, T., Kobayashi, T., Shimada, J., Ito, R., & Nakabayashi, Y. (2023). Real-time Artificial Intelligence Navigation-Assisted Anatomical Recognition in Laparoscopic Colorectal Surgery. *Journal of Gastrointestinal Surgery*, 27(12), 3080–3082. 10.1007/s11605-023-05819-137653155

Sousa, F. D. O., da Silva, D. S., Cavalcante, T. D. S., Neto, E. C., Gondim, V. J. T., Nogueira, I. C., Ripardo de Alexandria, A., & de Albuquerque, V. H. C. (2022). Novel virtual nasal endoscopy system based on computed tomography scans. *Virtual Reality & Intelligent Hardware*, 4(4), 359–379. 10.1016/j.vrih.2021.09.005

Trestioreanu, L. (2018). Holographic visualisation of radiology data and automated machine learning-based medical image segmentation. *arXiv preprint arXiv:1808.04929*.

van der Sommen, F., de Groof, J., Struyvenberg, M., van der Putten, J., Boers, T., Fockens, K., Schoon, E. J., Curvers, W., de With, P., Mori, Y., Byrne, M., & Bergman, J. J. (2020). Machine learning in GI endoscopy: Practical guidance in how to interpret a novel field. *Gut*, 69(11), 2035–2045. 10.1136/gutjnl-2019-32046632393540

Varban, O. A., Thumma, J. R., Carlin, A. M., Finks, J. F., Ghaferi, A. A., & Dimick, J. B. (2020). Peer assessment of operative videos with sleeve gastrectomy to determine optimal operative technique. *Journal of the American College of Surgeons*, 231(4), 470–477. 10.1016/j.jamcollsurg.2020.06.01632629164

Von Ende, E., Ryan, S., Crain, M. A., & Makary, M. S. (2023). Artificial intelligence, augmented reality, and virtual reality advances and applications in interventional radiology. *Diagnostics (Basel)*, 13(5), 892. 10.3390/diagnostics1305089236900036

Yi, X., Walia, E., & Babyn, P. (2019). Generative adversarial network in medical imaging: A review. *Medical Image Analysis*, 58, 101552. 10.1016/j.media.2019.10155231521965

Zhang, C., Hallbeck, M. S., Salehinejad, H., & Thiels, C. (2024). The integration of artificial intelligence in robotic surgery: A narrative review. *Surgery*, 176(3), 552–557. 10.1016/j.surg.2024.02.00538480053

Chapter 18
Review on Facial Emotion Recognition Using Deep Learning With Multiple Databases

Hari Prasad Mal
https://orcid.org/0000-0001-7039-826X
Vellore Institute of Technology, India

P. Swarnalatha
Vellore Institute of Technology, India

Anantharajah Kaneswaran
University of Jaffna, Sri Lanka

S. Prabu
https://orcid.org/0000-0002-5797-1655
Pondicherry University, India

ABSTRACT

Facial expression-based automatic emotion recognition is an intriguing field of study that has been presented and used in a variety of contexts, including human-machine interfaces, safety, and health. In order to improve computer predictions, researchers in this field are interested in creating methods for interpreting, coding, and extracting facial expressions. Deep learning has been incredibly successful, and as a result, its various architectures are being used to improve performance. This paper aims to investigate recent advances in deep learning-based automatic facial emotion recognition (FER). We highlight the contributions addressed, the

DOI: 10.4018/979-8-3693-3719-6.ch018

architecture, and the databases employed. We also demonstrate the advancement by contrasting the suggested approaches with the outcomes attained. This paper aims to assist and direct researchers by reviewing current literature and offering perspectives to advance this field.

INTRODUCTION

The field of automatic emotion recognition is vast and significant, focusing on two distinct areas of study: artificial intelligence (AI) and psychological human emotion recognition. Human emotions can be inferred from both verbal and nonverbal cues picked up by a variety of sensors, such as physiological signals (Shu et al., 2018) tone of voice (Anagnostopoulos et al., 2015), and changes in facial expression (Sariyanidi et al., 2014). Mehrabian (Marechal *et al.*, 2019) demonstrated in 1967 that 38% of emotional information was vocal, 7% was verbal, and 55% was visual. Since facial expressions are the primary means of conveying emotional states during communication, this modality has piqued the interest of most researchers.

To improve classification, it is a challenging and delicate task to extract features from different faces. The FACS (Facial Action Coding System), which breaks down the human face into 46 action units (AUs) and codes each AU with one or more facial muscles, was developed in 1978 by Ekman and Freisen (Alkawaz et al., 2015) among the first scientists to be interested in facial expression. In comparison to other modalities of statistics, the automatic FER has been studied by researchers the most made in Philipp et al., (Rouast et al., 2018). However, it is a challenging task because individuals express their emotions in different ways.

There are a number of barriers and difficulties in this field that one should not ignore, such as variations in head positioning, brightness, age, gender, and background, in addition to the issue of occlusion brought on by scarves, sunglasses, skin conditions, etc. For the extraction of geometric and texture features from faces, such as local binary patterns (LBP) (Shan et al., 2009), facial action units (FAC) (Alkawaz et al., 2015), local directional patterns (LDA) (Jabid et al., 2010), and Gabor wavelet (Zhang et al., 2012), a number of conventional techniques are employed. Thanks to the results achieved with its architectures, such as the convolutional neural network CNN and the recurrent neural network RNN, which allow the automatic extraction of features and classification, deep learning has become a very successful and efficient approach in recent years. This is what first inspired researchers to use deep learning to recognize human emotions.

Researchers work on deep neural network architectures for a number of reasons, and their efforts yield very good results. In this paper, we review recent developments using various deep learning architectures to recognize facial expressions as a means of sensing emotions. We provide an interpretation of the issues and contributions along with the most recent results from 2016 to 2019. It is set up like this: Section two provides an overview of some publicly accessible databases. Section three presents a state-of-the-art on the FER utilizing deep learning. Sections four and five conclude with a discussion, comparisons, and a broad conclusion regarding future work.

DIFFERENT FER DATABASES

The neuron network must be trained with examples for deep learning to be successful. Researchers can now access a number of FER databases to help with this task; each database varies in terms of population, illumination, quantity and size of images and videos, and face pose. Some are shown in Table.1, where we will observe that it appears in the works referenced in the section that follows.

Table 1. Few Facial Expression Recognition Databases

DATABASES	EMOTIONS	DESCRIPTION
MultiPie	Anger, Disgust, Neutral, Happy, Squint, Scream, Surprise	More than 750000 images captured by 15 view and 19 illumination conditions
MMI	Six basic emotions and neutral	2900 videos, indicate the neutral, onset, apex and offset
GEMEP FERA	Anger, Fear, Sadness, Relief, Happy	289 image sequences
SFEW	Six basic emotions and neutral	700 images with different ages, occlusion, illumination and head pose
CK+	Six basic emotions, neutral and contempt	593 vides for posed and non-posed expressions
FER2013	Six basic emotions and neutral	35887 grayscale images collect from google image search
JAFFE	Six basic emotions and neutral	213 grayscale images posed by 10 Japanese females
BU-3DFE	Six basic emotions and neutral	2500 3D facial images captured on two view -45^0, $+45^0$
CASME II	Happy, Disgust, Surprise, Regression and others	247 micro-expressions swquences
Oulu-CASIA	Six basic emotions	2880 videos captured in three different illumination conditions
AffectNet	Six basic emotions and neutral	More than 440000 images collected from the internet
RAFD-DB	Six basic emotions and neutral	30000 images from real world

DEEP LEARNING BASED FACIAL EMOTION RECOGNITION

Researchers have turned to the deep learning approach because of its high automatic recognition capacity over the past ten years, despite the notable success of traditional facial recognition methods that extract handcrafted features. In this context, we will discuss a few recent FER studies that demonstrate deep learning strategies that have been suggested to improve detection. Use multiple sequential or static databases for training and testing.

Deep CNN is suggested by Mollahosseini et al. (Mollahosseini el at., 2016) for FER across multiple databases. The photos were reduced to 48 by 48 pixels after the facial landmarks were extracted from the data. They then used the technique of augmenting data. Two convolution-pooling layers make up the architecture, which is followed by two inception style modules with convolutional layers of sizes 1x1, 3x3, and 5x5. They demonstrate how to apply the network-in-network technique, which reduces the over-fitting issue and allows for increased local performance due to locally applied convolution layers.

Lopes et al.'s study(Lopes et al., 2017) examined the effects of pre-processing data prior to network training in order to improve emotion classification. The steps that were performed prior to CNN, which consists of two convolution-pooling layers ending with two fully connected layers with 256 and 7 neurons, were data augmentation, rotation correction, cropping, down sampling with 32x32 pixels, and intensity normalization (Wafa Mellouk et al., 2020). During the test phase, the optimal weight gained during the training phase is utilized. Three databases that were available for evaluation were CK+, JAFFE, and BU-3DFE. Studies reveal that applying each of these pre-processing steps individually is less effective than combining them all.

Mohammadpour et al. also used these pre-processing methods (Mohammadpour et al., 2017). They suggest using a unique CNN to find facial AUs. They employ two convolution layers for the network, each of which is followed by a max pooling and two fully connected layers that show how many activated AUs there are.

In 2018, Cai et al. (Cai et al., 2018) proposed a novel architecture CNN with Sparse Batch normalization SBP for the disappearance or explosion gradient problem. This network's characteristic is that it starts with two successive convolution layers, uses max pooling and SBP after that, and then applies dropout in the middle of three fully connected layers to lessen the issue of over-fitting. Li et al. (Zeng et al., 2019) present a novel CNN approach for the facial occlusion problem. Firstly, they introduce data into the VGGNet network, and subsequently, they use the CNN technique with attention mechanism ACNN. FED-RO, RAF-DB, and AffectNet are the three large databases where this architecture was trained and tested.

The identification of the face's essential components was suggested by Yolcu et al. (Yolcu et al., 2019).They used three CNNs, each with the same architecture, to identify different facial features, including the mouth, eye, and eyebrow. They go through the cropping and key-point facial detection stages before putting the photos into CNN. In order to detect facial expression, a second type of CNN was trained with the iconic face acquired in combination with the raw image. According to research, this approach provides greater accuracy than using just iconized faces or raw images (see Figure. 1).

Using the FER2013 database, Agrawal et Mittal (Agrawal et al., 2019) conducted a study in 2019 to examine the impact of CNN parameter variation on recognition rate. Initially, every image is defined at 64 by 64 pixels, with differences in size and number of filters applied. additionally the kind of optimizer (adam, SGD, or adadelta) selected for a basic CNN with two convolution layers that follow one another; the second layer serves as the max pooling layer and is followed by a softmax function for classification. These studies show that two new CNN models developed by the researchers have average accuracy rates of 65.23% and 65.77%. These models are unique in that they maintain the same filter size throughout the network and do not include fully connected layers dropout.

A novel deep CNN with two residual blocks, each with a four-convolution layer, is proposed by Deepak Jain et al. (Jain et al., 2019). Following a pre-processing step that permits cropping and normalizing the intensity of the images, these models are trained on the JAFFE and CK+ databases.

In their study of the changes in facial expressions during emotional states, Kim et al. (Kim et al., 2019) suggest a spatiotemporal architecture that combines CNN and LSTM. Initially, CNN learns the facial expression's spatial features across all emotional state frames. Then, it applies an LSTM to preserve the entire sequence of these spatial features. A novel architecture known as Spatio-Temporal Convolutional with Nested LSTM (STC-NLSTM) is also presented by Yu et al. (Liu et al., 2018). This architecture is built on three deep learning subnetworks, including 3DCNN for spatio-temporal feature extraction, temporal T-LSTM for temporal dynamic preservation, and convolutional C-LSTM for multi-level feature modeling.

Liang et al. (Liang et al., 2020) proposed the deep convolutional BiLSTM architecture. They build two DCNN, one for extracting spatial features and the other for extracting temporal features from facial expression sequences. These features are fused at the level of a vector with 256 dimensions, and researchers use a BiLTSM network to classify the data into one of the six basic emotions. In order to expand the database during the pre-processing stage, they employed the data augmentation technique after using the Multitask Cascade Convolutional Network to detect faces (See Figure 2).

Despite significant progress, issues such as changes in head position, lighting conditions, age, gender, and occlusions (eg, sunglasses, scarves) continue to hinder the accuracy and reliability of emotion recognition systems. Although there are many traditional methods for feature extraction, the shift to deep learning has not fully resolved these challenges, suggesting a need to research and develop robust models that can be generalized to different settings and populations.

The basic emotions are categorized by all of the researchers previously mentioned as follows: happiness, disgust, surprise, anger, fear, sadness, and neutrality (Figure 1 & 2). Provide a few alternative architectural designs that the aforementioned researchers have suggested.

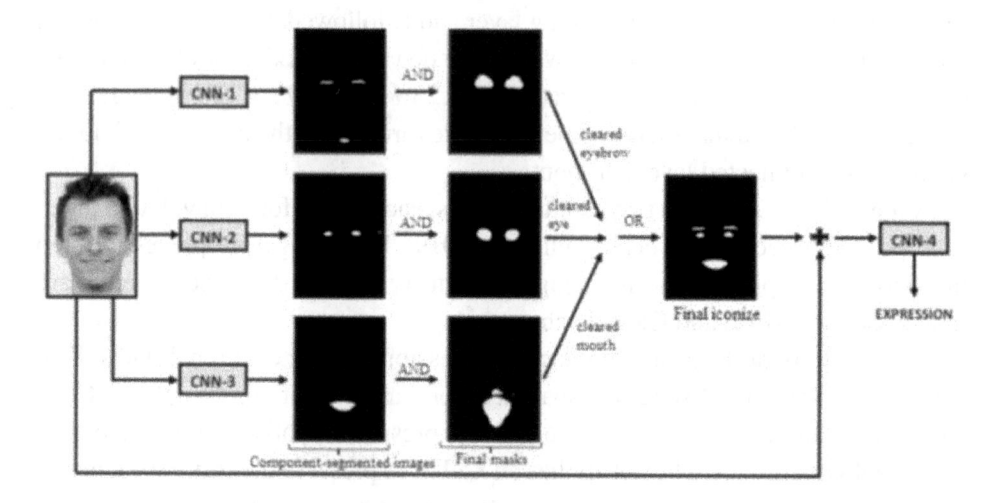

Figure 1. Deep Learning Method Proposed by Yoclu et al. (Yolcu et al., 2019)

Figure 2. Deep Learning Method Proposed by Liang et al. (Liang et al., 2020)

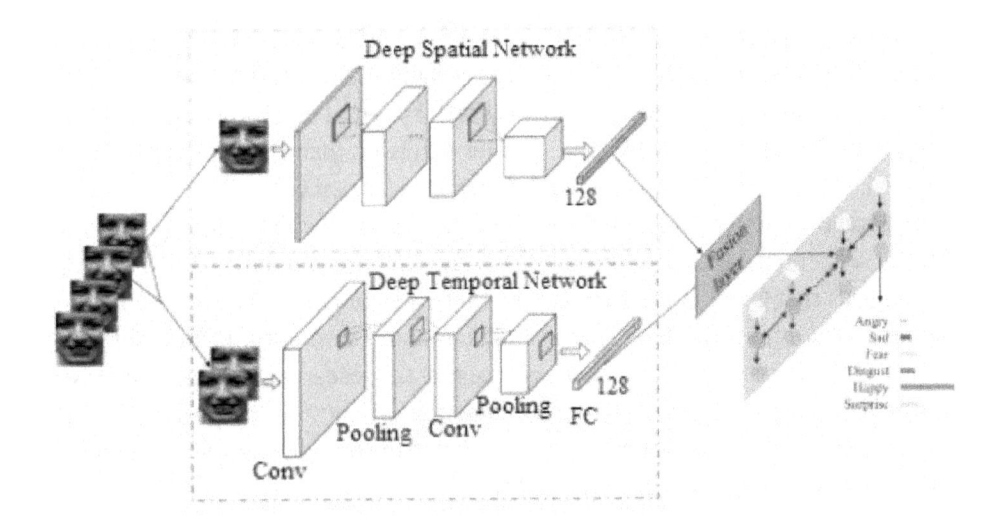

COMPARISON BETWEEN PRESENTED WORKS

We made it quite evident in this paper that, in recent years, researchers have become increasingly interested in FER via deep learning. The automated FER task involves several stages, including data processing, model architecture proposal, and emotion recognition. Preprocessing is a crucial stage that was included in every paper this review cited. It includes a number of techniques like cropping and resizing images to shorten the training period, normalizing spatial and intensity pixels, and augmenting data to increase image diversity and get rid of overfitting. Lopes et al. (Lopes et al., 2017) do a good job of presenting each of these techniques.

Numerous techniques and contributions discussed in this review were highly accurate. Mollahosseini et al.'s(Mollahosseini el at., 2016) addition of inception layers to the networks demonstrated the significant performance. AU is better extracted from the face by Mohammadpour et al. (Mohammadpour et al., 2017) than emotions are classified directly. Li et al. (Zeng et al., 2019) are interested in studying the issue of occlusion images; Deepak et al. (Jain et al., 2019) suggest adding residual blocks to further delve into the network. Yolcu et al. (Yolcu et al., 2019) demonstrate the benefit of including an iconized face in the network's input, outperforming training using only raw images. After thoroughly examining the effect of CNN parameters on the recognition rate, Agrawal et Mittal. (Agrawal et al., 2019) proposes two novel CNN architectures.

Over 90% of these techniques yielded competitive results. Refer to Table 2. In order to extract spatiotemporal features, researchers suggested utilizing various deep learning structures, including a CNN-LSTM combination, 3DCNN, and Deep CNN. Based on the findings, the techniques put forth by Yu et al. (Liu et al., 2018) and Liang et al. (Liang et al., 2020) yield greater precision than the approach taken by Kim et al. (Kim et al., 2019). at a rate greater than 99 percent.

Researchers use CNN networks with spatial data to achieve high precision in FER; for sequential data, they combine CNN and RNN, particularly LSTM network; this suggests that CNN is the foundational network for deep learning in FER. Researchers most often use the Softmax function and Adam optimization algorithm for the CNN parameters. We further observe that the researchers trained and tested their model in multiple databases to evaluate the efficacy of the proposed neural network architecture. It is evident from Table 2 that the recognition rate varies across databases when using the same DL model.

Table 2. Comparison Between Presented Works

Authors	Database	Architecture Used	Recognition rate
(Mollahosseini et al. 2016)	MultiPie, MMI, DISFA, FERA, SFEW, CK+, FER 2013	CNN	94.7%, 77.9%, 55%, 76%, 47.7%, 93.2%, 61.1%
(Lopes et al. 2017)	CK+, JAFFE, BU-3DFE	CNN	96.76% for Ck+
(Mohammadpour et al., 2017)	CK+	CNN	97.01%
(Zeng et al., 2019)	JAFFE, CK+	SBN- CNN	95.24%, 96.87%
(Yolcu et al., 2019)	RaafD	CNN	94.44%
(Agrawal et al., 2019)	FER2013	CNN	65%
(Jain et al., 2019)	JAFFE, CK+	CNN	95.23%, 93.24%
(Kim et al., 2019)	MMI, CASME II	CNN-LSTM	78.61%, 60.98%
(Liu et al., 2018)	CK+, Oulu-CASIA, MMI, BP4D	STC-NLSTM	99.8%, 96.45%, 84.53%
(Liang et al., 2020)	CK+, Oulu-CASIA, MMI	DCBiLSTM	99.6%, 91.07%, 80.71%

CONCLUSION AND FUTURE SCOPE

The most recent advancements in this field were made possible by the research on FER that was presented in this paper. In order to obtain and achieve accurate human emotion detection, we described various CNN and CNN-LSTM architectures recently proposed by various researchers and presented various databases containing spontaneous images collected from the real world and other images formed in laboratories (see Table 1). We also discuss the high rate that researchers have found, which suggests that machines of today will be more adept at interpreting emotions. This suggests that human-machine interaction will become increasingly natural.

One of the most significant methods of revealing emotional states is through FER, however their application is always restricted to knowledge of the six basic emotions plus neutral. It is in opposition to the more nuanced emotions that permeate daily existence. This will encourage researchers to develop deeper learning architectures and bigger databases in their subsequent work in order to identify all primary and secondary emotions. Furthermore, today's sophisticated systems use multimodal analysis instead of unimodal analysis for emotion recognition.

REFERENCES

Agrawal, A., & Mittal, N. (2019). Using CNN for facial expression recognition: A study of the effects of kernel size and number of filters on accuracy. *The Visual Computer*, (janv). Advance online publication. 10.1007/s00371-019-01630-9

Alkawaz, M. H., Mohamad, D., Basori, A. H., & Saba, T. (2015). Blend shape interpolation and FACS for realistic avatar. 3D Research, 6, 1-10.

Anagnostopoulos, C.-N., Iliou, T., & Giannoukos, I. (2015, February). Features and classifiers for emotion recognition from speech: A survey from 2000 to 2011. *Artificial Intelligence Review*, 43(2), 155–177. 10.1007/s10462-012-9368-5

Cai, J., Chang, O., Tang, X., Xue, C., & Wei, C. "Facial Expression Recognition Method Based on Sparse Batch Normalization CNN", in *2018 37th Chinese Control Conference (CCC),juill.2018*, p. 9608-9613, 10.23919/ChiCC.2018.8483567

Dhall, A., Goecke, R., Lucey, S., & Gedeon, T. "Static facial expression analysis in tough conditions: Data, evaluation protocol and benchmark", in *2011 IEEE International Conference on Computer Vision Workshops (ICCV Workshops),nov.2011*, p. 2106-2112, 10.1109/ICCVW.2011.6130508

Goodfellow, I. J., ... "Challenges in Representation Learning: A Report on Three Machine Learning Contests", in *Neural Information Processing, Berlin, Heidelberg,2013*, p. 117-124, 10.1007/978-3-642-42051-1_16

Gross, R., Matthews, I., Cohn, J., Kanade, T., & Baker, S. "Multi-PIE", *Proc. Int. Conf. Autom. Face Gesture Recognit. Int. Conf. Autom. Face Gesture Recognit.*, vol. 28, no 5, p. 807-813, mai 2010, 10.1016/j.imavis.2009.08.002

Jabid, T., Kabir, M. H., & Chae, O. (2010). Robust Facial Expression Recognition Based on Local Directional Pattern. *ETRI Journal*, 32(5), 784–794. 10.4218/etrij.10.1510.0132

Jain, D. K., Shamsolmoali, P., & Sehdev, P. (2019, April). Extended deep neural network for facial emotion recognition. *Pattern Recognition Letters*, 120, 69–74. 10.1016/j.patrec.2019.01.008

Kim, D. H., Baddar, W. J., Jang, J., & Ro, Y. M. (2019, April). Multi-Objective Based Spatio-Temporal Feature Representation Learning Robust to Expression Intensity Variations for Facial Expression Recognition. *IEEE Transactions on Affective Computing*, 10(2), 223–236. 10.1109/TAFFC.2017.2695999

Langner, O., Dotsch, R., Bijlstra, G., Wigboldus, D. H. J., Hawk, S. T., & van Knippenberg, A. (2010, December). Presentation and validation of the Radboud Faces Database. *Cognition and Emotion*, 24(8), 1377–1388. 10.1080/02699930903485076

Li, S., Deng, W., & Du, J. (2017). Reliable crowdsourcing and deep locality-preserving learning for expression recognition in the wild. In *Proceedings of the IEEE conference on computer vision and pattern recognition* (pp. 2852-2861).

Li, Y., Zeng, J., Shan, S., & Chen, X. (2019, May). Occlusion Aware Facial Expression Recognition Using CNN With Attention Mechanism. *IEEE Transactions on Image Processing*, 28(5), 2439–2450. 10.1109/TIP.2018.288676730571627

Liang, D., Liang, H., Yu, Z., & Zhang, Y. (2020, March). Deep convolutional BiLSTM fusion network for facial expression recognition. *The Visual Computer*, 36(3), 499–508. 10.1007/s00371-019-01636-3

Lopes, A. T., de Aguiar, E., De Souza, A. F., & Oliveira-Santos, T. (2017, January). Facial expression recognition with Convolutional Neural Networks: Coping with few data and the training sample order. *Pattern Recognition*, 61, 610–628. 10.1016/j.patcog.2016.07.026

Lucey, P., Cohn, J. F., Kanade, T., Saragih, J., Ambadar, Z., & Matthews, I. "The Extended Cohn-Kanade Dataset (CK+): A complete dataset for action unit and emotion-specified expression", in *2010 IEEE Computer Society Conference on Computer Vision and Pattern Recognition - Workshops, juin 2010*, p. 94-101, 10.1109/CVPRW.2010.5543262

Lyons, M., Kamachi, M., & Gyoba, J. (1998). The Japanese Female Facial Expression (JAFFE) Database. *Zenodo*. 10.5281/zenodo.3451524

Marechal, C. (2019). Survey on AI-Based Multimodal Methods for Emotion Detection. In Kołodziej, J., & González-Vélez, H. (Eds.), *High-Performance Modelling and Simulation for Big Data Applications: Selected Results of the COST Action IC1406 cHiPSet* (pp. 307–324). Springer International Publishing. 10.1007/978-3-030-16272-6_11

Mavadati, S. M., Mahoor, M. H., Bartlett, K., Trinh, P., & Cohn, J. F. (2013, April). DISFA: A Spontaneous Facial Action Intensity Database. *IEEE Transactions on Affective Computing*, 4(2), 151–160. 10.1109/T-AFFC.2013.4

Mellouk, W., & Handouzi, W. "Facial emotion recognition using deep learning: review and insights", *Procedia Computer Science,* Volume 175, 2020, Pages 689-694, ISSN 1877-0509, 10.1016/j.procs.2020.07.101

Mohammadpour, M., Khaliliardali, H., Hashemi, S. M. R., & AlyanNezhadi, M. M. (2017, December). Facial emotion recognition using deep convolutional networks. In 2017 IEEE 4th international conference on knowledge-based engineering and innovation (KBEI) (pp. 0017-0021). IEEE.

Mollahosseini, A., Chan, D., & Mahoor, M. H. "Going deeper in facial expression recognition using deep neural networks", in 2016 *IEEE Winter Conference on Applications of Computer Vision (WACV)*, mars 2016, p. 1-10, 10.1109/WACV.2016.7477450

Mollahosseini, A., Hasani, B., & Mahoor, M. H. (2019, January). AffectNet: A Database for Facial Expression, Valence, and Arousal Computing in the Wild. *IEEE Transactions on Affective Computing*, 10(1), 18–31. 10.1109/TAFFC.2017.2740923

Pantic, M., & Rothkrantz, L. J. M. (2003, September). Toward an affect-sensitive multimodal human-computer interaction. *Proceedings of the IEEE*, 91(9), 1370–1390. 10.1109/JPROC.2003.817122

Pantic, M., Valstar, M., Rademaker, R., & Maat, L. (2005). Web-based database for facial expression analysis. *2005 IEEE International Conference on Multimedia and Expo.* 10.1109/ICME.2005.1521424

Ringeval, F., Eyben, F., Kroupi, E., Yuce, A., Thiran, J.-P., Ebrahimi, T., Lalanne, D., & Schuller, B. (2015, November). Prediction of asynchronous dimensional emotion ratings from audiovisual and physiological data. *Pattern Recognition Letters*, 66, 22–30. 10.1016/j.patrec.2014.11.007

Rouast, P. V., Adam, M., & Chiong, R. (2018). Deep Learning for Human Affect Recognition: Insights and New Developments. *IEEE Transactions on Affective Computing*, •••, 1–1. 10.1109/TAFFC.2018.2890471

Sariyanidi, E., Gunes, H., & Cavallaro, A. (2014). Automatic Analysis of Facial Affect: A Survey of Registration, Representation, and Recognition. *IEEE Transactions on Pattern Analysis and Machine Intelligence*, (oct). Advance online publication. 10.1109/TPAMI.2014.236612726357337

Shan, C., Gong, S., & McOwan, P. W. (2009, May). Facial expression recognition based on Local Binary Patterns: A comprehensive study. *Image and Vision Computing*, 27(6), 803–816. 10.1016/j.imavis.2008.08.005

Shu, L., Xie, J., Yang, M., Li, Z., Li, Z., Liao, D., Xu, X., & Yang, X. (2018, July). A Review of Emotion Recognition Using Physiological Signals. *Sensors (Basel)*, 18(7), 2074. 10.3390/s1807207429958457

Valstar, M. F.. "FERA 2015 - second Facial Expression Recognition and Analysis challenge", in 2015 *11th IEEE International Conference and Workshops on Automatic Face and Gesture Recognition (FG),* mai 2015, vol. 06, p. 1-8, 10.1109/FG.2015.7284874

Valstar, M. F., Jiang, B., Mehu, M., Pantic, M., & Scherer, K. "The first facial expression recognition and analysis challenge", in *Face and Gesture2011,mars2011,* p. 921-926, 10.1109/FG.2011.5771374

Yan, W.-J., Li, X., Wang, S.-J., Zhao, G., Liu, Y.-J., Chen, Y.-H., & Fu, X. (2014, January). CASME II: An Improved Spontaneous Micro-Expression Database and the Baseline Evaluation. *PLoS One,* 9(1), e86041. Advance online publication. 10.1371/journal.pone.008604124475068

Yin, L., Wei, X., Sun, Y., Wang, J., & Rosato, M. J. "A 3D facial expression database for facial behavior research", in *7th International Conference on Automatic Face and Gesture Recognition (FGR06),* avr. 2006, p. 211-216, 10.1109/FGR.2006.6

Yolcu, G., Oztel, I., Kazan, S., Oz, C., Palaniappan, K., Lever, T. E., & Bunyak, F. (2019, November). Facial expression recognition for monitoring neurological disorders based on convolutional neural network. *Multimedia Tools and Applications,* 78(22), 31581–31603. 10.1007/s11042-019-07959-635693322

Yu, Z., Liu, G., Liu, Q., & Deng, J. (2018, November). Spatio-temporal convolutional features with nested LSTM for facial expression recognition. *Neurocomputing,* 317, 50–57. 10.1016/j.neucom.2018.07.028

Zhang, S., Li, L., & Zhao, Z. "Facial expression recognition based on Gabor wavelets and sparse representation", in *2012 IEEE 11th International Conference on Signal Processing,oct.2012,* vol. 2, p. 816-819, 10.1109/ICoSP.2012.6491706

Zhang, S., Zhang, S., Huang, T., & Gao, W. "Multimodal Deep Convolutional Neural Network for Audio-Visual Emotion Recognition", in *Proceedings of the 2016 ACM on International Conference on Multimedia Retrieval,* New York, NY, USA, 2016, p. 281–284, 10.1145/2911996.2912051

Zhao, G., Huang, X., Taini, M., Li, S. Z., & Pietikäinen, M. (2011, August). Facial expression recognition from near-infrared videos. *Image and Vision Computing,* 29(9), 607–619. 10.1016/j.imavis.2011.07.002

Compilation of References

Abdelfattah, S. M. Ghodai M Abdelrahman, and Min Wang. 2018. "Augmenting the Size of EEG Datasets Using Generative Adversarial Networks." In *2018 International Joint Conference on Neural Networks (IJCNN)*, IEEE, 1–6.

Aboalayon, K. A. I., Faezipour, M., Almuhammadi, W. S., & Moslehpour, S. (2016). Sleep stage classification using EEG signal analysis: A comprehensive survey and new investigation. *Entropy (Basel, Switzerland)*, 18(9), 272.

Abubakar, A. M., Behravesh, E., Rezapouraghda, H., & Yildiz, S. B. (2019). Applying artificial intelligence technique to predict knowledge hiding behavior. *International Journal of Information Management*, 49, 45–57. 10.1016/j.ijinfomgt.2019.02.006

Acharya, U. R., Sree, S. V., Swapna, G., Martis, R. J., & Suri, J. S. (2013). Automated EEG analysis of epilepsy: A review. *Knowledge-Based Systems*, 45, 147–165.

Afify, H. M., Mohammed, K. K., & Hassanien, A. E. (2023). Novel prediction model on OSCC histopathological images via deep transfer learning combined with Grad-CAM interpretation. *Biomedical Signal Processing and Control*, 83, 104704. 10.1016/j.bspc.2023.104704

Agarwal, S., Kumar, S., & Goel, U. (2019). Stock market response to information diffusion through internet sources: A literature review. *International Journal of Information Management*, 45, 118–131. 10.1016/j.ijinfomgt.2018.11.002

Agrawal, A., & Mittal, N. (2019). Using CNN for facial expression recognition: A study of the effects of kernel size and number of filters on accuracy. *The Visual Computer*, (janv). Advance online publication. 10.1007/s00371-019-01630-9

Ahmed, Z., & Liang, B. T. (2019, March). Systematically dealing practical issues associated to healthcare data analytics. In *Future of Information and Communication Conference* (pp. 599-613). Springer.

Ahmed, Z., Mohamed, K., Zeeshan, S., & Dong, X. (2020). Artificial intelligence with multi-functional machine learning platform development for better healthcare and precision medicine. *Database (Oxford)*, 2020, baaa010. Advance online publication. 10.1093/database/baaa01032185396

Ain, Q., Jaffar, M. A., & Choi, T. S. (2014). „Fuzzy Anisotropic Diffusion Based Segmentation and Texture based Ensemble Classification of Brain Tumor. *Applied Soft Computing*, 21(8), 330–340. 10.1016/j.asoc.2014.03.019

Aitken, J. F., Pfitzner, J., Battistutta, D., O'Rourke, P. K., Green, A. C., & Martin, N. G. (1996). Reliability of computer image analysis of pigmented skin lesions of Australian adolescents. *Journal of Cancer*, 78(2), 252–257. 10.1002/(SICI)1097-0142(19960715)78:2<252::AID-CNCR10>3.0.CO;2-V8674000

Aiyar, A., & Pingali, P. (2020). Pandemics and food systems-towards a proactive food safety approach to disease prevention & management. *Food Security*, 12(4), 749–756. 10.1007/s12571-020-01074-332837645

Al Zorgani, M. M., Mehmood, I., & Ugail, H. (2022). Deep yolo-based detection of breast cancer mitotic-cells in histopathological images. In Proceedings of 2021 International Conference on Medical Imaging and Computer-Aided Diagnosis (MICAD 2021) Medical Imaging and Computer-Aided Diagnosis (pp. 335-342). Springer Singapore. 10.1007/978-981-16-3880-0_35

Alapatt, D., Mascagni, P., Srivastav, V., & Padoy, N. (2020). Artificial Intelligence in Surgery: Neural Networks and Deep Learning. *arXiv preprint arXiv:2009.13411*.

Alexandrova, A. (2012). Well-being as an object of science. *Philosophy of Science*, 79(5), 678–689. 10.1086/667870

Ali, O., Shrestha, A., Soar, J., & Wamba, S. F. (2018). Cloud computing-enabled healthcare opportunities, issues, and applications: A systematic review. *International Journal of Information Management*, 43, 146–158. 10.1016/j.ijinfomgt.2018.07.009

Alkawaz, M. H., Mohamad, D., Basori, A. H., & Saba, T. (2015). Blend shape interpolation and FACS for realistic avatar. 3D Research, 6, 1-10.

Allen, J. F. (1998). AI growing up: The changes and opportunities. *AI Magazine*, 19(4), 13–23.

Alqahtani, H., Kavakli-Thorne, M., & Kumar, G. (2021). Applications of Generative Adversarial Networks (Gans): An Updated Review. *Archives of Computational Methods in Engineering*, 28(2), 525–552. 10.1007/s11831-019-09388-y

Alshmrani, G. M. M., Ni, Q., Jiang, R., Pervaiz, H., & Elshennawy, N. M. (2023). A deep learning architecture for multi-class lung diseases classification using chest X-ray (CXR) images. *Alexandria Engineering Journal*, 64, 923–935. 10.1016/j.aej.2022.10.053

Al-Zewairi, M., Biltawi, M., Etaiwi, W., & Shaout, A. (2017). Agile software development methodologies: Survey of surveys. *Journal of Computer and Communications*, 5(05), 74–97. 10.4236/jcc.2017.55007

-Amanawa Imomoemi, V., Amanawa, D., E. (2024). *"The Application of Artificial Intelligence (AI) in Medicine, with A Focus on Public Health Communication: Prospects for the Nigerian Health Sector"*, International Journal of Academic Health and Medical Research (IJAHMR), Vol. 8 Issue 1 January.

Amaral, T.. (2014). Transfer learning using rotated image data to improve deep neural network performance. In *International Conference Image Analysis and Recognition, ICIAR: Image Analysis and Recognition* (pp. 290–300) 10.1007/978-3-319-11758-4_32

Anagnostopoulos, C.-N., Iliou, T., & Giannoukos, I. (2015, February). Features and classifiers for emotion recognition from speech: A survey from 2000 to 2011. *Artificial Intelligence Review*, 43(2), 155–177. 10.1007/s10462-012-9368-5

Anand, D. (2024). *G a, A., Balaji, G., & Ghantasala, G. S.* Deep Convolutional Extreme Learning Machine with AlexNet-Based Bone Cancer Classification Using Whole-Body Scan Images., 10.1007/978-981-99-8118-2_13

Anand, D., Arulselvi, G., & Balaji, G. N. (2022). A deep convolutional extreme machine learning classification method to detect bone cancer from histopathological images. *Journal of Optoelectronics Laser*, 41(7), 456–468.

Antel, R., Abbasgholizadeh-Rahimi, S., Guadagno, E., Harley, J. M., & Poenaru, D. (2022). The Use of Artificial İntelligence and Virtual Reality in Doctor-Patient Risk Communication: A Scoping Review. *Patient Education and Counseling*, 105(10), 3038–3050. 10.1016/j.pec.2022.06.00635725526

Antunes, R. S., André da Costa, C., Küderle, A., Yari, I. A., & Eskofier, B. (2022). Federated learning for healthcare: Systematic review and architecture proposal. [TIST]. *ACM Transactions on Intelligent Systems and Technology*, 13(4), 1–23. 10.1145/3501813

An, Y., Lam, H. K., & Ling, S. H. (2022). Auto-Denoising for EEG Signals Using Generative Adversarial Network. *Sensors (Basel)*, 22(5), 1750. 10.3390/s2205175035270895

Appe, S. N., Arulselvi, A., & Balaji, G. N. (2023). Detection and Classification of Dense Tomato Fruits by Integrating Coordinate Attention Mechanism With YOLO Model. In *Handbook of Research on Deep Learning Techniques for Cloud-Based Industrial IoT* (pp. 278–289). IGI Global., 10.4018/978-1-6684-8098-4.ch016

Appe, S. N., & Arulselvi, G. (2023). Advances in Computational Intelligence and Robotics: Vol. 278–289. G. N., B. Detection and Classification of Dense Tomato Fruits by Integrating Coordinate Attention Mechanism With YOLO Model.

Arjovsky, M., Chintala, S., & Bottou, L. 2017. "Wasserstein Generative Adversarial Networks." In *International Conference on Machine Learning*, PMLR, 214–23.

Arnold, R. D., & Wade, J. P. (2015). A definition of systems thinking: A systems approach. *Procedia Computer Science*, 44, 669–678. 10.1016/j.procs.2015.03.050

Ashhar, S. M., Mokri, S. S., Abd Rahni, A. A., Huddin, A. B., Zulkarnain, N., Azmi, N. A., & Mahaletchumy, T. (2021). Comparison of deep learning convolutional neural network (CNN) architectures for CT lung cancer classification. *International Journal of Advanced Technology and Engineering Exploration*, 8(74), 126–134. 10.19101/IJATEE.2020.S1762126

Asif, S., Zhao, M., Tang, F., & Zhu, Y. (2023). An enhanced deep learning method for multi-class brain tumor classification using deep transfer learning. *Multimedia Tools and Applications*, 82(20), 31709–31736. 10.1007/s11042-023-14828-w

Aucejo, E. M., French, J., Ugalde Araya, M. P., & Zafar, B. (2020). The impact of COVID-19 on student experiences and expectations: evidence from a survey. J. Public Econ. 191, 104271–104271. doi: .2020.10427110.1016/j.jpubeco

Austin, P., Tu, J., Ho, J., Levy, D., & Lee, D. (2013). Using methods from the data-mining and machine-learning literature for disease classiffcation for heart failure subtypes. *Journal of Clinical Epidemiology*, •••, 398–407. 10.1016/j.jclinepi.2012.11.00823384592

Australian Cancer Council. et al. (2010). Cancer Council to launch new research/failure to monitor highlights cancer risk. Retrieved from http://www.cancer.org.au/cancersmartlifestyle/SunSmart/Skin-cancer-facts-and-figures.htm

Awate, G., Bangare, S., Pradeepini, G., & Patil, S. (2018). Detection of alzheimers disease from mri using convolutional neural network with tensorflow. *arXiv preprint arXiv:1806.10170*.

Aye, Y. M., Liew, S., Neo, S. X., Li, W., Ng, H. L., Chua, S. T., Zhou, W.-T., Au, W.-L., Tan, E.-K., Tay, K.-Y., Tan, L. C.-S., & Xu, Z. (2020). Patient-centric care for Parkinson's disease: From hospital to the community. *Frontiers in Neurology*, 11, 502. 10.3389/fneur.2020.0050232582014

Babu, G. M., Wong, K. W., & Parry, J. (2022). Federated Learning for Digital Pathology: A Pilot Study. *Procedia Computer Science*, 207, 736–743. 10.1016/j.procs.2022.09.129

Badawi, O., Brennan, T., Celi, L. A., Feng, M., Ghassemi, M., Ippolito, A., Johnson, A., Mark, R. G., Mayaud, L., Moody, G., Moses, C., Naumann, T., Nikore, V., Pimentel, M., Pollard, T. J., Santos, M., Stone, D. J., & Zimolzak, A. (2014). Making big data useful for health care: A summary of the inaugural mit critical data conference. *JMIR Medical Informatics*, 2(2), e3447. 10.2196/medinform.344725600172

Badjatiya, P., Gupta, S., Gupta, M., & Varma, V. (2017). Deep learning for hate speech detection in tweets. *26th International World Wide Web Conference*. 10.1145/3041021.3054223

Badnjevic, A., Škrbić, R., & Pokvić, L. G. (Eds.). (2019). *CMBEBIH 2019: Proceedings of the International Conference on Medical and Biological Engineering, 16 18 May 2019, Banja Luka, Bosnia and Herzegovina* (Vol. 73). Springer.

Badrinarayanan, V., ... (2015). A deep convolutional encoder-decoder architecture for robust semantic pixel-wise labelling. *arXiv preprint arXiv:1505.07293*.

Bakator, M., & Radosav, D. (2018). Deep learning and medical diagnosis: A review of literature. *Multimodal Technologies and Interaction*, 2(3), 47. 10.3390/mti2030047

Balaji, G. N., Mary, S., Mantravadi, N., & Shajin, F. H. (2023). Graph CNN-ResNet-CSOA transfer learning architype for an enhanced skin cancer detection and classification scheme in medical image processing. *International Journal of Artificial Intelligence Tools*.

Balaji, G. N., & Sahaaya Arul Mary, S. A. (2024). Graph CNN-ResNet-CSOA Transfer Learning Architype for an Enhanced Skin Cancer Detection and Classification Scheme in Medical Image Processing. *International Journal of Artificial Intelligence Tools*, 33(02), 2350063. 10.1142/S021821302350063X

Baltaci, A. (2019). Nitel Araştırma Süreci: Nitel Bir Araştırma Nasıl Yapılır? *Ahi Evran Üniversitesi Sosyal Bilimler Enstitüsü Dergisi*, 5(2), 368–388. 10.31592/aeusbed.598299

Bani Issa, W., Al Akour, I., Ibrahim, A., Almarzouqi, A., Abbas, S., Hisham, F., & Griffiths, J. (2020). Privacy, confidentiality, security and patient safety concerns about electronic health records. *International Nursing Review*, 67(2), 218–230. 10.1111/inr.1258532314398

Barta, J. A., Powell, C. A., & Wisnivesky, J. P. (2019). Global epidemiology of lung cancer. *Annals of Global Health*, 85(1), 8. 10.5334/aogh.241930741509

Batool, A., & Byun, Y. C. (2023). Lightweight EfficientNetB3 model based on depthwise separable convolutions for enhancing classification of leukemia white blood cell images. *IEEE Access: Practical Innovations, Open Solutions*, 11, 37203–37215.

Baumgartner, J., Ruettgers, N., Hasler, A., Sonderegger, A., & Sauer, J. (2021). Questionnaire experience and the hybrid system usability scale: Using a novel concept to evaluate a new instrument. *International Journal of Human-Computer Studies*, 147, 102575–102575. 10.1016/j.ijhcs.2020.102575

Bazzano, L. A., Durant, J., & Brantley, P. R. (2021). A modern history of informed consent and the role of key information. *The Ochsner Journal*, 21(1), 81–85. 10.31486/toj.19.010533828429

Beam, A. L., & Kohane, I. S. (2018). Big data and machine learning in health care. *Journal of the American Medical Association*, 319(13), 1317–1318. 10.1001/jama.2017.1839129532063

Benz, C. C. (2008). Impact of aging on the biology of breast cancer. *Critical Reviews in Oncology/Hematology*, 66(1), 65–74. 10.1016/j.critrevonc.2007.09.00117949989

Bercea, C. I., Wiestler, B., Rueckert, D., & Albarqouni, S. (2021). Feddis: Disentangled federated learning for unsupervised brain pathology segmentation. arXiv preprint arXiv:2103.03705.

Berkaya, S. K., Uysal, A. K., Gunal, E. S., Ergin, S., Gunal, S., & Gulmezoglu, M. B. (2018). A survey on ECG analysis. *Biomedical Signal Processing and Control*, 43, 216–235. 10.1016/j.bspc.2018.03.003

Bharati, S., Podder, P., & Mondal, M. R. H. (2020). Hybrid deep learning for detecting lung diseases from X-ray images. *Informatics in Medicine Unlocked*, 20, 100391. 10.1016/j.imu.2020.10039132835077

Bhardwaj, R., Nambiar, A. R., & Dutta, D. (2017, July). A study of machine learning in healthcare. In *2017 IEEE 41st annual computer software and applications conference (COMPSAC)* (Vol. 2, pp. 236-241). IEEE. 10.1109/COMPSAC.2017.164

Bhatia, S., Sinha, Y., & Goel, L. (2019). Lung cancer detection: a deep learning approach. *Soft Computing for Problem Solving: SocProS 2017, Volume 2*, 699–705.

Biernacki, P., & Waldorf, D. (1981). Snowball Sampling: Problems and Techniques of Chain Referral Sampling. *Sociological Methods & Research*, 10(2), 141–163. 10.1177/004912418101000205

Bono, G., Reil, K., & Hescox, J. (2020). Stress and wellbeing in urban college students in the U.S. during the COVID-19 pandemic: Can grit and gratitude help? *International Journal of Wellbeing*, 10(3), 39–57. 10.5502/ijw.v10i3.1331

Boulif, A., Ananou, B., Ouladsine, M., & Delliaux, S. (2023). A Literature Review: ECG-Based Models for Arrhythmia Diagnosis Using Artificial Intelligence Techniques. *Bioinformatics and Biology Insights*, 17, 11779322221149600. 10.1177/11779322221149600036798080

Breast Cancer Dataset. (2021b, July 17). Kaggle. Available: https://www.kaggle.com/datasets/anaselmasry/breast-cancer-dataset

Breast cancer statistics and resources: Breast Cancer Research Foundation: BCRF. Breast Cancer Research Foundation. Retrieved July 21, 2022,

Brevik, E. C., Slaughter, L., Singh, B. L., Steffan, J. J., Collier, D., Barnhart, P., & Pereira, P. (2020). Soil and Human Health: Current Status and Future Needs. *Air, Soil and Water Research*, 13. Advance online publication. 10.1177/1178622120934441

Brinker, T. J., Hekler, A., Enk, A. H., Berking, C., Hauschild, A., Ghoreschi, K., & von Kalle, C. (2019). Deep neural networks are superior to dermatologists in melanoma image classification. *European Journal of Cancer*, 119, 11–17. 10.1016/j.ejca.2019.05.02331401469

Brodeur, A., Clark, A. E., Fleche, S., & Powdthavee, N. (2021). COVID-19, lockdowns and well-being: Evidence from Google trends. *Journal of Public Economics*, 193, 104346–104346. 10.1016/j.jpubeco.2020.10434633281237

Brosch, T.. (2015). Deep convolutional encoder networks for multiple sclerosis lesion segmentation. In *International Conference on Medical Image Computing and Computer-Assisted Intervention – MICCAI* (Vol. 9351, pp. 3–11). 10.1007/978-3-319-24574-4_1

Bueno, G., Gonzalez-Lopez, L., Garcia-Rojo, M., Laurinavicius, A., & Deniz, O. (2020). Data for glomeruli characterization in histopathological images. *Data in Brief*, 29, 105314. 10.1016/j.dib.2020.10531432154349

-Bulut H, Kınoğlu NG, Karaduman B. (2024). *"The Fear of Artificial İntelligence: Dentists and the Anxiety of the Unknown"*, Journal of Advanced Research in Health Sciences, 7(1), https://doi.org/. 30.03.2024.10.26650/JARHS2024-1302739

Burns, D., Dagnall, N., & Holt, M. (2020). Assessing the impact of the COVID-19 pandemic on student wellbeing at universities in the United Kingdom: A conceptual analysis. *Frontiers in Education*, 5, 5. 10.3389/feduc.2020.582882

Burt, J. R., Torosdagli, N., Khosravan, N., RaviPrakash, H., Mortazi, A., Tissavirasingham, F., Hussein, S., & Bagci, U. (2018). Deep learning beyond cats and dogs: Recent advances in diagnosing breast cancer with deep neural networks. *The British Journal of Radiology*, 91(1089), 20170545. 10.1259/bjr.2017054529565644

Bustan, M. N., & Poerwanto, B. (2021). Logistic Regression Model of Relationship between Breast Cancer Pathology Diagnosis with Metastasis. *Journal of Physics: Conference Series*, 1752(1), 1752. 10.1088/1742-6596/1752/1/012026

Butler, J., & Kern, M. L. (2016). The PERMA-profiler: A brief multidimensional measure of flourishing. *International Journal of Wellbeing*, 6(3), 1–48. 10.5502/ijw.v6i3.526

Butow, P., & Hoque, E. (2020). Using Artificial İntelligence to Analyse and Teach Communication in Healthcare. *The Breast*, •••, 50.32007704

Cai, J., Chang, O., Tang, X., Xue, C., & Wei, C. "Facial Expression Recognition Method Based on Sparse Batch Normalization CNN", in *2018 37th Chinese Control Conference (CCC),juill.2018*, p. 9608-9613, 10.23919/ChiCC.2018.8483567

Can artificial intelligence help see cancer in new ways? (2022, March 22). National Cancer Institute. https://www.cancer.gov/news-events/cancer-currents-blog/2022/artificial-intelligence-cancer-imaging

Carrle, F. P., Hollenbenders, Y., & Reichenbach, A. (2023). Generation of Synthetic EEG Data for Training Algorithms Supporting the Diagnosis of Major Depressive Disorder. *Frontiers in Neuroscience*, 17, 1219133. 10.3389/fnins.2023.121913337849893

Carter, K., Banks, S., Armstrong, A., Kindon, S., & Burkett, I. (2013). Issues of disclosure and intrusion: Ethical challenges for a community researcher. *Ethics & Social Welfare*, 7(1), 92–100. 10.1080/17496535.2013.769344

Cervical Cancer largest dataset (SipakMed). (2021, March 12). Kaggle. Available: https://www.kaggle.com/datasets/prahladmehandiratta/cervical-cancer-largest-dataset-sipakmed

Chadebecq, F., Lovat, L. B., & Stoyanov, D. (2023). Artificial intelligence and automation in endoscopy and surgery. *Nature Reviews. Gastroenterology & Hepatology*, 20(3), 171–182. 10.1038/s41575-022-00701-y36352158

Chaloner, T. M., Gurr, S. J., & Bebber, D. P. (2021). Plant pathogen infection risk tracks global crop yields under climate change. *Nature Climate Change*, 11(8), 710–715. Advance online publication. 10.1038/s41558-021-01104-8

Chan, C. W., Law, B. M., So, W. K., Chow, K. M., & Waye, M. M. (2017). Novel strategies on personalized medicine for breast cancer treatment: An update. *International Journal of Molecular Sciences*, 18(11), 2423. 10.3390/ijms1811242329140300

Chang, Y., Stanley, R. J., Moss, R. H., & Van Stoecker, W. (2005). A systematic heuristic approach for feature selection for melanoma discrimination using clinical images. *Skin Research and Technology*, 11(3), 165–178. 10.1111/j.1600-0846.2005.00116.x15998327

Chan, L., Swain, V. D., Kelley, C., de Barbaro, K., Abowd, G. D., & Wilcox, L. (2018). Students' experiences with ecological momentary assessment tools to report on emotional well-being. *Proceedings of the ACM on Interactive, Mobile, Wearable and Ubiquitous Technologies*, 2(1), 1–20. 10.1145/3191735

Chaunzwa, T. L., Hosny, A., Xu, Y., Shafer, A., Diao, N., Lanuti, M., Christiani, D. C., Mak, R. H., & Aerts, H. J. W. L. (2021). Deep learning classification of lung cancer histology using CT images. *Scientific Reports*, 11(1), 5471. 10.1038/s41598-021-84630-x33727623

Cheng, J. (2017) Brain tumor dataset. *Figshare*. Available: https://figshare.com/articles/dataset/brain_tumor_dataset/1512427

Chi, B. W., & Hsu, C. C. (2012). A hybrid approach to integrate genetic algorithm into dual scoring model in enhancing the performance of credit scoring model. *Expert Systems with Applications*, 39(3), 2650–2661. 10.1016/j.eswa.2011.08.120

Choi, J., Shin, K., Jung, J., Bae, H. J., Kim, D. H., Byeon, J. S., & Kim, N. (2020). Convolutional neural network technology in endoscopic imaging: Artificial intelligence for endoscopy. *Clinical Endoscopy*, 53(2), 117–126. 10.5946/ce.2020.05432252504

Chow, J. C. L., Sanders, L., & Li, K. (2023). Impact of ChatGPT on medical chatbots as a disruptive technology". *Frontiers in Artificial Intelligence*, 6(1), 1–3. 10.3389/frai.2023.116601437091303

Çinar, A., & Yildirim, M. (2020). Detection of tumors on brain MRI images using the hybrid convolutional neural network architecture. *Medical Hypotheses*, 139, 109684. 10.1016/j.mehy.2020.10968432240877

Clifton, D. A., Gibbons, J., Davies, J., & Tarassenko, L. (2012, June). Machine learning and software engineering in health informatics. In 2012 first international workshop on realizing ai synergies in software engineering (raise) (pp. 37-41). IEEE. 10.1109/RAISE.2012.6227968

Cloutier, S., Ehlenz, M., & Afinowich, R. (2019). Cultivating community wellbeing: Guiding principles for research and practice. *International Journal of Community Well-being*, 2(3-4), 277–299. 10.1007/s42413-019-00033-x

Coburn, A., & Gormally, S. (2020). Defining well-being in community development from the ground up: A case study of participant and practitioner perspectives. *Community Development Journal: An International Forum*, 55(2), 237–257. 10.1093/cdj/bsy048

Codella, N. C., Rotemberg, V., Tschandl, P., Celebi, M. E., Dusza, S., Gutman, D., ... Halpern, A. (2019). Skin lesion analysis toward melanoma detection 2018: A challenge hosted by the International Skin Imaging Collaboration (ISIC). *arXiv preprint arXiv:1902.03368.*

Constant, I., & Sabourdin, N. (2012). The EEG Signal: A Window on the Cortical Brain Activity. *Paediatric Anaesthesia*, 22(6), 539–552. 10.1111/j.1460-9592.2012.03883.x22594406

Cooke, P. J., Melchert, T. P., & Connor, K. (2016). Measuring well-being: A review of instruments. *The Counseling Psychologist*, 44(5), 730–757. 10.1177/0011000016633507

Corley, I. A., & Huang, Y. 2018. "Deep EEG Super-Resolution: Upsampling EEG Spatial Resolution with Generative Adversarial Networks." In *2018 IEEE EMBS International Conference on Biomedical & Health Informatics (BHI)*, IEEE, 100–103. 10.1109/BHI.2018.8333379

Costanza-Chock, S. (2020). *Design justice: Community-led practices to build the worlds we need.* The MIT Press. 10.7551/mitpress/12255.001.0001

Crawford, D. N. (2020). Supporting student wellbeing during COVID-19. Tips from regional and remote Australia.

Creswell, J. W. (2021). *A Concise Introduction To Mixed Methods Research.* SAGE publications.

Crosby, D., Bhatia, S., Brindle, K. M., Coussens, L. M., Dive, C., Emberton, M., Esener, S., Fitzgerald, R. C., Gambhir, S. S., Kuhn, P., Rebbeck, T. R., & Balasubramanian, S. (2022). Early detection of cancer. *Science.* https://doi.org/aay9040

Cummins, M. R., Nachimuthu, S. K., Abdelrahman, S. E., Facelli, J. C., & Gouripeddi, R. (2023). Nonhypothesis-driven research: data mining and knowledge discovery. In *Clinical research informatics* (pp. 413–432). Springer International Publishing. 10.1007/978-3-031-27173-1_20

D'Alfonso, S. (2020). AI in mental health. *Current Opinion in Psychology*, 36, 112–117. 10.1016/j.copsyc.2020.04.00532604065

Daher, M., Carré, P. D., Jaramillo, A., Olivares, H., & Tomicic, A. (2017). Experience and meaning in qualitative research: a conceptual review and a methodological device proposal. Forum Qual. Sozialforschung 18. 10.17169/fqs-18.3.2696

Daryanto, S., Wang, L., & Jacinthe, P. A. (2016). Drought effects on root and tuber production: A meta-analysis. *Agricultural Water Management*, 176, 122–131. 10.1016/j.agwat.2016.05.019

Das, K., Bhattacharya, S., Sinha, R., & Paul, R. R. (2021). Artificial intelligence in dermatology: Recent developments and prospects. *Clinical Dermatology Review*, 5(3), 192–202. 10.4103/cdr.cdr_67_21

Dave, T., Athaluri, S. A., & Singh, S. (2023). Chatgpt in Medicine: An Overview of Its Applications, Advantages, Limitations, Future Prospects, and Ethical Considerations. *Frontiers in Artificial Intelligence*, 6, 1169595. 10.3389/frai.2023.116959537215063

De Pue, S., Gillebert, C., Dierckx, E., Vanderhasselt, M.-A., De Raedt, R., & Van den Bussche, E. (2021). The impact of the COVID-19 pandemic on wellbeing and cognitive functioning of older adults. *Scientific Reports*, 11(1), 4636. 10.1038/s41598-021-84127-733633303

Deepak, S., & Ameer, P. (2019). Brain tumor classification using deep CNN features via transfer learning. *Computers in Biology and Medicine*, 111, 103345. 10.1016/j.compbiomed.2019.10334531279167

Dejoux, C., & L'eon, E. (2018). *M´etamorphose des managers* (1st ed.). Pearson.

Delgado-Baquerizo, M., Guerra, C. A., Cano-Díaz, C., Egidi, E., Wang, J. T., Eisenhauer, N., Singh, B. K., & Maestre, F. T. (2020). The proportion of soil-borne pathogens increases with warming at the global scale. *Nature Climate Change*, 10(6), 550–554. 10.1038/s41558-020-0759-3

Demir, F. (2021). DeepBreastNet: A novel and robust approach for automated breast cancer detection from histopathological images. *Biocybernetics and Biomedical Engineering*, 41(3), 1123–1139. 10.1016/j.bbe.2021.07.004

Dennehy, D. (2020). Ireland post-pandemic: Utilizing AI to kick-start economic recovery. *Cutter Business Technology Journal*, 33(11), 22–27.

Desneux, N., Wajnberg, E., Wyckhuys, K. A., Burgio, G., Arpaia, S., Narváez-Vasquez, C. A., González-Cabrera, J., Ruescas, D. C., Tabone, E., Frandon, J., Pizzol, J., Poncet, C., Cabello, T., & Urbaneja, A. (2010). Biological invasion of European tomato crops by Tuta absoluta: Ecology, geographic expansion and prospects for biological control. *Journal of Pest Science*, 83(3), 197–215. 10.1007/s10340-010-0321-6

Devi, M., & Maheswaran, S. (2018). An efficient method for brain tumor detection using texture features and SVM classifier in MR images. Asian Pacific journal of cancer prevention. *APJCP*, 19(10), 2789.

Devkota, A. A., B, Prasad, PWC, Singh, AK & Elchouemi, A 2018, „Image Segmentation for Early Stage Brain Tumor Detection using Mathematical Morphological Reconstruction", Int. Conference on Smart Computing and Communications, Procedia Computer Science vol. 125, pp. 115–123. 10.1016/j.procs.2017.12.017

Dhall, A., Goecke, R., Lucey, S., & Gedeon, T. "Static facial expression analysis in tough conditions: Data, evaluation protocol and benchmark", in *2011 IEEE International Conference on Computer Vision Workshops (ICCV Workshops),nov.2011*, p. 2106-2112, 10.1109/ICCVW.2011.6130508

Diener, E., Emmons, R. A., Larsen, R., & Griffin, S. (1985). The satisfaction with life scale. *Journal of Personality Assessment*, 49(1), 71–75. 10.1207/s15327752jpa4901_1316367493

Diener, E., Suh, E. M., Lucas, R. E., & Smith, H. L. (1999). Subjective well-being: Three decades of progress. *Psychological Bulletin*, 125(2), 276–302. 10.1037/0033-2909.125.2.276

Dobermann, A., Bruulsema, T., Cakmak, I., Gerard, B., Majumdar, K., McLaughlin, M., Reidsma, P., Vanlauwe, B., Wollenberg, L., Zhang, F., & Zhang, X. (2022). Responsible plant nutrition: A new paradigm to support food system transformation. *Global Food Security*, 33, 100636. Advance online publication. 10.1016/j.gfs.2022.100636

Dodge, R., Daly, A., Huyton, J., & Sanders, L. (2012). The challenge of defining wellbeing. *International Journal of Wellbeing*, 2(3), 222–235. 10.5502/ijw.v2i3.4

Dooris, M., Farrier, A., & Froggett, L. (2018). Wellbeing: The challenge of 'operationalising' an holistic concept within a reductionist public health programme. *Perspectives in Public Health*, 138(2), 93–99. 10.1177/17579139177112042857430

Doppalapudi, S., Qiu, R. G., & Badr, Y. (2021). Lung cancer survival period prediction and understanding: Deep learning approaches. *International Journal of Medical Informatics*, 148, 104371. 10.1016/j.ijmedinf.2020.10437133461009

Dorigo, M., Birattari, M., & Stutzle, T. (2006). Ant colony optimization. *IEEE Computational Intelligence Magazine*, 1(4), 28–39. 10.1109/MCI.2006.329691

Dubberly, H., & Pangaro, P. (2019). Cybernetics and design: Conversations for action. *Design Research Foundations*, 85–99. 10.1007/978-3-030-18557-2_4

Dubberly, H., & Pangaro, P. (2007). Cybernetics and service-craft: Language for behavior-focused design. *Kybernetes*, 36(9/10), 1301–1317. 10.1108/03684920710827319

Duffy, FD, Gordon, GH, Whelan, G, Cole-Kelly, K, & Frankel, R. (2004). Assessing competence in communication and interpersonal skills: The Kalamazoo II report. *Academic Medicine*, •••, 79.15165967

Duleba, A. J., & Olive, D. L. (1996). Regression analysis and multivariate analysis. *Seminars in Reproductive Endocrinology*, 14(2), 139–153. 10.1055/s-2007-10163228796937

Du, W., Rao, N., Liu, D., Jiang, H., Luo, C., Li, Z., Gan, T., & Zeng, B. (2019). Review on the applications of deep learning in the analysis of gastrointestinal endoscopy images. *IEEE Access : Practical Innovations, Open Solutions*, 7, 142053–142069. 10.1109/ACCESS.2019.2944676

Dwivedi, Y.K. (2023). Opinion Paper: "So What if Chatgpt Wrote İt?" Multidisciplinary Perspectives on Opportunities, Challenges and İmplications of Generative Conversational aI For Research, Practice and Policy. *International Journal of Information Management*. Advance online publication. 10.1016/j.ijinfomgt.2023.102642 26.03.2024

El-Bendary, N., & Belal, N. A. (2020). A feature-fusion framework of clinical, genomics, and histopathological data for METABRIC breast cancer subtype classification. *Applied Soft Computing*, 91, 106238. 10.1016/j.asoc.2020.106238

El-Hagrassy, M. M., Duarte, D., Thibaut, A., Lucena, M. F., & Fregni, F. (2018). Principles of designing a clinical trial: Optimizing chances of trial success. *Current Behavioral Neuroscience Reports*, 5(2), 143–152. 10.1007/s40473-018-0152-y30467533

-Else, H. (2023). *"Abstracts Written by Chatgpt Fool Scientists"*, 423-423 Nature, *613* (7944). https://doi.org/.10.1038/d41586-023-00056-7

Erkal, B., Başak, S., Çiloğlu, A., & Şener, D. D. (2020, November). Multiclass classification of brain cancer with machine learning algorithms. In *2020 Medical Technologies Congress (TIPTEKNO)* (pp. 1-4). IEEE. 10.1109/TIPTEKNO50054.2020.9299233

Esmaeili, M., & Kiani, K. (2023). Generating Personalized Facial Emotions Using Emotional EEG Signals and Conditional Generative Adversarial Networks. *Multimedia Tools and Applications*, 83(12), 1–26. 10.1007/s11042-023-17018-w

Esteva, A., Kuprel, B., Novoa, R. A., Ko, J., Swetter, S. M., Blau, H. M., & Thrun, S. (2017). Dermatologist-level classification of skin cancer with deep neural networks. *Nature*, 542(7639), 115–118. 10.1038/nature2105628117445

European Commission. (2019). A definition of artificial intelligence: Main capabilities and scientific disciplines. Shaping Europe's digital future. Retrieved from https://digital-strategy.ec.europa.eu/en/library/definition-artificial-intelligence-main-capabilities-and-scientific-disciplines

Farabet, C., Couprie, C., Najman, L., & LeCun, Y. (2013). Learning hierarchical features for scene labeling. *IEEE Transactions on Pattern Analysis and Machine Intelligence*, 35(8), 1915–1929. 10.1109/TPAMI.2012.23123787344

Farina, E., Nabhen, J. J., Dacoregio, M. I., Batalini, F., & Moraes, F. Y. (2022, February 10). An overview of artificial intelligence in oncology. *Future Science OA*, 8(4), FSO787. Advance online publication. 10.2144/fsoa-2021-007435369274

Fassihi, N.. (2011). Melanoma diagnosis by the use of wavelet analysis based on morphological operators. In *Proceedings of the International MultiConference of Engineers and Computer Scientists* (pp. 16–18).

Fawaz, M., & Samaha, A. (2021). E-learning: Depression, anxiety, and stress symptomatology among Lebanese university students during COVID-19 quarantine. *Nursing Forum*, 56(1), 52–57. 10.1111/nuf.1252133125744

Fayyad, U., Piatetsky-Shapiro, G., & Smyth, P. (1996). From data mining to knowledge discovery in databases. *AI Magazine*, 17(3), 37–37.

Ferroni, P., Zanzotto, F. M., Riondino, S., Scarpato, N., Guadagni, F., & Roselli, M. (2019). Breast Cancer Prognosis Using a Machine Learning Approach. *Cancers (Basel)*, 11(3), 328. 10.3390/cancers1103032830866535

Figueroa, M., Hammond-Kosack, K. E., & Solomon, P. S. (2018). A review of wheat diseases—A field perspective. *Molecular Plant Pathology*, 19(6), 1523–1536. 10.1111/mpp.1261829045052

Fioramonti, L., Coscieme, L., Costanza, R., Kubiszewski, I., Trebeck, K., Wallis, S., Roberts, D., Mortensen, L. F., Pickett, K. E., Wilkinson, R., Ragnarsdottír, K. V., McGlade, J., Lovins, H., & De Vogli, R. (2022). Wellbeing economy: An effective paradigm to mainstream post-growth policies? *Ecological Economics*, 192, 107261. 10.1016/j.ecolecon.2021.107261

Fokkinga, S. F., Desmet, P. M. A., & Hekkert, P. (2020). Impact-centered design: Introducing an integrated framework of the psychological and behavioral effects of design. *International Journal of Design*, 14(2), 97–116.

Frisch, M. B., Cornell, J., Villanueva, M., & Retzlaff, P. J. (1992). Clinical validation of the quality of life inventory: A measure of life satisfaction for use in treatment planning and outcome assessment. *Psychological Assessment*, 4(1), 92–101. 10.1037/1040-3590.4.1.92

Fu, B., Li, F., Niu, Y., Wu, H., Li, Y., & Shi, G. (2021). Conditional Generative Adversarial Network for EEG-Based Emotion Fine-Grained Estimation and Visualization. *Journal of Visual Communication and Image Representation*, 74, 102982. 10.1016/j.jvcir.2020.102982

Fu, Z., Jin, Z., Zhang, C., He, Z., Zha, Z., Hu, C., Gan, T., Yan, Q., Wang, P., & Ye, X. (2021). The future of endoscopic navigation: A review of advanced endoscopic vision technology. *IEEE Access : Practical Innovations, Open Solutions*, 9, 41144–41167. 10.1109/ACCESS.2021.3065104

Gallego, J., Pedraza, A., Lopez, S., Steiner, G., Gonzalez, L., Laurinavicius, A., & Bueno, G. (2018). Glomerulus classification and detection based on convolutional neural networks. *Journal of Imaging*, 4(1), 20. 10.3390/jimaging4010020

Galvez-Nino, M., Ruiz, R., Pinto, J. A., Roque, K., Mantilla, R., Raez, L. E., & Mas, L. (2020). Lung cancer in the young. *Lung*, 198(1), 195–200. 10.1007/s00408-019-00294-531773258

Garg, A., Venkataramani, V. V., Karthikeyan, A., & Priyakumar, U. D. (2022, January). Modern AI/ML methods for healthcare: Opportunities and challenges. In *International Conference on Distributed Computing and Internet Technology* (pp. 3-25). Cham: Springer International Publishing. 10.1007/978-3-030-94876-4_1

Genç, E., & Arslan, G. (2021). Optimism and dispositional hope to promote college students' subjective well-being in the context of the COVID-19 pandemic. *Journal of Positive School Psychology*, 5(2), 87–96. 10.47602/jpsp.v5i2.255

Gensheimer, M. F., Henry, A. S., Wood, D. J., Hastie, T. J., Aggarwal, S., Dudley, S. A., Pradhan, P., Banerjee, I., Cho, E., Ramchandran, K., Pollom, E., Koong, A. C., Rubin, D. L., & Chang, D. T. (2019). Automated Survival Prediction in Metastatic Cancer Patients Using High-Dimensional Electronic Medical Record Data. *Journal of the National Cancer Institute*, 111(6), 568–574. 10.1093/jnci/djy17830346554

Getzen, E., Ungar, L., Mowery, D., Jiang, X., & Long, Q. (2023). Mining for equitable health: Assessing the impact of missing data in electronic health records. *Journal of Biomedical Informatics*, 139, 104269. 10.1016/j.jbi.2022.10426936621750

Gillespie, T. (2014). The relevance of algorithms. In Gillespie, T., Boczkowski, P. J., & Foot, K. A. (Eds.), *Media Technologies* (pp. 167–194). The MIT Press. 10.7551/mitpress/9042.003.0013

Glanville, R. (2009). Article. *System Science and Cybernetics*, 3, 59–86.

Golan, R., Reddy, R., & Ramasamy, R. (2024). The Rise of Artificial İntelligence-Driven Health Communication. *Translational Andrology and Urology*, 13(2), 356–358. 10.21037/tau-23-55638481858

Goodfellow, I. J., ... "Challenges in Representation Learning: A Report on Three Machine Learning Contests", in *Neural Information Processing, Berlin, Heidelberg,2013*, p. 117-124, 10.1007/978-3-642-42051-1_16

Goodfellow, I.. (2014). Generative Adversarial Nets. *Advances in Neural Information Processing Systems*, •••, 27.

Gracious, L. A., Jasmine, R. M., Pooja, E., Anish, T. P., Johncy, G., & Subramanian, R. S. (2023, October). Machine Learning and Deep Learning Transforming Healthcare: An Extensive Exploration of Applications, Algorithms, and Prospects. In 2023 4th IEEE Global Conference for Advancement in Technology (GCAT) (pp. 1-6). IEEE.

Graham, S., Depp, C., Lee, E. E., Nebeker, C., Tu, X., Kim, H.-C., & Jeste, D. V. (2019). Artificial intelligence for mental health and mental illnesses: An overview. *Current Psychiatry Reports*, 21(11), 116. 10.1007/s11920-019-1094-031701320

Green, A., Martin, N., Pfitzner, J., O'Rourke, M., & Knight, N. (1994). Computer image analysis in the diagnosis of melanoma. *Journal of the American Academy of Dermatology*, 31(5), 958–964. 10.1016/S0190-9622(94)70264-07962777

Green, N., Rubinelli, S., Scott, D., & Visser, A. (2013). Health Communication Meets Artificial İntelligence. *Patient Education and Counseling*, 92(2), 139–141. 10.1016/j.pec.2013.06.01323866991

Gregory, T., Engelhardt, D., Lewkowicz, A., Luddy, S., Guhn, M., Gadermann, A., Schonert-Reichl, K., & Brinkman, S. (2019). Validity of the middle years development instrument for population monitoring of student wellbeing in Australian school children. *Child Indicators Research*, 12(3), 873–899. 10.1007/s12187-018-9562-3

Gross, R., Matthews, I., Cohn, J., Kanade, T., & Baker, S. "Multi-PIE", *Proc. Int. Conf. Autom. Face Gesture Recognit. Int. Conf. Autom. Face Gesture Recognit.*, vol. 28, no 5, p. 807-813, mai 2010, 10.1016/j.imavis.2009.08.002

Gulrajani, I.. (2017). Improved Training of Wasserstein Gans. *Advances in Neural Information Processing Systems*, •••, 30.

H. Li, Y. Cao, S. Li, J. Zhao and Y. Sun, "XGBoost Model and Its Application to Personal Credit Evaluation," in IEEE Intelligent Systems, vol. 35, no. 3, 52-61, 1 May-June 2020, .10.1109/MIS.2020.2972533

Habashi, A. G., Azab, A. M., Eldawlatly, S., & Aly, G. M. (2023). Generative Adversarial Networks in EEG Analysis: An Overview. *Journal of Neuroengineering and Rehabilitation*, 20(1), 40. 10.1186/s12984-023-01169-w37038142

Haenssle, H. A., Fink, C., Schneiderbauer, R., Toberer, F., Buhl, T., Blum, A., Kalloo, A., Hassen, A. B. H., Thomas, L., Enk, A., Uhlmann, L., Alt, C., Arenbergerova, M., Bakos, R., Baltzer, A., Bertlich, I., Blum, A., Bokor-Billmann, T., Bowling, J., & Zalaudek, I.Reader Study Level-I Group. (2018). Man against machine: Diagnostic performance of a deep learning convolutional neural network for dermoscopic melanoma recognition in comparison to 58 dermatologists. *Annals of Oncology : Official Journal of the European Society for Medical Oncology*, 29(8), 1836–1842. 10.1093/annonc/mdy16629846502

Hagey, K., & Horwitz, J. (2021). Facebook tried to make its platform a healthier place. It got angrier instead. *Wall Street Journal*, 1–16.

Hancock, M. C., & Magnan, J. F. (2019). Level set image segmentation with velocity term learned from data with applications to lung nodule segmentation. *ArXiv Preprint ArXiv:1910.03191*.

Hartmann, K. G., Schirrmeister, R. T., & Ball, T. 2018. "EEG-GAN: Generative Adversarial Networks for Electroencephalograhic (EEG) Brain Signals." *arXiv preprint arXiv:1806.01875*.

Hashemzadeh, H., Shojaeilangari, S., Allahverdi, A., Rothbauer, M., Ertl, P., & Naderi-Manesh, H. (2021). A combined microfluidic deep learning approach for lung cancer cell high throuhput screening toward automatic cancer screening applications. *Scientific Reports*, 11(1), 9804. 10.1038/s41598-021-89352-833963232

Havaei, M.. (2014). Brain tumor segmentation with deep neural networks. In *Proceedings of the BRATS-MICCAI*.

Heisler, M, Bouknight, RR, Hayward, RA, Smith, DM, & Kerr, EA. (2002). The relative importance of physician communication, participatory decision-making, and patient understanding in diabetes self-management. *Journal of General Internal Medicine*, •••, 17.11972720

Hekkert, P., & van Dijk, M. (2011). *Vision in design - a guidebook for innovators*. BIS Publishers.

Helm, J. E., Alaeddini, A., Stauffer, J. M., Bretthauer, K. M., & Skolarus, T. A. (2016). Reducing hospital readmissions by integrating empirical prediction with resource optimization. *Production and Operations Management*, 25(2), 233–257. 10.1111/poms.12377

Helwig, N. E. (2017). *Multivariate Linear Regression*. University of Minnesota.

Hemmatirad, K., Babaie, M., Afshari, M., Maleki, D., Saiadi, M., & Tizhoosh, H. R. (2022, June). Quality Control of Whole Slide Images using the YOLO Concept. In 2022 IEEE 10th International Conference on Healthcare Informatics (ICHI) (pp. 282-287). IEEE. 10.1109/ICHI54592.2022.00049

Hersh, W. R., Crabtree, M. K., Hickam, D. H., Sacherek, L., Friedman, C. P., Tidmarsh, P., & Kraemer, D. (2002). Factors associated with success in searching MEDLINE and applying evidence to answer clinical questions. *Journal of the American Medical Informatics Association : JAMIA*, 9(3), 283–293. 10.1197/jamia.M099611971889

Histopathologic Oral Cancer Detection using CNNs. (2021, July 21). Kaggle. Available: https://www.kaggle.com/datasets/ashenafifasilkebede/dataset

Hohenstein, J., Kizilcec, R. F., DiFranzo, D., Aghajari, Z., Mieczkowski, H., Levy, K., Naaman, M., Hancock, J., & Jung, M. F. (2023). Artificial Intelligence in Communication Impacts Language and Social Relationships". *Scientific Reports*, 13(1), 5487. 10.1038/s41598-023-30938-937015964

Hong, X., Lin, R., Yang, C., Zeng, N., Cai, C., Gou, J., & Yang, J. (2019). Predicting Alzheimer's disease using LSTM. *IEEE Access : Practical Innovations, Open Solutions*, 7, 80893–80901. 10.1109/ACCESS.2019.2919385

Hossain, L., Kam, D., Kong, F., Wigand, R. T., & Bossomaier, T. (2016). Social media in Ebola outbreak. *Epidemiology and Infection*, 144(10), 2136–2143. 10.1017/S095026881600039X26939535

Howlader, N., Cronin, K. A., Kurian, A. W., & Andridge, R. (2018). Differences in Breast Cancer Survival by Molecular Subtypes in the United States. *Cancer Epidemiology, Biomarkers & Prevention*, 27(6), 619–626. 10.1158/1055-9965. EPI-17-062729593010

Huang, S., Wang, P., Yamaji, N., & Ma, J. F. (2020). Plant Nutrition for Human Nutrition: Hints from Rice Research and Future Perspectives. *Molecular Plant*, 13(6), 825–835. 10.1016/j.molp.2020.05.00732434072

Hu, C., Chen, C., & Dong, X.-P. (2021). Impact of COVID-19 pandemic on patients with neurodegenerative diseases. *Frontiers in Aging Neuroscience*, 13, 664965. 10.3389/fnagi.2021.66496533897410

Hueman, M. T., Wang, H., Yang, C. Q., Sheng, L., Henson, D. E., Schwartz, A. M., & Chen, D. (2018). Creating prognostic systems for cancer patients: A demonstration using breast cancer. *Cancer Medicine*, 7(8), 3611–3621. 10.1002/cam4.162929968970

Hu, Y. (2015). Health Communication Research in the Digital Age: A Systematic Review. *Journal of Communication in Healthcare*, 8(4), 260–288. 10.1080/17538068.2015.1107308

Ibrahim, D. M., Elshennawy, N. M., & Sarhan, A. M. (2021). Deep-chest: Multi-classification deep learning model for diagnosing COVID-19, pneumonia, and lung cancer chest diseases. *Computers in Biology and Medicine*, 132, 104348. 10.1016/j.compbiomed.2021.10434833774272

Islam, J., & Zhang, Y. (2018). Brain MRI analysis for Alzheimer's disease diagnosis using an ensemble system of deep convolutional neural networks. *Brain Informatics*, 5(2), 1–14. 10.1186/s40708-018-0080-329881892

Islam, M. N., Hasan, M., Hossain, M. K., Alam, M. G. R., Uddin, M. Z., & Soylu, A. (2022). Vision transformer and explainable transfer learning models for auto detection of kidney cyst, stone and tumor from CT-radiography. *Scientific Reports*, 12(1), 11440. 10.1038/s41598-022-15634-435794172

Jabid, T., Kabir, M. H., & Chae, O. (2010). Robust Facial Expression Recognition Based on Local Directional Pattern. *ETRI Journal*, 32(5), 784–794. 10.4218/etrij.10.1510.0132

Jain, A. K., & Farrokhnia, F. (1991). Unsupervised texture segmentation using Gabor filters. *Pattern Recognition*, 24(12), 1167–1186. 10.1016/0031-3203(91)90143-S

Jain, D. K., Shamsolmoali, P., & Sehdev, P. (2019, April). Extended deep neural network for facial emotion recognition. *Pattern Recognition Letters*, 120, 69–74. 10.1016/j.patrec.2019.01.008

Jawarkar, J., Solanki, N., Vaishnav, M., Vichare, H., & Degadwala, S. (2021). Multistage lung cancer detection and prediction using deep learning. *International Journal of Scientific Research in Science, Engineering and Technology*, •••, 54–60. 10.32628/IJSRSET218217

Jiang, F., Jiang, Y., Zhi, H., Dong, Y., Li, H., Ma, S., Wang, Y., Dong, Q., Shen, H., & Wang, Y. (2017). Artificial intelligence in healthcare: Past, present and future. *Stroke and Vascular Neurology*, 2(4), 230–243. 10.1136/svn-2017-00010129507784

Jiang, P., Ergu, D., Liu, F., Cai, Y., & Ma, B. (2022). A Review of Yolo Algorithm Developments. *Procedia Computer Science*, 199, 1066–1073. 10.1016/j.procs.2022.01.135

Jiang, W., Zeng, G., Wang, S., Wu, X., & Xu, C. (2022). Application of deep learning in lung cancer imaging diagnosis. *Journal of Healthcare Engineering*, 2022, 2022. 10.1155/2022/610794035028122

Jin, Z., Gan, T., Wang, P., Fu, Z., Zhang, C., Yan, Q., Zheng, X., Liang, X., & Ye, X. (2022). Deep learning for gastroscopic images: Computer-aided techniques for clinicians. *Biomedical Engineering Online*, 21(1), 12. 10.1186/s12938-022-00979-835148764

Ji, X., Bossé, Y., Landi, M. T., Gui, J., Xiao, X., Qian, D., Joubert, P., Lamontagne, M., Li, Y., Gorlov, I., de Biasi, M., Han, Y., Gorlova, O., Hung, R. J., Wu, X., McKay, J., Zong, X., Carreras-Torres, R., Christiani, D. C., & Amos, C. I. (2018). Identification of susceptibility pathways for the role of chromosome 15q25. 1 in modifying lung cancer risk. *Nature Communications*, 9(1), 3221. 10.1038/s41467-018-05074-y30104567

Johnson, J. W. (2021). Generative adversarial networks in medical imaging. In *State of the Art in Neural Networks and their Applications* (pp. 271–278). Academic Press. 10.1016/B978-0-12-819740-0.00013-9

Joris, P., Develter, W., Van De Voorde, W., Suetens, P., Maes, F., Vandermeulen, D., & Claes, P. (2018). „PreProcessing of Heteroscedastic Medical Images". *IEEE Access : Practical Innovations, Open Solutions*, 6(2), 26047–26058. 10.1109/ACCESS.2018.2833286

Kabiraj, S., ... "Breast Cancer Risk Prediction using XGBoost and Random Forest Algorithm," 2020 11th International Conference on Computing, Communication and Networking Technologies (ICCCNT), Kharagpur, India, 2020,1-4 10.1109/ICCCNT49239.2020.9225451

Kalaivani, N., Manimaran, N., Sophia, S., & Devi, D. D. (2020). Deep learning based lung cancer detection and classification. *IOP Conference Series. Materials Science and Engineering*, 994(1), 012026. 10.1088/1757-899X/994/1/012026

Kamala, S. P. R., Gayathri, S., Pillai, N. M., Gracious, L. A., Varun, C. M., & Subramanian, R. S. (2023, July). Predictive Analytics for Heart Disease Detection: A Machine Learning Approach. In 2023 4th International Conference on Electronics and Sustainable Communication Systems (ICESC) (pp. 1583-1589). IEEE.

Kang, K., ... (2014). Fully convolutional neural networks for crowd segmentation. *arXiv preprint arXiv:1411.4464*. Retrieved from https://arxiv.org/abs/1411.4464

Kanwal, M., Ding, X., & Cao, Y. (2017). Familial risk for lung cancer. *Oncology Letters*, 13(2), 535–542. 10.3892/ol.2016.551828356926

Karuna, M., & Joshi, A. (2013). AUTOMATIC DETECTION AND SEVERITY ANALYSIS OF BRAIN TUMORS USING GUI IN MATLAB. *International Journal of Research in Engineering and Technology*, 02(10), 586–594. 10.15623/ijret.2013.0210092

Kathamuthu, N. D., Subramaniam, S., Le, Q. H., Muthusamy, S., Panchal, H., Sundararajan, S. C. M., Alrubaie, A. J., & Zahra, M. M. A. (2023). A deep transfer learning-based convolution neural network model for COVID-19 detection using computed tomography scan images for medical applications. *Advances in Engineering Software*, 175, 103317. 10.1016/j.advengsoft.2022.10331736311489

Kavitha, G., Sudha, K., Jayasutha, D., Sivaraman, V., Nalini, M., & Subramanian, R. S. (2023, November). Accelerating Alzheimer's Research with Machine Learning Models for Improved Detection. In 2023 7th International Conference on Electronics, Communication and Aerospace Technology (ICECA) (pp. 855-862). IEEE.

Kawahara, J., BenTaieb, A., & Hamarneh, G. (2016). Deep features to classify skin lesions. In 2016 IEEE 13th International Symposium on Biomedical Imaging (ISBI) (pp. 1397-1400). IEEE. https://doi.org/10.1109/ISBI.2016.7493528

Kawazoe, Y., Shimamoto, K., Yamaguchi, R., Shintani-Domoto, Y., Uozaki, H., Fukayama, M., & Ohe, K. (2018). Faster R-CNN-based glomerular detection in multistained human whole slide images. *Journal of Imaging*, 4(7), 91. 10.3390/jimaging4070091

Keesstra, S. D., Bouma, J., Wallinga, J., Tittonell, P., Smith, P., Cerdà, A., Montanarella, L., Quinton, J. N., Pachepsky, Y., Putten, W. H., Bardgett, R. D., Moolenaar, S., Mol, G., Jansen, B., & Fresco, L. O. (2016). The significance of soils and soil science towards realization of the United Nations Sustainable Development Goals. *Soil (Göttingen)*, 2(2), 111–128. 10.5194/soil-2-111-2016

Khademi, S., Heidarian, S., Afshar, P., Naderkhani, F., Oikonomou, A., Plataniotis, K. N., & Mohammadi, A. (2023). Spatio-Temporal Hybrid Fusion of CAE and SWin Transformers for Lung Cancer Malignancy Prediction. *ICASSP 2023-2023 IEEE International Conference on Acoustics, Speech and Signal Processing (ICASSP)*, 1–5.

Khan, I., Shah, D., & Shah, S. S. (2021). COVID-19 pandemic and its positive impacts on environment: An updated review. *International Journal of Environmental Science and Technology*, 18(2), 521–530. 10.1007/s13762-020-03021-333224247

Khatri, K., & Sharma, A. (2020). ECG Signal Analysis for Heart Disease Detection Based on Sensor Data Analysis with Signal Processing by Deep Learning Architectures. Research Journal of Computer Systems and Engineering, 1(1), 06-10.

Kidney Cancer - statistics. (2023, May 23). Cancer.Net. Available: https://www.cancer.net/cancer-types/kidney-cancer/statistics

Kim, D. H., Baddar, W. J., Jang, J., & Ro, Y. M. (2019, April). Multi-Objective Based Spatio-Temporal Feature Representation Learning Robust to Expression Intensity Variations for Facial Expression Recognition. *IEEE Transactions on Affective Computing*, 10(2), 223–236. 10.1109/TAFFC.2017.2695999

Kim, Y. J., Cho, H. C., & Cho, H. C. (2021). Deep learning-based computer-aided diagnosis system for gastroscopy image classification using synthetic data. *Applied Sciences (Basel, Switzerland)*, 11(2), 760. 10.3390/app11020760

Kitchenham, B. (2004). Procedures for performing systematic reviews. *Keele, UK, Keele University, 33*(2004), 1–26.

Kitchenham, B., Brereton, O. P., Budgen, D., Turner, M., Bailey, J., & Linkman, S. (2009). Systematic literature reviews in software engineering–a systematic literature review. *Information and Software Technology*, 51(1), 7–15. 10.1016/j.infsof.2008.09.009

Kjell, O. N. E., & Diener, , E. (2020). Abbreviated Three-Item Versions of the Satisfaction with Life Scale and the Harmony in Life Scale Yield as Strong Psychometric Properties as the Original Scales. *Journal of Personality Assessment*, 0, 1–2. 10.1080/00223891.2020.173709332167788

Klenke, K. (2016). *Qualitative Research In The Study Of Leadership*. Emerald Group Publishing Limited.

-Koçyiğit, A., Darı, A.B., (2023), *"Yapay Zekâ İletişiminde ChatGPT: İnsanlaşan Dijitalleşmenin Geleceği"*, Stratejik ve Sosyal Araştırmalar Dergisi, C.7, S.2, S..427-438.

Kohli, P. S., & Arora, S. (2018, December). Application of machine learning in disease prediction. In 2018 4th International conference on computing communication and automation (ICCCA) (pp. 1-4). IEEE. 10.1109/CCAA.2018.8777449

Kolbjørnsrud, V., Amico, R., & Thomas, R. J. (2017). Partnering with AI: How organizations can win over skeptical managers. *Strategy and Leadership*, 45(1), 37–43. 10.1108/SL-12-2016-0085

Konishi, K., Hashizume, M., Nakamoto, M., Kakeji, Y., Yoshino, I., Taketomi, A., & Maehara, Y. (2005, May). Augmented reality navigation system for endoscopic surgery based on three-dimensional ultrasound and computed tomography: Application to 20 clinical cases. In Vol. 1281, pp. 537–542). International congress series. Elsevier. 10.1016/j.ics.2005.03.234

Kourou, K., Exarchos, T. P., Exarchos, K. P., Karamouzis, M. V., & Fotiadis, D. I. (2014). Machine learning applications in cancer prognosis and prediction. *Computational and Structural Biotechnology Journal*, 13, 8–17. 10.1016/j.csbj.2014.11.00525750696

Kowalski, P. A., & Łukasik, S. (2015). Experimental study of selected parameters of the krill herd algorithm. In *Intelligent Systems' 2014:Proceedings of the 7th IEEE International Conference Intelligent Systems IS'2014, September 24-26, 2014, Warsaw, Poland,* Volume 1*: Mathematical Foundations, Theory, Analyses* (pp. 473-485). Springer International Publishing. 10.1007/978-3-319-11313-5_42

Kreps, G. L., & Neuhauser, L. (2013). Artificial intelligence and immediacy: Designing health communication to personally engage consumers and providers. *Patient Education and Counseling*, 92(2), 205–210.

Kriegsmann, M., Haag, C., Weis, C.-A., Steinbuss, G., Warth, A., Zgorzelski, C., Muley, T., Winter, H., Eichhorn, M. E., Eichhorn, F., Kriegsmann, J., Christopoulos, P., Thomas, M., Witzens-Harig, M., Sinn, P., von Winterfeld, M., Heussel, C., Herth, F., Klauschen, F., & Kriegsmann, K. (2020). Deep learning for the classification of small-cell and non-small-cell lung cancer. *Cancers (Basel)*, 12(6), 1604. 10.3390/cancers1206160432560475

Kumar, S., & Raman, S. (2020). Lung nodule segmentation using 3-dimensional convolutional neural networks. *Soft Computing for Problem Solving: SocProS 2018, Volume 1*, 585–596.

Kumar, S., Dikshit, H. K., Mishra, G. P., Singh, A., Aski, M. & Virk, P. S. (2022). Biofortification of Staple Crops: Present Status and Future Strategies. *Biofortification of Staple Crops*, 1-30. 10.1007/978-981-16-3280-8_1

Kumar, K., Kumar, V., Seema, , Sharma, M. K., Khan, A. A., & Idrisi, M. J. (2024). *"A Systematic Review of Blockchain Technology Assisted with Artificial Intelligence Technology for Networks and Communication Systems"*, Hindawi. *Journal of Computer Networks and Communications*, 2024, 9979371. Advance online publication. 10.1155/2024/9979371

Kumar, N., & Kumar, D. (2021, August). Machine learning based heart disease diagnosis using non-invasive methods: A review. []. IOP Publishing.]. *Journal of Physics: Conference Series*, 1950(1), 012081. 10.1088/1742-6596/1950/1/012081

Kumar, S., Dikshit, H. K., Mishra, G. P., & Singh, A. (2022). *Biofortification of Staple Crops*. Springer Nature Singapore Pte. Ltd., 10.1007/978-981-16-3280-8

Kumar, V., & Bakariya, B. (2021). Classification of malignant lung cancer using deep learning. *Journal of Medical Engineering & Technology*, 45(2), 85–93. 10.1080/03091902.2020.185383733448905

Kurzweil, R. (2005). *The singularity is near*. Viking.

Labovitz, D. L., Shafner, L., Reyes Gil, M., Virmani, D., & Hanina, A. (2017). Using artificial intelligence to reduce the risk of nonadherence in patients on anticoagulation therapy. *Stroke*, 48(5), 1416–1419. 10.1161/STROKEAHA.116.01628128386037

Lacity, M., Willcocks, L., & Andrew, C. (2015). *Robotic process automation: Mature capabilities in the energy sector*. LSE Research Online Documents on Economics.

Lai, Y.-H., Chen, W.-N., Hsu, T.-C., Lin, C., Tsao, Y., & Wu, S. (2020). Overall survival prediction of non-small cell lung cancer by integrating microarray and clinical data with deep learning. *Scientific Reports*, 10(1), 4679. 10.1038/s41598-020-61588-w32170141

Langley, P. (2011). Artificial Intelligence. *AISB Quarterly*.

Langner, O., Dotsch, R., Bijlstra, G., Wigboldus, D. H. J., Hawk, S. T., & van Knippenberg, A. (2010, December). Presentation and validation of the Radboud Faces Database. *Cognition and Emotion*, 24(8), 1377–1388. 10.1080/02699930903485076

LeCun, Y., Bengio, Y., & Hinton, G. (2015). Deep Learning.Nature, 521, 436–444.

Leidner, D., & Kayworth, T. (2006). A review of culture in information systems research: Toward a theory of information technology culture conflict. *Management Information Systems Quarterly*, 30(2), 357–399.

LeCun, Y., Bottou, L., Bengio, Y., & Haffner, P. (1998). Gradient-based learning applied to document recognition. *Proceedings of the IEEE*, 86(11), 2278–2324. 10.1109/5.726791

Lee, G., Nho, K., Kang, B., Sohn, K. A., Kim, D., Weiner, M. W., Aisen, P., Petersen, R., Jack, C. R.Jr, Jagust, W., Trojanowki, J. Q., Toga, A. W., Beckett, L., Green, R. C., Saykin, A. J., Morris, J., Shaw, L. M., Khachaturian, Z., Sorensen, G., & Fargher, K. (2019). Predicting Alzheimer's disease progression using multi-modal deep learning approach. *Scientific Reports*, 9(1), 1952. 10.1038/s41598-018-37769-z30760848

Lee, H. C. (1994). *Skin cancer diagnosis using hierarchical neural networks and fuzzy logic*. Department of Computer Science, University of Missouri.

Leng, G., & Hall, J. (2019). Crop yield sensitivity of global major agricultural countries to droughts and the projected changes in the future. *The Science of the Total Environment*, 654, 811–821. 10.1016/j.scitotenv.2018.10.43430448671

Leone, J. P., & Leone, B. A. (2015). Breast cancer brain metastases: The last frontier. *Experimental Hematology & Oncology*, 4(1), 33. 10.1186/s40164-015-0028-826605131

Leukemia, A. L. (2021, April 30). Kaggle. Available: https://www.kaggle.com/datasets/mehradaria/leukemia

Li, D., ... 2019. "MAD-GAN: Multivariate Anomaly Detection for Time Series Data with Generative Adversarial Networks." In *International Conference on Artificial Neural Networks*, Springer, 703–16. 10.1007/978-3-030-30490-4_56

Liang, D., Liang, H., Yu, Z., & Zhang, Y. (2020, March). Deep convolutional BiLSTM fusion network for facial expression recognition. *The Visual Computer*, 36(3), 499–508. 10.1007/s00371-019-01636-3

Li, B., Dai, C., Wang, L., Deng, H., Li, Y., Guan, Z., & Ni, H. (2020). A novel drug repurposing approach for non-small cell lung cancer using deep learning. *PLoS One*, 15(6), e0233112. 10.1371/journal.pone.023311232525938

Liew, X. Y., Hameed, N., & Clos, J. (2021). An investigation of XGBoost-based algorithm for breast cancer classification. *Machine Learning with Applications*, 6, 100154. 10.1016/j.mlwa.2021.100154

Li, J., Zhou, Z., Dong, J., Fu, Y., Li, Y., Luan, Z., & Peng, X. (2021). Predicting breast cancer 5-year survival using machine learning: A systematic review. *PLoS One*, 16(4), e0250370. 10.1371/journal.pone.025037033861809

Li, M., Ruan, B., Yuan, C., Song, Z., Dai, C., Fu, B., Qiu, J., Maseleno, A., Yuan, X., & Balas, V. E. (2020). Intelligent system for predicting breast tumors using machine learning. *Journal of Intelligent & Fuzzy Systems*, 39(4), 4813–4822. 10.3233/JIFS-179967

Lim, H., & Dewaraja, Y. (2019). *Y-90 patients PET/CT & SPECT/CT and corresponding contours dataset*. University of Michigan-Deep Blue.

Lim, S., & Schmälzle, R. (2023). Artificial İntelligence for Health Message Generation: An Empirical Study Using A Large Language Model (LLM) and Prompt Engineering. *Frontiers in Communication*, 8, 1129082. 10.3389/fcomm.2023.1129082

Li, R., Niu, Y., Scott, S. R., Zhou, C., Lan, L., Liang, Z., & Li, J. (2021). Using electronic medical record data for research in a Healthcare Information and Management Systems Society (HIMSS) Analytics Electronic Medical Record Adoption Model (EMRAM) stage 7 hospital in Beijing: Cross-sectional study. *JMIR Medical Informatics*, 9(8), e24405. 10.2196/2440534342589

Li, S., Deng, W., & Du, J. (2017). Reliable crowdsourcing and deep locality-preserving learning for expression recognition in the wild. In *Proceedings of the IEEE conference on computer vision and pattern recognition* (pp. 2852-2861).

Liu, F., Wee, C. Y., Chen, H., & Shen, D. (2014). Inter-modality relationship constrained multi-modality multi-task feature selection for Alzheimer's Disease and mild cognitive impairment identification. *NeuroImage*, 84, 466–475. 10.1016/j.neuroimage.2013.09.01524045077

Liu, X., Li, M., Hao, F., Zhang, G., Wang, C., & Zhou, X. (2020, October). GLO-YOLO: a dynamic glomerular detecting and slicing model in whole slide images. In *Proceedings of the 2020 Conference on Artificial Intelligence and Healthcare* (pp. 229-233). 10.1145/3433996.3434038

Liu, Y., Jain, A., Eng, C., Way, D. H., Lee, K., Bui, P., Kanada, K., de Oliveira Marinho, G., Gallegos, J., Gabriele, S., Gupta, V., Singh, N., Natarajan, V., Hofmann-Wellenhof, R., Corrado, G. S., Peng, L. H., Webster, D. R., Ai, D., Huang, S. J., & Coz, D. (2020). A deep learning system for differential diagnosis of skin diseases. *Nature Medicine*, 26(6), 900–908. 10.1038/s41591-020-0842-332424212

Li, Y., Zeng, J., Shan, S., & Chen, X. (2019, May). Occlusion Aware Facial Expression Recognition Using CNN With Attention Mechanism. *IEEE Transactions on Image Processing*, 28(5), 2439–2450. 10.1109/TIP.2018.288676730571627

Li, Z., Wang, S., Yu, H., Zhu, Y., Wu, Q., Wang, L., Wu, Z., Gan, Y., Li, W., Qiu, B., & Tian, J. (2022). A novel deep learning framework based mask-guided attention mechanism for distant metastasis prediction of lung cancer. *IEEE Transactions on Emerging Topics in Computational Intelligence*, 7(2), 330–341. 10.1109/TETCI.2022.3171311

Li, Z., & Yu, Y. 2020. "Improving EEG-Based Motor Imagery Classification with Conditional Wasserstein GAN." In *2020 International Conference on Image, Video Processing and Artificial Intelligence*, SPIE, 437–43. 10.1117/12.2581328

Long, E. S.. (2015). Fully convolutional networks for semantic segmentation. In *Proceedings of the IEEE Conference on Computer Vision and Pattern Recognition (CVPR)* (pp. 3431–3440).

Lopes, A. T., de Aguiar, E., De Souza, A. F., & Oliveira-Santos, T. (2017, January). Facial expression recognition with Convolutional Neural Networks: Coping with few data and the training sample order. *Pattern Recognition*, 61, 610–628. 10.1016/j.patcog.2016.07.026

Lucey, P., Cohn, J. F., Kanade, T., Saragih, J., Ambadar, Z., & Matthews, I. "The Extended Cohn-Kanade Dataset (CK+): A complete dataset for action unit and emotion-specified expression", in *2010 IEEE Computer Society Conference on Computer Vision and Pattern Recognition - Workshops, juin 2010*, p. 94-101, 10.1109/CVPRW.2010.5543262

Lu, M. Y., Chen, R. J., Kong, D., Lipkova, J., Singh, R., Williamson, D. F., Chen, T. Y., & Mahmood, F. (2022). Federated learning for computational pathology on gigapixel whole slide images. *Medical Image Analysis*, 76, 102298. 10.1016/j.media.2021.10229834911013

Lung and colon cancer. (2021, November 24). Kaggle. Available: https://www.kaggle.com/datasets/biplobdey/lung-and-colon-cancer

Luo, Y., & Lu, B.-L. 2018. "EEG Data Augmentation for Emotion Recognition Using a Conditional Wasserstein GAN." In *2018 40th Annual International Conference of the IEEE Engineering in Medicine and Biology Society (EMBC)*, IEEE, 2535–38. 10.1109/EMBC.2018.8512865

Lutnick, B., Manthey, D., Becker, J. U., Zuckerman, J. E., Rodrigues, L., Jen, K. Y., & Sarder, P. (2022). A tool for federated training of segmentation models on whole slide images. *Journal of Pathology Informatics*, 13, 100101. 10.1016/j.jpi.2022.10010135910077

Lyons, M., Kamachi, M., & Gyoba, J. (1998). The Japanese Female Facial Expression (JAFFE) Database. *Zenodo*. 10.5281/zenodo.3451524

Maalem, S., Bouhamed, M. M., & Gasmi, M. (2022). A deep-based compound model for lung cancer detection. *2022 4th International Conference on Pattern Analysis and Intelligent Systems (PAIS)*, 1–4.

Maheshwari, U., Kiranmayee, B. V., & Suresh, C. (2022, December). *Diagnose Colon and Lung Cancer Histopathological Images Using Pre-Trained Machine Learning Model. In 2022 5th International Conference on Contemporary Computing and Informatics (IC3I)*. IEEE. https://ieeexplore.ieee.org/abstract/document/10073184/

Mahlein, A. K. (2016). Plant disease detection by imaging sensors–parallels and specific demands for precision agriculture and plant phenotyping. *Plant Disease*, 100(2), 241–251. 10.1094/PDIS-03-15-0340-FE30694129

Mamun, M., Farjana, A., Al Mamun, M., & Ahammed, M. S. (2022). Lung cancer prediction model using ensemble learning techniques and a systematic review analysis. *2022 IEEE World AI IoT Congress (AIIoT)*, 187–193.

Mamun, M., Mahmud, M. I., Meherin, M., & Abdelgawad, A. (2023). Lcdctcnn: Lung cancer diagnosis of ct scan images using cnn based model. *2023 10th International Conference on Signal Processing and Integrated Networks (SPIN)*, 205–212.

Manickavasagam, R., Selvan, S., & Selvan, M. (2022). CAD system for lung nodule detection using deep learning with CNN. *Medical & Biological Engineering & Computing*, 60(1), 221–228. 10.1007/s11517-021-02462-334811644

-Marchetti, D., Lanzola, G., Stefanelli, M. (2001). In S. Quaglini, P. Barahona, & S. Andreassen (Eds.), An AI-Based Approach to Support Communication in Health Care Organizations (pp. 384–394). AIME., LNAI 2101.

Marechal, C. (2019). Survey on AI-Based Multimodal Methods for Emotion Detection. In Kołodziej, J., & González-Vélez, H. (Eds.), *High-Performance Modelling and Simulation for Big Data Applications: Selected Results of the COST Action IC1406 cHiPSet* (pp. 307–324). Springer International Publishing. 10.1007/978-3-030-16272-6_11

Martínez-Murcia, F. J., Górriz, J. M., Ramírez, J., Castillo-Barnes, D., Segovia, F., Salas-Gonzalez, D., & Ortiz, A. (2018, November). A deep decomposition of MRI to explore neurodegeneration in Alzheimer's disease. In *2018 IEEE Nuclear Science Symposium and Medical Imaging Conference Proceedings (NSS/MIC)* (pp. 1-3). IEEE. 10.1109/NSSMIC.2018.8824320

Masood, A., Al-Jumaily, A. A., & Anam, K. (2015). Self-supervised learning model for skin cancer diagnosis. In 2015 7th International IEEE/EMBS Conference on Neural Engineering (NER) (pp. 1010-1013). IEEE. https://doi.org/10.1109/NER.2015.7146798

Mavadati, S. M., Mahoor, M. H., Bartlett, K., Trinh, P., & Cohn, J. F. (2013, April). DISFA: A Spontaneous Facial Action Intensity Database. *IEEE Transactions on Affective Computing*, 4(2), 151–160. 10.1109/T-AFFC.2013.4

McCarthy, J. (1988). Mathematical logic in arti

cial intelligence. *Daedalus*, 117(1), 297–311.

McCorduck, P. (2004). *Machines who think: A personal inquiry into the history and prospects artificial intelligence* (2nd ed.). A. K. Peters. 10.1201/9780429258985

Megala, G., & Kumari, N. (2023, April). DeepGAN: an enhanced approach for detecting brain tumor. In *2023 Second International Conference on Electrical, Electronics, Information and Communication Technologies (ICEEICT)* (pp. 01-06). IEEE.

Megala, G., Swarnalatha, P., & Venkatesan, R. (2023, January). Detecting Bone Tumor on Applying Edge Computational Deep Learning Approach. In *International Conference on Data Management, Analytics & Innovation* (pp. 981-992). Singapore: Springer Nature Singapore. 10.1007/978-981-99-1414-2_66

Megala, G., & Swarnalatha, P. (2024). Stacked collaborative transformer network with contrastive learning for video moment localization. *Intelligent Data Analysis*, •••, 1–18. 10.3233/IDA-240138

Mehrotra, R., & Yadav, K. (2022). Breast cancer in India: Present scenario and the challenges ahead. *World Journal of Clinical Oncology*, 13(3), 209–218. 10.5306/wjco.v13.i3.20935433294

Mellouk, W., & Handouzi, W. "Facial emotion recognition using deep learning: review and insights", *Procedia Computer Science,* Volume 175, 2020, Pages 689-694, ISSN 1877-0509, 10.1016/j.procs.2020.07.101

Mena, P., & Angelino, D. (2020). Plant Food, Nutrition and Human Health. *Nutrients*, 12(7), 2157. Advance online publication. 10.3390/nu1207215732698451

Menichetti, J., Hillen, M. A., Papageorgiou, A., & Pieterse, A. H. (2023). How Can Chatgpt be Used to Support Healthcare Communication Research? *Patient Education and Counseling*, 115, 107947. 10.1016/j.pec.2023.107947

-Metz, A. (2022). *"6 Exciting Ways to Use Chatgpt – From Coding to Poetry"*. TechRadar. htt ps://www.techradar.com/features/6-exciting-ways-to-use-chatgpt -from-coding-to -poetry Accessed: 26.03.2024.

Miao, K. H., & Miao, J. H. (2018). Coronary heart disease diagnosis using deep neural networks. international journal of advanced computer science and applications, 9(10).

Mirza, M., & Osindero, S. 2014. "Conditional Generative Adversarial Nets." *arXiv preprint arXiv:1411.1784*.

Mishra, G. P., & Dikshit, H. K. Priti, Kukreja, B., Aski, M., Yadava, D. K., ... & Kumar, S. (2022). Historical overview of biofortification in crop plants and its implications. In Biofortification of Staple Crops (pp. 31-61). Singapore: Springer Singapore.

Mishra, R., Sharma, K., Jha, R. R., & Bhavsar, A. (2023). NeuroGAN: Image Reconstruction from EEG Signals via an Attention-Based GAN. *Neural Computing & Applications*, 35(12), 9181–9192.

Mohammadpour, M., Khaliliardali, H., Hashemi, S. M. R., & AlyanNezhadi, M. M. (2017, December). Facial emotion recognition using deep convolutional networks. In 2017 IEEE 4th international conference on knowledge-based engineering and innovation (KBEI) (pp. 0017-0021). IEEE.

Mollahosseini, A., Chan, D., & Mahoor, M. H. "Going deeper in facial expression recognition using deep neural networks", in 2016 *IEEE Winter Conference on Applications of Computer Vision (WACV)*, mars 2016, p. 1-10, 10.1109/WACV.2016.7477450

Mollahosseini, A., Hasani, B., & Mahoor, M. H. (2019, January). AffectNet: A Database for Facial Expression, Valence, and Arousal Computing in the Wild. *IEEE Transactions on Affective Computing*, 10(1), 18–31. 10.1109/TAFFC.2017.2740923

Moreb, M., Mohammed, T. A., & Bayat, O. (2020). A novel software engineering approach toward using machine learning for improving the efficiency of health systems. *IEEE Access : Practical Innovations, Open Solutions*, 8, 23169–23178. 10.1109/ACCESS.2020.2970178

Multi Cancer Dataset. (2022, April 6). Kaggle. Available: https://www.kaggle.com/datasets/obulisainaren/multi-cancers

Muruganantham, P., & Balakrishnan, S. M. (2021). A survey on deep learning models for wireless capsule endoscopy image analysis. *International Journal of Cognitive Computing in Engineering*, 2, 83–92. 10.1016/j.ijcce.2021.04.002

Myrden, A., & Chau, T. (2017). A Passive EEG-BCI for Single-Trial Detection of Changes in Mental State. *IEEE Transactions on Neural Systems and Rehabilitation Engineering*, 25(4), 345–356. 10.1109/TNSRE.2016.264195628092565

Nadarzynski, T., Miles, O., Cowie, A., & Ridge, D. (2019). Acceptability of Artificial İntelligence (AI)-led Chatbot Services in Healthcare: A Mixed-Methods Study. *Digital Health*, 5, 1–12. journals.sagepub.com/home/dhj. 10.1177/205520 7619871808314676 82

Nandhini, J. M., Joshi, S., & Anuratha, K. (2022, November). Federated learning based prediction of chronic kidney diseases. In 2022 1st International Conference on Computational Science and Technology (ICCST) (pp. 1-6). IEEE. 10.1109/ICCST55948.2022.10040317

Nasr-Esfahani, M., Samavi, S., Karimi, N., Najarian, K., & Soroushmehr, S. M. (2016). Melanoma detection by analysis of clinical images using a convolutional neural network. In 2016 38th Annual International Conference of the IEEE Engineering in Medicine and Biology Society (EMBC) (pp. 1373-1376). IEEE. https://doi.org/10.1109/EMBC.2016.7590963

Naylor, C. D. (2018). On the prospects for a (deep) learning health care system. *Journal of the American Medical Association*, 320(11), 1099–1100. 10.1001/jama.2018.1110330178068

Nie, Y., Sommella, P., O'Nils, M., Liguori, C., & Lundgren, J. (2019). *Automatic Detection of Melanoma with Yolo Deep Convolutional Neural Networks. 2019 E-Health and Bioengineering Conference*. EHB.

Nithya, T., Kumar, V. N., Gayathri, S., Deepa, S., Varun, C. M., & Subramanian, R. S. (2023, August). A comprehensive survey of machine learning: Advancements, applications, and challenges. In *2023 Second International Conference on Augmented Intelligence and Sustainable Systems (ICAISS)* (pp. 354-361). IEEE. 10.1109/ICAISS58487.2023.10250547

Norori, N., Hu, Q., Aellen, F. M., Faraci, F. D., & Tzovara, A. (2021). Addressing bias in big data and AI for health care: A call for open science. *Patterns (New York, N.Y.)*, 2(10), 100347. 10.1016/j.patter.2021.10034734693373

Nsoesie, E. O., Kraemer, M. U., Golding, N., Pigott, D. M., Brady, O. J., Moyes, C. L., Johansson, M. A., Gething, P. W., Velayudhan, R., Khan, K., Hay, S. I., & Brownstein, J. S. (2016). Global distribution and environmental suitability for chikungunya virus, 1952 to 2015. *Eurosurveillance*, 21(20), 30234. 10.2807/1560-7917. ES.2016.21.20.3023427239817

Octaviani, L., & Rustam, Z. (2019). Random forest for breast cancer prediction. *AIP Conference Proceedings*, 2168, 020050. 10.1063/1.5132477

Omar, L. T., Hussein, J. M., Omer, L. F., Qadir, A. M., & Ghareb, M. I. (2023, May). Lung And Colon Cancer Detection Using Weighted Average Ensemble Transfer Learning. In *2023 11th International Symposium on Digital Forensics and Security (ISDFS)* (pp. 1-7). IEEE.(https://ieeexplore.ieee.org/abstract/document/10131836/)

Orlov, N. V., Chen, W. W., Eckley, D. M., Macura, T. J., Shamir, L., Jaffe, E. S., & Goldberg, I. G. (2010). Automatic classification of lymphoma images with transform-based global features. *IEEE Transactions on Information Technology in Biomedicine*, 14(4), 1003–1013. 10.1109/TITB.2010.205069520659835

Panesar, A. (2019). *Machine learning and AI for healthcare*. Apress. 10.1007/978-1-4842-3799-1

Pantic, M., & Rothkrantz, L. J. M. (2003, September). Toward an affect-sensitive multimodal human-computer interaction. *Proceedings of the IEEE*, 91(9), 1370–1390. 10.1109/JPROC.2003.817122

Pantic, M., Valstar, M., Rademaker, R., & Maat, L. (2005). Web-based database for facial expression analysis. *2005 IEEE International Conference on Multimedia and Expo*. 10.1109/ICME.2005.1521424

Panwar, S., Rad, P., Quarles, J., & Huang, Y. 2019. "Generating EEG Signals of an RSVP Experiment by a Class Conditioned Wasserstein Generative Adversarial Network." In *2019 IEEE International Conference on Systems, Man and Cybernetics (SMC)*, IEEE, 1304–10. 10.1109/SMC.2019.8914492

Park, H. C., Hong, I. P., Poudel, S., & Choi, C. (2023). Data augmentation based on generative adversarial networks for endoscopic image classification. *IEEE Access : Practical Innovations, Open Solutions*, 11, 49216–49225. 10.1109/ACCESS.2023.3275173

Park, Y. T., & Atalag, K. (2015). Current national approach to healthcare ICT standardization: Focus on progress in New Zealand. *Healthcare Informatics Research*, 21(3), 144–151. 10.4258/hir.2015.21.3.14426279950

Perez-Ramirez, U., Arana, E., & Moratal, D. (2016). „Brain Metastases Detection on MR by means of Three-Dimensional Tumor Appearance Template Matching". *Journal of Magnetic Resonance Imaging*, 44(3), 642–652. 10.1002/jmri.2520726934581

Perrottelli, A., Giordano, G. M., Brando, F., Giuliani, L., & Mucci, A. (2021). EEG-Based Measures in at-Risk Mental State and Early Stages of Schizophrenia: A Systematic Review. *Frontiers in Psychiatry*, 12, 653642. 10.3389/fpsyt.2021.65364234017273

Pham, T. C., Tran, D. H., Dang, T. T., & Nguyen, D. T. (2019). A comparative study for classification of skin cancer. In *2019 International Conference on Advanced Computing and Applications (ACOMP)* (pp. 1-6). IEEE. https://doi.org/10.1109/ICSSE.2019.8823124

Pillai, V., Koohpayegani, S. A., Ouligian, A., Fong, D., & Pirsiavash, H. (2021). Consistent Explanations by Contrastive Learning. *2022 IEEE/CVF Conference on Computer Vision and Pattern Recognition (CVPR)*, 10203-10212.

Pinheiro, P.. (2014). Recurrent convolutional neural networks for scene labeling. In *Proceedings of the 31st International Conference on Machine Learning* (pp. 82–90).

Polesel, J., Franceschi, S., Talamini, R., Negri, E., Barzan, L., Montella, M., & La Vecchia, C. (2006). Tobacco smoking and the risk of upper aerodigestive tract cancers: A reanalysis of case-control studies using spline models. *International Journal of Cancer*, 122(10), 2398–2402. 10.1002/ijc.2338518224689

Poornachandra, S., & Naveena, C. (2017). *Pre-processing of MR Images for Efficient Quantitative Image Analysis using Deep Learning Techniques", Recent Advances in Electronics and Communication Technology*. ICRAECT.

Pradhan, K. S., Chawla, P., & Tiwari, R. (2023). HRDEL: High ranking deep ensemble learning-based lung cancer diagnosis model. *Expert Systems with Applications*, 213, 118956. 10.1016/j.eswa.2022.118956

Praveen, G. B. & Anita Agarwal 2015, „Hybrid Approach for Brain Tumor Detection and Classification in Magnetic Resonance Images", International Conference on Communication, Control and Intelligent Systems (CCIS). Balaji, G. N., & Parthasarathy, G. (2024, March). A modified convolutional neural network for tumor segmentation in multimodal brain magnetic resonance images. In *AIP Conference Proceedings* (Vol. 2919, No. 1). AIP Publishing.

Pyšek, P., Hulme, P. E., Simberloff, D., Bacher, S., Blackburn, T. M., Carlton, J. T., Dawson, W., Essl, F., Foxcroft, L. C., Genovesi, P., Jeschke, J. M., Kühn, I., Liebhold, A. M., Mandrak, N. E., Meyerson, L. A., Pauchard, A., Pergi, J., Roy, H. E., Seebens, H., & Richardson, D. M. (2020). Scientists' warning on invasive alien species. *Biological Reviews of the Cambridge Philosophical Society*, 95(6), 1511–1534. 10.1111/brv.1262732588508

Qian, X., & Yuan, S. (2014). AI-Powered Mental Health Communication: Examining the Effects of Affection Expectations on Health Behavioral İntentions. *Patient Education and Counseling*, 122, •••. www.journals.elsevier.com/patient-education-and-counseling38237529

-Radford A., Narasimhan K., Salimans T., Sutskever I. (2018). *"Improving Language Understanding by Generative Pre-Training"*, [Google Akademik], 26.03.2024

Radford, A., Metz, L., & Chintala, S. 2015. "Unsupervised Representation Learning with Deep Convolutional Generative Adversarial Networks." *arXiv preprint arXiv:1511.06434*.

Raghupathi, V. (2019). An empirical investigation of chronic diseases: A visualization approach to medicare in the United States. *International Journal of Healthcare Management*, 12(4), 327–339. 10.1080/20479700.2018.1472849

Raghupathi, W., & Raghupathi, V. (2014). Big data analytics in healthcare: Promise and potential. *Health Information Science and Systems*, 2(1), 1–10. 10.1186/2047-2501-2-325825667

Rahman, Md. M. (2021). *A Deep Learning Approach to Detect Lung Cancer Using Alexnet and kNN*. Daffodil International University.

Rajendran, T., Rajathi, S. A., Balakrishnan, C., Aswini, J., Prakash, R. B., & Subramanian, R. S. (2023, December). Risk Prediction Modeling for Breast Cancer using Supervised Machine Learning Approaches. In 2023 2nd International Conference on Automation, Computing and Renewable Systems (ICACRS) (pp. 702-708). IEEE. 10.1109/ICACRS58579.2023.10404482

Rajkomar, A., Dean, J., & Kohane, I. (2019). Machine learning in medicine. *The New England Journal of Medicine*, 380(14), 1347–1358. 10.1056/NEJMra181425930943338

Rajkumar, K., Ramoju, R. T. S., Balelly, T., Ashadapu, S., Prasad, C. R., & Srikanth, Y. (2023, April). Kidney Cancer Detection using Deep Learning Models. In *2023 7th International Conference on Trends in Electronics and Informatics (ICOEI)* (pp. 1197-1203). IEEE. https://ieeexplore.ieee.org/abstract/document/10125589/

Rajput, A., & Subasi, A. (2023). Lung cancer detection from histopathological lung tissue images using deep learning. In *Applications of Artificial Intelligence in Medical Imaging* (pp. 51–74). Elsevier. 10.1016/B978-0-443-18450-5.00008-6

Rana, M., & Bhushan, M. (2023). Classifying breast cancer using transfer learning models based on histopathological images. *Neural Computing & Applications*, 35(19), 14243–14257. 10.1007/s00521-023-08484-2

Rani, M., Bakshi, A., & Gupta, A. (2020, March). Prediction of Heart Disease Using Naïve bayes and Image Processing. In *2020 International Conference on Emerging Smart Computing and Informatics (ESCI)* (pp. 215-219). IEEE. 10.1109/ESCI48226.2020.9167537

Razavi, F., Tarokh, M. J., & Alborzi, M. (2019). An intelligent Alzheimer's disease diagnosis method using unsupervised feature learning. *Journal of Big Data*, 6(1), 32. 10.1186/s40537-019-0190-7

Redmon, J., Divvala, S., Girshick, R., & Farhadi, A. (2016). *You Only Look Once: Unified*. Real-Time Object Detection.

-Reed, L. (2022). *"Chatgpt For Automated Testing: From Conversation to Code"*. Sauce Labs. https://saucelabs.com/blog/chatgpt-automated-testing-conversation-to-code Accessed: February 20, 2023.

Rehman, A., Naz, S., Razzak, M. I., Akram, F., & Imran, M. (2019). A Deep Learning-Based Framework for Automatic Brain Tumors Classification Using Transfer Learning. *Circuits, Systems, and Signal Processing*, 39(2), 757–775. 10.1007/s00034-019-01246-3

Ren, S., He, K., Girshick, R., & Sun, J. (2017). Faster R-CNN: Towards real-time object detection with region proposal networks. *IEEE Transactions on Pattern Analysis and Machine Intelligence*, 39(6), 1137–1149. 10.1109/TPAMI.2016.257703127295650

Renzi, C, Abeni, D, Picardi, A, Agostini, E, Melchi, CF, Pasquini, P, Prudu, P, & Braga, M. (2001). Factors associated with patient satisfaction with care among dermatological outpatients". *British Journal of Dermatology*, •••, 145.11703289

Ringeval, F., Eyben, F., Kroupi, E., Yuce, A., Thiran, J.-P., Ebrahimi, T., Lalanne, D., & Schuller, B. (2015, November). Prediction of asynchronous dimensional emotion ratings from audiovisual and physiological data. *Pattern Recognition Letters*, 66, 22–30. 10.1016/j.patrec.2014.11.007

Rjoub, G., Wahab, O. A., Bentahar, J., & Bataineh, A. S. (2021, August). Improving autonomous vehicles safety in snow weather using federated YOLO CNN learning. In *International Conference on Mobile Web and Intelligent Information Systems* (pp. 121-134). Cham: Springer International Publishing. 10.1007/978-3-030-83164-6_10

Ronneberger, O., ... (2015). U-net: Convolutional networks for biomedical image segmentation. In *Proceedings of the 18th International Conference on Medical Image Computing and Computer-Assisted Intervention (MICCAI)* (p. 8). Huang, J., & et al. (2013). Deep and wide multiscale recursive networks for robust image labeling. *arXiv preprint arXiv:1310.0354*. 10.1007/978-3-319-24574-4_28

Rouast, P. V., Adam, M., & Chiong, R. (2018). Deep Learning for Human Affect Recognition: Insights and New Developments. *IEEE Transactions on Affective Computing*, •••, 1–1. 10.1109/TAFFC.2018.2890471

Roy, S., Dora, S., McCreadie, K., & Prasad, G. 2020. "MIEEG-GAN: Generating Artificial Motor Imagery Electroencephalography Signals." In *2020 International Joint Conference on Neural Networks (IJCNN)*, IEEE, 1–8. 10.1109/IJCNN48605.2020.9206942

Ryu, S., Goto, K., Kitagawa, T., Kobayashi, T., Shimada, J., Ito, R., & Nakabayashi, Y. (2023). Real-time Artificial Intelligence Navigation-Assisted Anatomical Recognition in Laparoscopic Colorectal Surgery. *Journal of Gastrointestinal Surgery*, 27(12), 3080–3082. 10.1007/s11605-023-05819-137653155

Safran, DG, Taira, D, Rogers, WH, Kosinski, M, Ware, JE, & Tarlov, AR. (1998). Linking primary care performance to outcomes of care. *The Journal of Family Practice*, 47(3).9752374

Sah, S., Shringi, A., Ptucha, R., Burry, A., & Loce, R. (2017). Video redaction: A survey and comparison of enabling technologies. *Journal of Electronic Imaging*, 26(5), 51406. 10.1117/1.JEI.26.5.051406

Sallam, M., Salim, N. A., Al-Tammemi, A. B., Barakat, M., Fayyad, D., Hallit, S., Harapan, H., Hallit, R., & Mahafzah, A. (2023). ChatGPT Output Regarding Compulsory Vaccination and COVID-19 Vaccine Conspiracy: A Descriptive Study at the Outset of a Paradigm Shift in Online Search for Information. *Cureus*, 15(2), e35029. 10.7759/cureus.3502936819954

Salvador-Meneses, J., Ruiz-Chavez, Z., & Garcia-Rodriguez, J. (2019). Compressed kNN: K-Nearest Neighbors with Data Compression. *Entropy (Basel, Switzerland)*, 21(3), 234. 10.3390/e2103023433266949

Salvagno, M., Taccone, F. S., & And Gerlı, A. G. (2023). Can Artificial Intelligence Help For Scientific Writing? *Critical Care*, 27(1).

Sanchez, S. A., Romero, H. J., & Morales, A. D. (2020). A review: Comparison of performance metrics of pretrained models for object detection using the TensorFlow framework. *IOP Conference Series. Materials Science and Engineering*, 844, 12024. 10.1088/1757-899X/844/1/012024

Sanei, S., & Chambers, J. A. (2013). *EEG signal processing*. John Wiley & Sons.

Saraswathi, T., & Bhaskaran, V. M. (2023, February). Classification of Oral Squamous Carcinoma Histopathological images using Alex Net. In *2023 International Conference on Intelligent Systems for Communication, IoT and Security (ICISCoIS)* (pp. 637-643). IEEE.(https://ieeexplore.ieee.org/abstract/document/10100510/)

Saraswat, M. A., & Kalra, B. (2021). Identification and classification of brain tumors with optimized neural network and canny edge detection algorithm. *Annals of the Romanian Society for Cell Biology*, •••, 5651–5660.

Sariyanidi, E., Gunes, H., & Cavallaro, A. (2014). Automatic Analysis of Facial Affect: A Survey of Registration, Representation, and Recognition. *IEEE Transactions on Pattern Analysis and Machine Intelligence*, (oct). Advance online publication. 10.1109/TPAMI.2014.236612726357337

Sava, J. (2023, April 27). Current applications of artificial intelligence in Oncology. Targeted Oncology. https://www.targetedonc.com/view/current-applications-of-artificial-intelligence-in-oncology

Savic, M., Ma, Y., Ramponi, G., Du, W., & Peng, Y. (2021). Lung nodule segmentation with a region-based fast marching method. *Sensors (Basel)*, 21(5), 1908. 10.3390/s2105190833803297

Schiavon, M., Nardi, S., Vecchia, F. D., & Ertani, A. (2020). Selenium biofortification in the 21st century: Status and challenges for healthy human nutrition. *Plant and Soil*, 453(1-2), 245–270. 10.1007/s11104-020-04635-932836404

Schmidhuber, J. (2015). Deep learning in neural networks: An overview. *Neural Networks*, 61, 85–117. 10.1016/j.neunet.2014.09.00325462637

Sebetci, Ö. (2024). *Yapay Zeka ile Sağlık Sistemlerden Uygulamalara*. Kodlab Basın Yayın.

Seddik, F., & Shawky, D. M. "Logistic regression model for breast cancer automatic diagnosis," *2015 SAI Intelligent Systems Conference (IntelliSys)*, London, UK, 2015, 150-154 10.1109/IntelliSys.2015.7361138

Seladi-Schulman, J. (2022, February 21). When breast cancer metastasizes to the brain. Available: https://www.healthline.com/health/breast-cancer/breast-cancer-metastasis-to-brain#overview

Serj, M. F., Lavi, B., Hoff, G., & Valls, D. P. (2018). A deep convolutional neural network for lung cancer diagnostic. *ArXiv Preprint ArXiv:1804.08170.*

Shailaja, K., Seetharamulu, B., & Jabbar, M. A. (2018, March). Machine learning in healthcare: A review. In 2018 Second international conference on electronics, communication and aerospace technology (ICECA) (pp. 910-914). IEEE. 10.1109/ICECA.2018.8474918

Shan, C., Gong, S., & McOwan, P. W. (2009, May). Facial expression recognition based on Local Binary Patterns: A comprehensive study. *Image and Vision Computing*, 27(6), 803–816. 10.1016/j.imavis.2008.08.005

Shandilya, S., & Nayak, S. R. (2022). Analysis of lung cancer by using deep neural network. *Innovation in Electrical Power Engineering, Communication, and Computing Technology:Proceedings of Second IEPCCT 2021*, 427–436.

Shankar, K., Lakshmanaprabu, S. K., Khanna, A., Tanwar, S., Rodrigues, J. J., & Roy, N. R. (2019). Alzheimer detection using Group Grey Wolf Optimization based features with convolutional classifier. *Computers & Electrical Engineering*, 77, 230–243. 10.1016/j.compeleceng.2019.06.001

Sharma, D., Jamra, G., Singh, U. M., Sood, S., & Kumar, A. (2017). Calcium Biofortification: Three Pronged Molecular Approaches for Dissecting Complex Trait of Calcium Nutrition in Finger Millet (Eleusine coracena) for Devising Strategies of Enrichment of Food Crops. *Frontiers in Plant Science*, 7. Advance online publication. 10.3389/fpls.2016.0202828144246

Sharma, S., Fulzele, P., & Sreedevi, I. (2020). Hybrid model for lung nodule segmentation based on support vector machine and k-nearest neighbor. *2020 Fourth International Conference on Computing Methodologies and Communication (ICCMC)*, 170–175. 10.1109/ICCMC48092.2020.ICCMC-00034

She, Y., Jin, Z., Wu, J., Deng, J., Zhang, L., Su, H., Jiang, G., Liu, H., Xie, D., Cao, N., Ren, Y., & Chen, C. (2020). Development and validation of a deep learning model for non–small cell lung cancer survival. *JAMA Network Open*, 3(6), e205842–e205842. 10.1001/jamanetworkopen.2020.584232492161

She, Z., Liu, Y., & Damatoa, A. (2007). Combination of features from skin pattern and ABCD analysis for lesion classification. *Skin Research and Technology*, 13(1), 25–33. 10.1111/j.1600-0846.2007.00181.x17250529

Shreve, J., Khanani, S., & Haddad, T. C. (2022). Artificial intelligence in Oncology: Current capabilities, future opportunities, and ethical considerations. *American Society of Clinical Oncology Educational Book*, 42(42), 842–851. 10.1200/EDBK_35065235687826

Shrot, S., Salhov, M., Dvorski, N., Konen, E., Averbuch, A., & Hoffmann, C. (2019). Application of MR morphologic, diffusion tensor, and perfusion imaging in the classification of brain tumors using machine learning scheme. *Neuroradiology*, 61(7), 757–765. 10.1007/s00234-019-02195-z30949746

Shu, L., Xie, J., Yang, M., Li, Z., Li, Z., Liao, D., Xu, X., & Yang, X. (2018, July). A Review of Emotion Recognition Using Physiological Signals. *Sensors (Basel)*, 18(7), 2074. 10.3390/s1807207429958457

Sidoti, E., Paolini, G., & Tringali, G. (2008). Skin surveillance attitudes and behaviors about skin checks for early signs of skin cancer in a sample of secondary school students and teachers in Palermo, Western Sicily. *Italian Journal of Public Health*, 5(4). Advance online publication. 10.2427/5818

Simberloff, D., Martin, J. L., Genovesi, P., Maris, V., Wardle, D. A., Aronson, J., Courchamp, F., Galil, B., García-Berthou, E., Pascal, M., Pyšek, P., Sousa, R., Tabacchi, E., & Vilà, M. (2013). Impacts of biological invasions: What's what and the way forward. *Trends in Ecology & Evolution*, 28(1), 58–66. 10.1016/j.tree.2012.07.01322889499

Siva, S. R., Sudha, K., Pooja, E., Maheswari, B., & Girija, P. (2024). Revolutionizing Healthcare Delivery: Applications and Impact of Cutting-Edge Technologies. *AI and IoT Technology and Applications for Smart Healthcare Systems*, 75-91.

Soltaninejad, M., Yang, G., Lambrou, T., Allinson, N., Jones, T. L., Barrick, T. R., Howe, F. A., & Ye, X. (2016). Automated brain tumour detection and segmentation using superpixel-based extremely randomized trees in FLAIR MRI. *International Journal of Computer Assisted Radiology and Surgery*, 12(2), 183–203. 10.1007/s11548-016-1483-327651330

Sori, W. J., Feng, J., Godana, A. W., Liu, S., & Gelmecha, D. J. (2021). DFD-Net: Lung cancer detection from denoised CT scan image using deep learning. *Frontiers of Computer Science*, 15(2), 1–13. 10.1007/s11704-020-9050-z

Sousa, F. D. O., da Silva, D. S., Cavalcante, T. D. S., Neto, E. C., Gondim, V. J. T., Nogueira, I. C., Ripardo de Alexandria, A., & de Albuquerque, V. H. C. (2022). Novel virtual nasal endoscopy system based on computed tomography scans. *Virtual Reality & Intelligent Hardware*, 4(4), 359–379. 10.1016/j.vrih.2021.09.005

Spanos, A., & Hendry, D. (2011). The multivariate linear regression model. *Statistical Foundations of Econometric Modeling*, 571–607.

Stein, A. J. (2010). Global impacts of human mineral malnutrition. *Plant and Soil*, 335(1-2), 133–154. 10.1007/s11104-009-0228-2

-Stokel-Walker, C. J. N. (2023). *"Chatgpt Listed As Author On Research Papers: Many Scientists Disapprove."* Nature, *613*, 620–621. 26.03.2024.10.1038/d41586-023-00107-z

Subarna, T. G., & Sukumar, P. (2022). Detection and classification of cervical cancer images using CEENET deep learning approach. *Journal of Intelligent & Fuzzy Systems*, 43(3), 3695–3707. 10.3233/JIFS-220173

Subramanian, M., Cho, J., Sathishkumar, V. E., & Naren, O. S. (2023). Multiple Types of Cancer Classification Using CT/MRI Images Based on Learning Without Forgetting Powered Deep Learning Models. *IEEE Access : Practical Innovations, Open Solutions*, 11, 10336–10354. 10.1109/ACCESS.2023.3240443

Subramanian, R. R., Mourya, R. N., Reddy, V. P. T., Reddy, B. N., & Amara, S. (2020). Lung cancer prediction using deep learning framework. *International Journal of Control and Automation*, 13(3), 154–160.

Subramanian, R. S., Yamini, B., Sudha, K., & Sivakumar, S. (2024). Ensemble-based deep learning techniques for customer churn prediction model. *Kybernetes*. Advance online publication. 10.1108/K-08-2023-1516

Sudha, K., Ambhika, C., Maheswari, B., Girija, P., & Nalini, M. (2023). AI and IoT Applications in Medical Domain Enhancing Healthcare Through Technology Integration. In AI and IoT-Based Technologies for Precision Medicine (pp. 280-294). IGI Global.

Sudha, K., Lakshmipriya, C., Pajila, P. B., Venitha, E., & Anita, M. (2024, January). Enhancing Diabetes Prediction and Management through Machine Learning: A Comparative Study. In *2024 Fourth International Conference on Advances in Electrical, Computing, Communication and Sustainable Technologies (ICAECT)* (pp. 1-6). IEEE.

Sullivan, LM, Stein, MD, Savetsky, JB, & Samet, JH. (2000). The doctor-patient relationship and HIV-infected patients' satisfaction with primary care physicians". *Journal of General Internal Medicine*, •••, 15.10940132

Szerement, J., Szatanik-Kloc, A., Mokrzycki, J., & Mierzwa-Hersztek, M. (2022). Agronomic Biofortification with Se, Zn and Fe: An Effective Strategy to Enhance Crop Nutritional Quality and Stress Defense-A Review. *Journal of Soil Science and Plant Nutrition*, 22(1), 1129–1159. 10.1007/s42729-021-00719-2

Szilagyi, L. Laszlo Lefkovits & Balázs Benyo 2015, „Automatic Brain Tumor Segmentation in multispectral MRI vol.s using a fuzzy c means cascade algorithm", *12th International Conference on Fuzzy Systems and Knowledge Discovery (FSKD)*, DOI: . 2015. 7381955.10.1109/FSKD

Szurhaj, W., Lamblin, M.-D., Kaminska, A., & Sediri, H. (2015). "EEG Guidelines in the Diagnosis of Brain Death." *Neurophysiologie Clinique. Clinical Neurophysiology*, 45(1), 97–104. 10.1016/j.neucli.2014.11.00525687591

Talukder, M. A., Islam, M. M., Uddin, M. A., Akhter, A., Hasan, K. F., & Moni, M. A. (2022). Machine learning-based lung and colon cancer detection using deep feature extraction and ensemble learning. *Expert Systems with Applications*, 205, 117695. 10.1016/j.eswa.2022.117695

Thibodeau, R., Jorgensen, R. S., & Kim, S. (2006). Depression, Anxiety, and Resting Frontal EEG Asymmetry: A Meta-Analytic Review. *Journal of Abnormal Psychology*, 115(4), 715–729. 10.1037/0021-843X.115.4.71517100529

Torre, L. A., Siegel, R. L., & Jemal, A. (2016). Lung cancer statistics. *Lung Cancer and Personalized Medicine: Current Knowledge and Therapies*, 1–19.

Torre, L. A., Bray, F., Siegel, R. L., Ferlay, J., Lortet-Tieulent, J., & Jemal, A. (2015). Global cancer statistics, 2012. *CA: a Cancer Journal for Clinicians*, 65(2), 87–108. 10.3322/caac.2126225651787

Trestioreanu, L. (2018). Holographic visualisation of radiology data and automated machine learning-based medical image segmentation. *arXiv preprint arXiv:1808.04929.*

Tschandl, P., Rosendahl, C., & Kittler, H. (2019). The HAM10000 dataset, is a large collection of multi-source dermatoscopic images of common pigmented skin lesions. *Scientific Data*, 5(1), 180161. 10.1038/sdata.2018.16130106392

Turing, A. M. (1950). *I.—Computing machinery and intelligence.Mind, LIX, 433–460. U.S. National Science and Technology Council. (2016).Preparing for the future artificial intelligence.* Government Printing Office.

Upadhyay, A. K., & Khandelwal, K. (2019). Artificial intelligence-based training learning from application. *Development and Learning in Organizations*, 33(2), 20–23. Advance online publication. 10.1108/DLO-05-2018-0058

Ura, K., Alkire, S., & Zangmo, T. (2012). *GNH and GNH Index*. Centre for Bhutan Studies.

Urban, B.. (2014). Multi-modal brain tumor segmentation using deep convolutional neural networks. In *Proceedings of the BRATS-MICCAI*.

Uysal, G., & Ozturk, M. (2020, November). Classifying early and late mild cognitive impairment stages of Alzheimer's disease by analyzing different brain areas. In *2020 Medical Technologies Congress (TIPTEKNO)* (pp. 1-4). IEEE.

Vallabhaneni, R. B., & Rajesh, V. (2018). „Brain tumor detection using mean shift clustering and GLCM features with edge adaptive total variation denoising technique". *Alexandria Engineering Journal*, 57(4), 2387–2392. 10.1016/j.aej.2017.09.011

Valstar, M. F., Jiang, B., Mehu, M., Pantic, M., & Scherer, K. "The first facial expression recognition and analysis challenge", in *Face and Gesture2011,mars2011*, p. 921-926, 10.1109/FG.2011.5771374

Valstar, M. F.. "FERA 2015 - second Facial Expression Recognition and Analysis challenge", in 2015 *11th IEEE International Conference and Workshops on Automatic Face and Gesture Recognition (FG)*, mai 2015, vol. 06, p. 1-8, 10.1109/FG.2015.7284874

van der Sommen, F., de Groof, J., Struyvenberg, M., van der Putten, J., Boers, T., Fockens, K., Schoon, E. J., Curvers, W., de With, P., Mori, Y., Byrne, M., & Bergman, J. J. (2020). Machine learning in GI endoscopy: Practical guidance in how to interpret a novel field. *Gut*, 69(11), 2035–2045. 10.1136/gutjnl-2019-32046632393540

Van Dis, E. A., Bollen, J., Zuidema, W., Van Rooij, R., & Bockting, C. L. (2023). ChatGPT: Five priorities for research. *Nature*, 614(7947), 224–226.

VanderWeele, T. J. (2019). Measures of community well-being: A template. *International Journal of Community Well-being*, 2(3-4), 253–275. 10.1007/s42413-019-00036-8

Varban, O. A., Thumma, J. R., Carlin, A. M., Finks, J. F., Ghaferi, A. A., & Dimick, J. B. (2020). Peer assessment of operative videos with sleeve gastrectomy to determine optimal operative technique. *Journal of the American College of Surgeons*, 231(4), 470–477. 10.1016/j.jamcollsurg.2020.06.01632629164

-Veisdal, J. (2019). "The birthplace of ai, "Cantor's paradise,", https://www.cantorsparadise.com/the-birthplace-of-ai-9ab7d4e5fb00, View at: Google Scholar

Velazquez, M., Anantharaman, R., Velazquez, S., & Lee, Y., & Alzheimer's Disease Neuroimaging Initiative. (2019, November). RNN-based Alzheimer's disease prediction from prodromal stage using diffusion tensor imaging. In *2019 IEEE International Conference on Bioinformatics and Biomedicine (BIBM)* (pp. 1665-1672). IEEE. 10.1109/BIBM47256.2019.8983391

Venkatesan, R., & Balaji, G. N. (2024). Balancing composite motion optimization using R-ERNN with plant disease. *Applied Soft Computing*, 154, 111288. Advance online publication. 10.1016/j.asoc.2024.111288

Von Ende, E., Ryan, S., Crain, M. A., & Makary, M. S. (2023). Artificial intelligence, augmented reality, and virtual reality advances and applications in interventional radiology. *Diagnostics (Basel)*, 13(5), 892. 10.3390/diagnostics13050892 36900036

Wang, J., Lin, L., Zhao, S., Wu, X., & Wu, S. (2019). Research progress on computed tomography image detection and classification of pulmonary nodule based on deep learning. *Sheng Wu Yi Xue Gong Cheng Xue Za Zhi= Journal of Biomedical Engineering= Shengwu Yixue Gongchengxue Zazhi*, 36(4), 670–676.

Wang, F., Kaushal, R., & Khullar, D. (2020). Should health care demand interpretable artificial intelligence or accept "black box" medicine? *Annals of Internal Medicine*, 172(1), 59–60. 10.7326/M19-2548 31842204

Wang, F., Su, Q., & Li, C. (2022). Identidication of novel biomarkers in non-small cell lung cancer using machine learning. *Scientific Reports*, 12(1), 16693. 10.1038/s41598-022-21050-5 36202977

Wang, X., Chen, H., Gan, C., Lin, H., Dou, Q., Tsougenis, E., Huang, Q., Cai, M., & Heng, P.-A. (2019). Weakly supervised deep learning for whole slide lung cancer image analysis. *IEEE Transactions on Cybernetics*, 50(9), 3950–3962. 10.1109/TCYB.2019.2935141 31484154

Wasi, S., Alam, S. B., Rahman, R., Amin, M. A., & Kobashi, S. (2023, May). Kidney Tumor Recognition from Abdominal CT Images using Transfer Learning. In *2023 IEEE 53rd International Symposium on Multiple-Valued Logic (ISMVL)* (pp. 54-58). IEEE. https://ieeexplore.ieee.org/abstract/document/10153815/

Webster, J., & Watson, R. T. (2002). Analyzing the past to prepare for the future: Writing a literature review. *Management Information Systems Quarterly*, •••, xiii–xxiii.

Weth, F. R., Hoggarth, G. B., Weth, A. F., Paterson, E., White, M. P., Tan, S. T., Peng, L., & Gray, C. (2024). Unlocking hidden potential: Advancements, approaches, and obstacles in repurposing drugs for cancer therapy. *British Journal of Cancer*, 130(5), 703–715. 10.1038/s41416-023-02502-938012383

White, P. J., & Brown, P. H. (2010). Plant nutrition for sustainable development and global health. *Annals of Botany*, 105(7), 1073–1080. 10.1093/aob/mcq08520430785

Wolpaw, J. R., Birbaumer, N., Heetderks, W. J., McFarland, D. J., Peckham, P. H., Schalk, G., Donchin, E., Quatrano, L. A., Robinson, C. J., & Vaughan, T. M. (2000). Brain-Computer Interface Technology: A Review of the First International Meeting. *IEEE Transactions on Rehabilitation Engineering*, 8(2), 164–173. 10.1109/TRE.2000.84780710896178

Wurts, A., Oakley, D. H., Hyman, B. T., & Samsi, S. (2020, July). Segmentation of tau stained Alzheimers brain tissue using convolutional neural networks. In *2020 42nd Annual International Conference of the IEEE Engineering in Medicine & Biology Society (EMBC)* (pp. 1420-1423). IEEE. 10.1109/EMBC44109.2020.9175832

Xie, J., Siyu, C., Zhang, Y., Gao, D., & Liu, T. (2021). Combining Generative Adversarial Networks and Multi-Output CNN for Motor Imagery Classification. *Journal of Neural Engineering*, 18(4), 46026. 10.1088/1741-2552/abecc533821808

Xu, F., Rong, F., Leng, J., Sun, T., Zhang, Y., Siddharth, S., & Jung, T.-P. (2021). Classification of Left-versus Right-Hand Motor Imagery in Stroke Patients Using Supplementary Data Generated by CycleGAN. *IEEE Transactions on Neural Systems and Rehabilitation Engineering*, 29, 2417–2424. 10.1109/TNSRE.2021.312396934710045

-Yağar, S.D., (2023). *"Chatgpt'nin Sağlık Alanındaki Potansiyel Kullanımına İlişkin Çıkarımlar"*, bmij 11 (3): 1226-1240, doi: https://doi.org/10.15295/bmij.v11i3.2264

Yaman, O., & Tuncer, T. (2022). Exemplar pyramid deep feature extraction based cervical cancer image classification model using pap-smear images. *Biomedical Signal Processing and Control*, 73, 103428. 10.1016/j.bspc.2021.103428

Yamini, B., Kaneti, V. R., Nalini, M., & Subramanian, S. (2023). Machine Learning-driven PCOS prediction for early detection and tailored interventions. *SSRG International Journal of Electrical and Electronics Engineering*, 10(9), 61–75. 10.14445/23488379/IJEEE-V10I9P106

Yang, J., Yu, H., Shen, T., Song, Y., & Chen, Z. (2021). 4-Class Mi-Eeg Signal Generation and Recognition with Cvae-Gan. *Applied Sciences (Basel, Switzerland)*, 11(4), 1798. 10.3390/app11041798

Yang, Y., Yang, J., Liang, Y., Liao, B., Zhu, W., Mo, X., & Huang, K. (2021). Identification and validation of the efficacy of immunological therapy for lung cancer from histopathological images based on deep learning. *Frontiers in Genetics*, 12, 642981. 10.3389/fgene.2021.64298133633793

Yan, W.-J., Li, X., Wang, S.-J., Zhao, G., Liu, Y.-J., Chen, Y.-H., & Fu, X. (2014, January). CASME II: An Improved Spontaneous Micro-Expression Database and the Baseline Evaluation. *PLoS One*, 9(1), e86041. Advance online publication. 10.1371/journal.pone.008604124475068

Yeh, M. C.-H., Wang, Y.-H., Yang, H.-C., Bai, K.-J., Wang, H.-H., & Li, Y.-C. J. (2021). Correction: Artificial Intelligence–Based Prediction of Lung Cancer Risk Using Nonimaging Electronic Medical Records: Deep Learning Approach. *Journal of Medical Internet Research*, 23(10), e33519–e33519. 10.2196/3351934653015

-Yıldız M.S., Alper A. (2023). *"Potential Functions of Artificial İntelligence Chatbot Chatgpt in Health Management: Scoping Review"*, Turk Hijyen ve Biyoloji Dergisi, 80(4).

-Yıldız, İ.,İmik Tanyıldızı, N. (2015). *"Türkiye'de 2012 Yılında Sağlık Haberlerinin Ulusal Yazılı Basında Yer Alış Biçimleri Ve Bilgilendirme Düzeyleri (Habertürk, Hürriyet, Posta, Sabah, Sözcü Ve Zaman Gazeteleri Örneği)"*, Sosyal Bilimler Dergisi / The Journal of Social Science / SOBİDER, Yıl: 2, Sayı: 2

Yin, J.. (2023). A GAN Guided Parallel CNN and Transformer Network for EEG Denoising. *IEEE Journal of Biomedical and Health Informatics*.37220036

Yin, L., Wei, X., Sun, Y., Wang, J., & Rosato, M. J. "A 3D facial expression database for facial behavior research", in *7th International Conference on Automatic Face and Gesture Recognition (FGR06)*, avr. 2006, p. 211-216, 10.1109/FGR.2006.6

Yi, X., Walia, E., & Babyn, P. (2019). Generative adversarial network in medical imaging: A review. *Medical Image Analysis*, 58, 101552. 10.1016/j.media.2019.10155231521965

Yolcu, G., Oztel, I., Kazan, S., Oz, C., Palaniappan, K., Lever, T. E., & Bunyak, F. (2019, November). Facial expression recognition for monitoring neurological disorders based on convolutional neural network. *Multimedia Tools and Applications*, 78(22), 31581–31603. 10.1007/s11042-019-07959-635693322

YOLO. YOLO Dataset. 2022. (2022).

Yue, L., Gong, X., Li, J., Ji, H., Li, M., & Nandi, A. K. (2019). Hierarchical feature extraction for early Alzheimer's disease diagnosis. *IEEE Access : Practical Innovations, Open Solutions*, 7, 93752–93760. 10.1109/ACCESS.2019.2926288

Yu, L., Chen, H., Dou, Q., Qin, J., & Heng, P. A. (2016). Automated melanoma recognition in dermoscopy images via very deep residual networks. *IEEE Transactions on Medical Imaging*, 36(4), 994–1004. 10.1109/TMI.2016.264283928026754

Yu, Z., Liu, G., Liu, Q., & Deng, J. (2018, November). Spatio-temporal convolutional features with nested LSTM for facial expression recognition. *Neurocomputing*, 317, 50–57. 10.1016/j.neucom.2018.07.028

Zacharaki, E. I., Wang, S., Chawla, S., Soo Yoo, D., Wolf, R., Melhem, E. R., & Davatzikos, C. (2009). Classification of brain tumor type and grade using MRI texture and shape in a machine learning scheme. *Magnetic Resonance in Medicine*, 62(6), 1609–1618. 10.1002/mrm.2214719859947

-Zachariae R, Pederson CG, Jensen AB, Ehrnrooth E, Rossen PB, Von der Maase H. (2003). *"Association of Perceived Physician Communication Style With Patient Satisfaction, Distress, Cancer-Related Self-Efficacy, and Perceived Control Over the Disease"*. Br J Canc,88.

Zappa, C., & Mousa, S. A. (2016). Non-small cell lung cancer: Current treatment and future advances. *Translational Lung Cancer Research*, 5(3), 288–300. 10.21037/tlcr.2016.06.0727413711

Zayani, H. M., Ammar, I., Ghodhbani, R., Maqbool, A., Saidani, T., Ben Slimane, J., Kachoukh, A., Kouki, M., Kallel, M., Alsuwaylimi, A. A., & Alenezi, S. M. (2024). Deep Learning for Tomato Disease Detection with YOLOv8. *Engineering, Technology &. Applied Scientific Research*, 14(2), 13584–13591.

Zeiler, M. D., & Fergus, R. (2014). Visualizing and understanding convolutional networks. In *European Conference on Computer Vision* (pp. 818-833). Springer. https://doi.org/10.1007/978-3-319-10590-1_53

Zhang, S., Li, L., & Zhao, Z. "Facial expression recognition based on Gabor wavelets and sparse representation", in *2012 IEEE 11th International Conference on Signal Processing,oct.2012*, vol. 2, p. 816-819, 10.1109/ICoSP.2012.6491706

Zhang, C., Hallbeck, M. S., Salehinejad, H., & Thiels, C. (2024). The integration of artificial intelligence in robotic surgery: A narrative review. *Surgery*, 176(3), 552–557. 10.1016/j.surg.2024.02.00538480053

Zhang, K., Xu, G., Han, Z., Ma, K., Zheng, X., Chen, L., Duan, N., & Zhang, S. (2020). Data Augmentation for Motor Imagery Signal Classification Based on a Hybrid Neural Network. *Sensors (Basel)*, 20(16), 1–20. 10.3390/s2016448532796607

Zhang, M., & Li, J. (2021). A commentary of GPT-3 in MIT Technology Review 2021. *Fundamental Research (Beijing)*, 1(6), 831–833. 10.1016/j.fmre.2021.11.011

Zhang, S., Zhang, S., Huang, T., & Gao, W. "Multimodal Deep Convolutional Neural Network for Audio-Visual Emotion Recognition", in *Proceedings of the 2016 ACM on International Conference on Multimedia Retrieval,* New York, NY, USA, 2016, p. 281–284, 10.1145/2911996.2912051

Zhang, X., Lu, Z., & Li, H. (2021). Realizing the Application of EEG Modeling in BCI Classification: Based on a Conditional GAN Converter. *Frontiers in Neuroscience,* 15, 727394. 10.3389/fnins.2021.72739434867150

Zhang, Y., Malzahn, A. A., Sretenovic, S., & Qi, Y. (2019). The emerging and uncultivated potential of CRISPR technology in plant science. *Nature Plants,* 5(8), 778–794. 10.1038/s41477-019-0461-531308503

Zhao, G., Huang, X., Taini, M., Li, S. Z., & Pietikäinen, M. (2011, August). Facial expression recognition from near-infrared videos. *Image and Vision Computing,* 29(9), 607–619. 10.1016/j.imavis.2011.07.002

Zhao, Y., Ma, B., Jiang, P., Zeng, D., Wang, X., & Li, S. (2020). Prediction of Alzheimer's disease progression with multi-information generative adversarial network. *IEEE Journal of Biomedical and Health Informatics,* 25(3), 711–719. 10.1109/JBHI.2020.300692532750952

Zheng, C., Xia, Y., Pan, Y., & Chen, J. (2016). Automated identification of dementia using medical imaging: A survey from a pattern classification perspective. *Brain Informatics,* 3(1), 17–27. 10.1007/s40708-015-0027-x27747596

Zhong, Y., She, Y., Deng, J., Chen, S., Wang, T., Yang, M., Ma, M., Song, Y., Qi, H., Wang, Y., Shi, J., Wu, C., Xie, D., & Chen, C. (2022). Deep learning for prediction of N2 metastasis and survival for clinical stage I non–small cell lung cancer. *Radiology,* 302(1), 200–211. 10.1148/radiol.2021211090234698568

Zhou, S., & Peng, F. (2020). Patterns of metastases in cervical cancer: A population-based study. *International Journal of Clinical and Experimental Pathology,* 13(7), 1615.

Zhou, Y., Zhao, L., Zhou, N., Zhao, Y., Marino, S., Wang, T., Sun, H., Toga, A. W., & Dinov, I. D. (2019). Predictive big data analytics using the UK Biobank data. *Scientific Reports,* 9(1), 1–10. 10.1038/s41598-019-41634-y30979917

Zhu, J.-Y., Park, T., & Isola, P., and Alexei A Efros. 2017. "Unpaired Image-to-Image Translation Using Cycle-Consistent Adversarial Networks." In *Proceedings of the IEEE International Conference on Computer Vision,* 2223–32. 10.1109/ICCV.2017.244

Zikic, I.. (2014). Segmentation of brain tumor tissues with convolutional neural networks. In *Proceedings of the BRATS-MICCAI*.

About the Contributors

Swarnalatha Purushotham is a Professor, in the School of Computer Science and Engineering, Vellore Institute of Technology at Vellore, India. She pursued her Ph.D degree in Image Processing and Intelligent Systems. She has published more than 130+ papers in International Journals/International Conference Proceedings/National Conferences. She is having 23+ years of teaching experiences. She has filed two Patents and also awarded with Dr. APJ Abdul Kalam Award for Teaching Excellence. She is a senior member of IACSIT, CSI, ACM, IACSIT, IEEE (WIE), ACEEE. She is an Editorial board member/reviewer of reputed International/National Journals and Conferences. Her current research interest includes Image Processing, Ai, Deep Learning, Blockchain Technology, Cloud Computing, GIS, Software Engineering, Human Computer Interaction, IoT, Deep Learning

Prabu Sevugan is a Certified Blockchain Associate, completed B.Engg., in CSE and Did double M.Tech's and double Ph.D.'s in Remote Sensing and CSE respectively. He was a Post-Doctoral Fellow at the Department of Computer Science and Engineering, Indian Institute of Technology Bombay. He has more than 120 publications in peer-reviewed journals and conferences, Edited 3 Books, and published 12 book chapters, and 1 patent. He has organized 3 International Conferences, which include one IEEE Conference as chair and also participated in many workshops and seminars. He is a member of many professional bodies and a senior member of IEEE. He has 19+ years of experience in teaching and research. He worked as a Professor and Head Department of Information Security, the School of Computer Science and Engineering, Vellore Institute of Technology Vellore. Currently, serving as an Associate Professor in the Department of Banking Technology, Pondicherry University, Puducherry, India.

***

Ponmalar A. is an Associate Professor at R.M.K. Engineering College. She excels in her field, contributing significantly through impactful research and dedicated teaching. Her commitment to academic excellence and innovation is pivotal to the institution's success.

Dennis Ananth is currently working as a Senior Assistant Professor at School of Computing, SASTRA Deemed University, Thanjavur. He has been in the teaching & research field for a span of 17 years. He did his B.Tech in Information Technology from Anna University, Chennai and M.Tech in Software Engineering from JNTU Hyderabad. He has completed his Ph.D from Anna University, Chennai in the area of Deep Learning. His research interests include Machine Learning, Deep Learning and Big Data Analytics. He has published many papers in refereed journals and has been a reviewer for many national and international journals. He has been a member in various professional societies in India and abroad. He was conferred with "Promising Engineer Award" by Institution of Engineers (India) in the year 2012.

Maheswari B. working as an Assistant Professor In RMK Engineering College, Puduvoyal, Tamilnadu, India, in the department of Computer Science and Engineering. She received the B.E degree in Computer Science and Engineering and M.E degree in Software Engineering from Anna University, India. She is currently pursuing PhD in computer science and engineering from Anna University, Chennai. Her area of interest is Internet of things and Big Data.

Yamini B. (Yamini Bhavani Shankar) is an Associate Professor in the Department of Networking and Communications at the School of Computing, SRM Institute of Science and Technology (SRMIST), Kattankulathur. She excels in both teaching and research, significantly contributing to the academic and technological advancements at SRMIST.

Shiva Chaithanya Goud Bollipelly is a student in the School of Computing Science and Engineering at Vellore Institute of Technology in Vellore, India. He is pursuing a Bachelor of Technology degree in Computer Science Engineering. His current research interests include Data Science, Image Processing, Blockchain Technology, Machine Learning, and Artificial Intelligence.

Megala G. received B.E. and M.E. degrees in Computer Science and Engineering from Anna University in 2009 and 2013 respectively. She is currently pursuing her Ph.D. degree in Computer Science and Engineering from Vellore Institute of Technology, Vellore. She has 8 years of teaching experience and 3 years of research associate. Her field of specialization is cryptosystems, computational theory and compilers. Her research interests include multimedia security, lightweight cryptography, image and video processing, cloud computing and deep learning.

Balaji G.N., is an Associate Professor from the School of Computer Science and Engineering, Vellore Institute of Technology, Vellore. He worked as an Assistant Professor in the Department of IT, CVR College of Engineering, Hyderabad. He graduated from Annamalai University and post-graduated with M.Tech from SRM University. He completed his doctoral research in the Department of CSE, Faculty of Engineering and Technology, Annamalai University under the guidance of Dr. T. S. Subashini and his area of research is Medical Image Analysis. He published his papers in 35 international journals and conferences, including Springer, Elsevier, and Taylor & Francis. He coordinated a UGC-funded research project, Computer Aided Detection and Diagnosis of Diaphyseal Femur Fracture. He is an active editorial member in Austin Cardiology Journal, USA, and in professional bodies like IEEE, ACM, IAENG, ISTE, and EAI. His research interest includes Image Processing, Pattern Recognition, and Computer Vision. He has organized two National workshops and faculty development programs. He is regularly invited to deliver lectures in various programs to impart skills in research methodology to students.

Nural Imik Tanyildizi She is working in Firat University. She works on public relations, political communication, communication and artificial intelligence. She currently has over 50 articles and studies.

Maithili K. is an Assistant Professor in the Department of Computer Science and Engineering at Veltech Rangarajan Dr Sagunthala R&D Institute of Science and Technology, Chennai, Tamil Nadu, India. Her work emphasizes research and development, making significant contributions to the academic community

Anantharajah Kaneswaran obtained his BSc Eng degree specializing in Electrical and Electronic Engineering with a First Class Honors (CGPA 3.70/4.0) from University of Peradeniya and Doctor of Philosophy degree from Queensland University of Technology, Australia. He has been recognized as Professional Engineer by Engineers Australia. He is a member of IEEE, and Associate Member of IESL. He has been a reviewer for several International Conferences and reviewer of the IET Biometrics Journal. He was instrumental in the development of the department of Computer Engineering as a head of the department at University of Jaffna. He is the chairman of the Academic Development and Planning Committee (ADPC) of the faculty of Engineering. He served as track convener of the first international conference on Engineering 2022 (ICE 2022). Further, he served as finance co-chair for International Conference on Information and Automation for Sustainability (ICIAfS) 2018. His current research interest includes Machine Learning, Computer Vision, and Computer vision application for precision agriculture.

Karthikeyan M is an esteemed member of the faculty at RMK College of Engineering and Technology, located in Puduvoyal, Tamil Nadu. His professional focus includes computer science and engineering, with expertise in areas such as computer network, artificial intelligence, machine learning, and software development.

Rajakumaran M. received his B.E. degree in Computer Science and Engineering from Anna University, Tiruchirappalli, in 2011, ME degree in Computer Science and Engineering from Anna University, Chennai, in 2014 and Ph.D degree in Computer Science and Engineering from Anna University, Chennai, Tamilnadu, India in 2022. He is currently working as an Assistant Professor Grade III in the department of Computer Science and Engineering, School of Computing at SASTRA Deemed University. His areas of interest are Cyber Security, Network & Wireless Sensor Networks. He has published 10 papers in International Journals, 10 papers in National and International Conferences and 3 Patents. He is a life member of Indian Society for Technical Education.

Mal Hari Prasad is a Research Scholar, in the School of Computing Science and Engineering, Vellore Institute of Technology at Vellore, India. He has received M.Tech degree from Chaitanya Barathi Institute of Technology, Hyderabad in 2008 and B.Tech degree from Scient Institute of Technology, Hyderabad in 2006. He has 14 years of teaching experience. He has published 5 papers. His research interests include image and video processing, programming languages, design and analysis of algorithms

Kirti Nayak is a passionate researcher and developer with a strong foundation in software engineering. She is currently pursuing a Master's degree in Artificial Intelligence & Machine Learning (M.Tech) at VIT Vellore, further developing her expertise in data science and machine learning. Prior to her academic pursuits, Kirti leveraged her programming skills for over 3 years as a Software Development Engineer (SDE), primarily using Java. During this time, a curiosity for machine learning and deep learning concepts emerged. This sparked a desire to not only develop solutions but also to understand the underlying principles through research. Now, as a Data Science Enthusiast and Aspiring Researcher, Kirti is actively applying her technical foundation and research mindset to the world of data science. She is eager to contribute her skills, learn from experienced professionals, and contribute to advancements in the field through research.

Immaculate Rexi Jenifer received Bachelor of Technology degree in Information Technology from E.G.S.Pillay Engineering College, Nagapattinam in 2010 and Master of Engineering in Computer Science and Engineering from Anna University, BIT-Campus Trichy in 2014. and completed her doctoral degree in Anna University, Chennai Tamilnadu, India in 2023. Her current research includes Deep Learning, Machine Learning, She is an Assistant Professor Grade II in School of Computing, SASTRA Deemed University, Thanjavur. She has published 5 papers in International Journals, 10 papers in National and International Conferences.

Maheswari R. has completed her Graduation Bachelor of Computer Applications from Kongu Arts and Science College, Erode and secured University Gold Medal. She did her Post Graduation Master of Business Administration at Kongu Arts and Science College, Erode. Secured University 8th Rank. NET Qualified faculty. Completed PhD in Management from Bharathiar University, Coimbatore. She has teaching experience of 11 years and presently working as Assistant Professor at Kongu Engineering College, Erode. She also has Industrial Experience of 2 years and Entrepreneurial Experience of 3 years. She holds 2 patents. She is author of various book chapters and has published articles in various academic journals. She has cleared NISM Equity and Derivatives trader certification and Mutual Funds Distributor certification. She has conducted Management Development Faculty for various organizations across the state. She is a Motivational Speaker and Trainer for various organizations and institutions. Posted articles in her Blog and Facebook Page. Certified Trainer at Lions Club International and JCI. She has completed Neuro Linguistic Program(NLP)–Basic level and Certified Adolescencestudents'handler.

Siva Subramanian R is an esteemed member of the faculty at RMK College of Engineering and Technology, located in Puduvoyal, Tamil Nadu. His professional focus includes computer science and engineering, with expertise in areas such as artificial intelligence, machine learning, and software development. Mr. Siva Subramanian is committed to academic excellence and actively contributes to the advancement of technology education within his institution.

Venkatesan R. received Ph.D. degree in Computer Science and Engineering from VIT University: Vellore Institute of Technology, Vellore. He has more than 30 publications in national and international journals and conferences. He has more than 17+ years of experience in teaching and 9 years of experience in research. His current research includes satellite image processing and neural networks. Currently, he is an Assistant Professor in the School of Computing, SASTRA University, Thanjavur.

Gokila R.G. received his M.E degree in Software Engineering from Easwari Engineering College, Chennai in 2012 and Ph.D degree in Computer Science and Engineering from Anna University, Chennai, Tamilnadu, India in 2024. She is currently working as a Assistant Professor in the department of Computer Science and Engineering, School of Computing at SASTRA Deemed University, Thanjavur. Her areas of interest are Machine Learning and Applications, Data Mining, Cyber Security. She has published 6 papers in International Journals, 10 papers in National and International Conferences . She is a life member of Indian Society for Technical Education.

Markkandeyan S. received his M.E degree in Computer Science and Engineering from Vinayaka Mission University, Salem, in 2007 and Ph.D degree in Computer Science and Engineering from Anna University, Chennai, Tamilnadu, India in 2016. He is currently working as a Senior Assistant Professor in the department of Computer Science and Engineering, School of Computing at SASTRA Deemed University, Thanjavur. His areas of interest are Machine Learning and Applications, Data Mining, Web Mining and Text Mining. He has published 17 papers in International Journals, 15 papers in National and International Conferences and 2 Patents. He is a life member of Indian Society for Technical Education.

Evin Şahin Sadık is an Assistant Professor in the Department of Electrical and Electronics Engineering at Dumlupınar University, Turkey. She completed her Ph.D. in Electrical and Electronics Engineering with a focus on Biomedical Signal Processing. Dr. Sadık's current research interests include Artificial Intelligence, Deep Learning, Biomedical Signal Processing, and related technologies.

Vetrivel S.C. is a faculty member in the Department of Management Studies, Kongu Engineering College (Autonomous), Perundurai, Erode Dt. Having experience in Industry 20 years and Teaching 16 years. Awarded with Doctoral Degree in Management Sciences in Anna University, Chennai. He has organized various workshops and Faculty Development Programmes. He is actively involved in research and consultancy works. He acted as a resource person to FDPs & MDPs to various industries like, SPB ltd, Tamilnadu Police, DIET, Rotary school and many. His areas of interest include Entrepreneurship, Business Law, Marketing and Case writing. Articles published more than 100 International and National Journals. Presented papers in more than 30 National and International conferences including IIM Bangalore, IIM Kozhikode, IIM Kashipur and IIM Indore. He was a Chief Co-ordinator of Entrepreneurship and Management Development Centre (EMDC) of Kongu Engineering College, he was instrumental in organizing various Awareness Camps, FDP, and TEDPs to aspiring entrepreneurs which was funded by NSTEDB – DST/GoI

Singaravelan Shanmugasundaram received B.E in Electronics and Communication Engineering Degree from FX Engineering College , Tirunelveli , india in 2004 and his M.E., Computer Science and Engineering Degree form Manonmaniam Sundaranar University ,Tirunelveli , India in 2007. He completed Doctoral Research in Computer Science and Engineering Degree form Manonmaniam Sundaranar University, Tirunelveli , India in 2016. His Research interest in Image Processing , Data Mining , Artificial Intelligence , Data Analysis.

Anish T.P. is an esteemed member of the faculty at RMK College of Engineering and Technology, located in Puduvoyal, Tamil Nadu. His professional focus includes computer science and engineering, with expertise in areas such as artificial intelligence, machine learning, and software development. Mr. Anish T P is committed to academic excellence and actively contributes to the advancement of technology education within his institution.

Sanjay V. Received his B.E Computer science and Engineering Degree from Adithya Institute of Technology, Coimbatore,India in 2019 and his M.E. Computer science and Engineering Degree from Kumaraguru College of Technology, Coimbatore,India in 2021.He is currently pursuing his Doctoral Research in School of Computer Science and Engineering at Vellore Institute of Technology, Vellore, India.His research interest includes Medical Image processing, Deep Learning and computer vision. Email: sanjay.researcher@gmail.com

Selvakumar V is an Associate Professor in CSE Department.

Ragupathyraj Valluvan obtained his BSc Eng degree specializing in Electrical and Electronic Engineering with a First Class Honors (CGPA 3.90/4.0) from University of Peradeniya and MSc degree in Electrical Engineering specializing in Telecommunication Engineering from UT Dallas. He was graduate research assistant at UC Irvine focusing on Machine Learning on Graphical Models before joining University of Jaffna as a Lecturer. He co-authored two peer-reviewed journal publication, seven (07) peer-reviewed conference publications, six (06) abstracts and extended abstracts, one published international patent (PCT- the very first one for University Jaffna), one published national patent and three (03) national patent filing under review together with one US copyright. Further, he has successfully secured a total of 1.13 million LKR as PI from external sources and contributed to securing nearly 60 million LKR as Co-PI. He is having 13+ years of teaching experience. He has mentored several successful research projects resulting in National and Internal Recognition, notably IEEE SA Telehealth Solutions Pitch Competition where the project "Multi-purpose Healthcare Monitoring Bracelet" obtained in first place in student/academia category. He is a member of IEEE, and Associate Member of IESL. He has been a reviewer for several National and International Conferences. He was instrumental in the establishment of University Business Linkage of University of Jaffna, drafting and implementation of IP Policy, and the establishment of the National Incubation Center at University of Jaffna. His current research interest includes Machine Learning, Communication Systems (IoT) and Innovation Management and Technology Commercialization.

Arun V.P. is a driven and accomplished professional with a diverse educational background and extensive hands-on experience across various industries. Graduating with honors, Arun earned his Master of Business Administration (M.B.A) with a specialization in Human Resources and Marketing from the renowned Sona School of Management in Salem in 2018, where he excelled academically with an impressive 8.3 Cumulative Grade Point Average (CGPA). Before pursuing his MBA, Arun laid a solid foundation by obtaining a Bachelor of Engineering degree from Kongu Engineering College in 2014. Throughout his academic journey, Arun displayed an unwavering commitment to learning and personal growth, actively seeking opportunities to expand his knowledge and skills beyond the confines of traditional education. He sought practical experiences to complement his theoretical understanding, such as a 45-day summer internship focused on conducting a feasibility study for R-Doc Sustainability in the market. Additionally, Arun broadened his horizons through a 7-day industrial visit to Malaysia and Singapore, immersing himself in diverse cultural and professional environments. Arun's academic pursuits were further enriched by his involvement in hands-on projects, including a comprehensive study on Employee Job Satisfaction at Roots Cast Private Limited.

Index

A

algorithm bias 18
Artificial Intelligence (AI) 2, 11, 16, 18, 20, 37, 61, 62, 63, 70, 74, 76, 78, 80, 81, 83, 84, 85, 86, 88, 89, 90, 93, 94, 95, 96, 98, 99, 101, 113, 115, 116, 117, 118, 119, 120, 121, 122, 123, 124, 125, 126, 129, 130, 131, 132, 133, 134, 135, 136, 137, 143, 151, 155, 169, 182, 225, 226, 249, 250, 251, 278, 282, 301, 303, 306, 310, 322, 323, 324, 326, 337, 339, 340, 341, 346, 348, 350, 351, 353, 365, 366, 367, 370, 378

B

Brain 9, 73, 155, 220, 221, 253, 254, 255, 256, 258, 259, 261, 262, 263, 264, 265, 266, 267, 269, 272, 274, 276, 277, 278, 279, 281, 282, 283, 287, 288, 300, 301, 302, 303, 306, 318, 319, 320, 321, 322, 323, 324, 325, 326, 330, 331, 333, 334, 335, 336, 337, 338, 339, 340, 341, 342, 366
Breast Cancer 21, 37, 41, 42, 43, 44, 47, 56, 57, 58, 59, 73, 155, 282, 284, 288, 301, 302, 303

C

Chat GPT 117, 137
clinical data 7, 68, 80, 235, 248
Computer-Aided Diagnosis 155, 226, 255, 261, 263, 354, 358, 365

D

data augmentation 169, 173, 174, 236, 266, 269, 322, 324, 325, 333, 336, 341, 343, 366, 372, 373
data balancing 333
data harmonization 333
data privacy 3, 18, 33, 63, 71, 75, 84, 85, 140, 141, 143, 144, 145, 146, 147, 148, 149, 150, 151, 152, 244
Data security 12, 31, 36, 65, 70, 79, 139, 140, 148, 149, 150, 151, 152, 153, 154, 245, 336
deep learning 5, 6, 7, 10, 18, 20, 21, 22, 56, 57, 61, 72, 73, 78, 97, 98, 101, 115, 116, 118, 141, 142, 146, 165, 170, 171, 172, 182, 183, 207, 223, 225, 228, 229, 233, 242, 246, 247, 248, 249, 250, 251, 253, 254, 255, 258, 259, 261, 262, 263, 264, 266, 267, 278, 279, 281, 284, 300, 301, 302, 303, 305, 306, 308, 314, 318, 324, 326, 330, 345, 346, 347, 348, 351, 352, 361, 364, 365, 366, 369, 370, 371, 372, 373, 374, 375, 376, 379, 380
Densenet 229, 264, 283, 284, 285, 286, 294
dermatology 134, 171, 172, 174, 182, 220
dermoscopic images 172, 185
Detection and diagnosis 71, 174, 225
Dice coefficient 186, 346
Digital pathology 139, 140, 142, 143, 144, 145, 146, 148, 149, 150, 151, 152, 153, 154, 155
disease detection 20, 21, 61, 62, 84, 166, 279, 316
disease management 76
Disease Prediction 1, 4, 21, 71, 73, 78, 79, 305, 319
Drug Discovery 28, 36, 71, 73, 80, 81, 232

E

EEG 9, 321, 322, 323, 324, 325, 326, 327, 328, 329, 330, 331, 332, 333, 334, 335, 336, 337, 338, 339, 340, 341, 342, 343
Esteva 171, 182

F

Facial emotion recognition 369, 372, 378, 379, 380
facial expression 324, 369, 370, 371, 373, 378, 379, 380, 381

feature extraction 6, 171, 175, 191, 194, 195, 197, 208, 214, 225, 232, 254, 255, 264, 269, 284, 285, 294, 303, 304, 307, 320, 346, 347, 354, 356, 373, 374

Federated learning 34, 35, 37, 104, 139, 140, 141, 142, 143, 144, 145, 146, 147, 148, 149, 150, 151, 152, 153, 154, 155, 156, 223, 236, 244

functional magnetic resonance imaging 337

G

Generative Adversarial Network 320, 324, 325, 330, 334, 335, 340, 341, 342, 346, 355, 356, 364, 367

Generator and Discriminator 326, 330, 354, 355, 356

Glomeruli detection 139, 140, 141, 142, 143, 145, 146, 147, 148, 149, 150, 152, 153, 154

Gradient boosting 43, 48, 50

H

healthcare 1, 2, 3, 4, 5, 6, 7, 8, 9, 10, 11, 12, 14, 15, 16, 17, 18, 19, 20, 21, 22, 23, 24, 26, 27, 28, 30, 33, 35, 36, 37, 38, 39, 41, 45, 61, 62, 63, 64, 65, 66, 67, 68, 69, 70, 71, 72, 74, 75, 76, 77, 78, 79, 80, 81, 82, 83, 84, 85, 86, 115, 117, 118, 119, 122, 125, 128, 129, 132, 133, 135, 136, 140, 141, 142, 144, 145, 146, 148, 149, 152, 153, 154, 155, 169, 172, 180, 225, 226, 229, 242, 244, 245, 247, 251, 328, 338, 346, 347, 348, 351, 352

healthcare costs 8, 10, 27, 65, 172

Healthcare Informatics 1, 7, 38, 155

Health Communication 117, 118, 119, 120, 121, 122, 123, 124, 125, 126, 127, 128, 129, 130, 131, 132, 133, 134, 135, 137

I

image classification 170, 182, 207, 219, 242, 267, 293, 304, 365, 366

Image Processing 2, 12, 13, 14, 21, 76, 171, 206, 215, 217, 255, 278, 282, 293, 340, 364, 379

Immunotherapy 225, 243

J

Jaccard index 186, 358

L

Lung Cancer 223, 224, 225, 226, 228, 229, 230, 231, 232, 233, 234, 235, 236, 239, 241, 242, 243, 244, 245, 246, 247, 248, 249, 250, 251, 302

M

Machine Learning (ML) 1, 2, 4, 5, 6, 7, 10, 18, 20, 21, 22, 43, 56, 57, 58, 61, 62, 63, 70, 71, 72, 73, 74, 77, 78, 80, 81, 83, 85, 86, 87, 90, 98, 101, 102, 109, 110, 111, 112, 114, 133, 140, 143, 164, 171, 172, 174, 178, 215, 218, 221, 223, 225, 228, 232, 233, 236, 250, 251, 257, 263, 279, 283, 284, 296, 302, 303, 318, 321, 322, 323, 336, 338, 340, 348, 350, 352, 353, 366, 378

Medical image analysis 6, 139, 144, 145, 149, 151, 152, 155, 241, 262, 346, 352, 364, 367

medical imaging 2, 5, 6, 13, 14, 62, 68, 70, 71, 77, 84, 143, 145, 148, 150, 151, 152, 155, 184, 228, 232, 244, 249, 253, 254, 262, 263, 319, 320, 350, 351, 353, 364, 365, 367

Medical Signal Processing 10

melanoma 27, 170, 171, 172, 177, 178, 180, 182, 183, 184, 186, 188, 189, 190, 191, 192, 195, 196, 197, 214, 219, 220, 264, 278

METABRIC 42, 47, 56, 57

MRI Images 253, 254, 262, 263, 264, 286, 301, 303

N

noise removal 203, 206, 332, 333, 334

O

Object Detection 71, 139, 141, 145, 146, 148, 151, 183, 207, 217, 261, 262, 263, 264, 267, 268, 269, 270, 271, 277, 278, 279, 293

P

patient engagement 63, 67, 75, 81
patient outcomes 1, 5, 7, 18, 29, 61, 63, 67, 70, 71, 73, 74, 75, 76, 77, 81, 84, 85, 122, 152, 154, 169, 170, 174, 181, 226, 228, 232, 242, 244, 262, 263, 277, 347, 348, 364
personalized medicine 25, 27, 37, 61, 62, 63, 68, 70, 71, 79, 83, 228, 249, 282, 283
plant health 157, 158, 159, 162, 163, 164
positron emission tomography 13
precision agriculture 163, 166
predictive analytics 3, 11, 20, 63, 70, 73, 77, 78, 79, 85, 100, 102, 104, 108, 110, 111, 114
Pretrained models 279, 283, 284

R

Regularized Convolutional Neural Network 253, 258
Resource Optimization 38, 78

S

Semantic Segmentation 221, 253
Skin lesion segmentation 185, 192, 193
Smart Healthcare 21, 251, 346, 347, 348, 351
softmax 207, 212, 257, 263, 281, 293, 294, 373, 376
synthetic data generation 236, 323

T

transfer learning 171, 175, 220, 261, 262, 263, 264, 278, 279, 301, 302, 303, 304, 308, 336, 337, 340
Tumor Detection 76, 228, 232, 255, 259, 262, 263, 264, 277, 278

V

virtual health assistants 63, 81, 82

W

Watershed segmentation 345, 352, 353, 355, 356, 357, 358, 364

X

Xception 169, 175, 229, 263, 264, 285, 286
XGBoost 41, 42, 43, 44, 48, 52, 53, 58, 233

Y

YOLO 141, 145, 155, 156, 165, 261, 262, 264, 267, 269, 273, 278, 279
YOLOv3 139, 140, 143, 145, 146, 147, 148, 149, 150, 151, 152

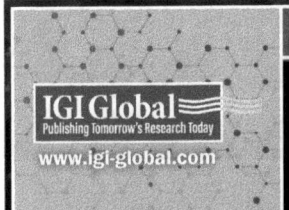

Publishing Tomorrow's Research Today

IGI Global
www.igi-global.com

Uncover Current Insights and Future Trends in Scientific, Technical, & Medical (STM)
with IGI Global's Cutting-Edge Recommended Books

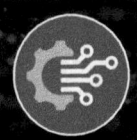

Print Only, E-Book Only, or Print + E-Book.
Order direct through IGI Global's Online Bookstore at www.igi-global.com or through your preferred provider.

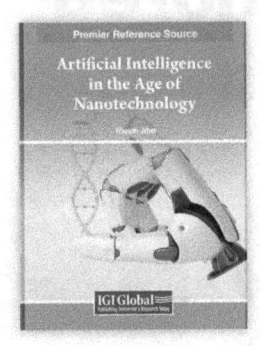

Artificial Intelligence in the Age of Nanotechnology
ISBN: 9798369303689
© 2024; 299 pp.
List Price: US$ 300

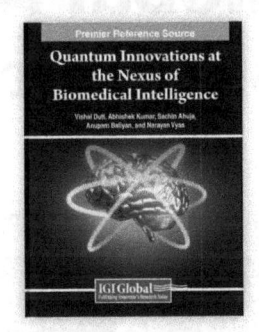

Quantum Innovations at the Nexus of Biomedical Intelligence
ISBN: 9798369314791
© 2024; 287 pp.
List Price: US$ 330

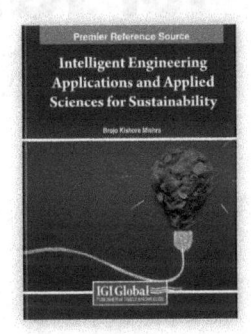

Intelligent Engineering Applications and Applied Sciences for Sustainability
ISBN: 9798369300442
© 2023; 542 pp.
List Price: US$ 270

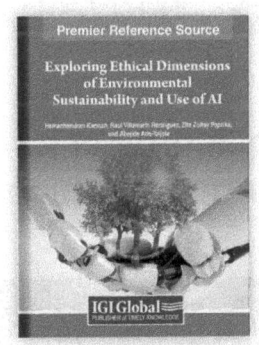

Exploring Ethical Dimensions of Environmental Sustainability and Use of AI
ISBN: 9798369308929
© 2024; 426 pp.
List Price: US$ 265

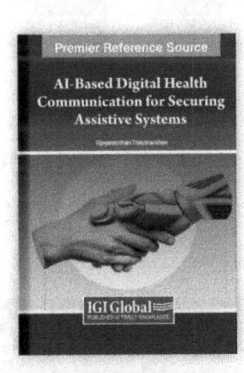

AI-Based Digital Health Communication for Securing Assistive Systems
ISBN: 9781668489383
© 2023; 299 pp.
List Price: US$ 325

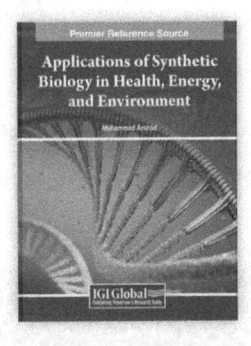

Applications of Synthetic Biology in Health, Energy, and Environment
ISBN: 9781668465776
© 2023; 454 pp.
List Price: US$ 325

Do you want to stay current on the latest research trends, product announcements, news, and special offers? Join IGI Global's mailing list to receive customized recommendations, exclusive discounts, and more.
Sign up at: www.igi-global.com/newsletters.

Scan the QR Code here to view more related titles in STM.

www.igi-global.com | Sign up at www.igi-global.com/newsletters | facebook.com/igiglobal | twitter.com/igiglobal | linkedin.com/igiglobal

Ensure Quality Research is Introduced to the Academic Community

Become a Reviewer for IGI Global Authored Book Projects

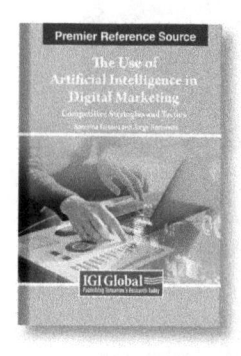

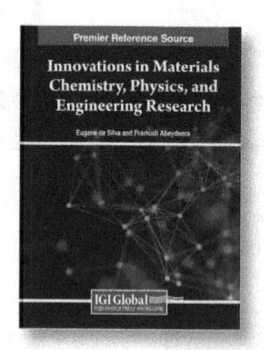

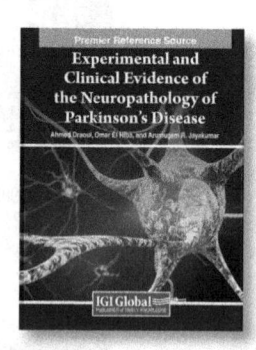

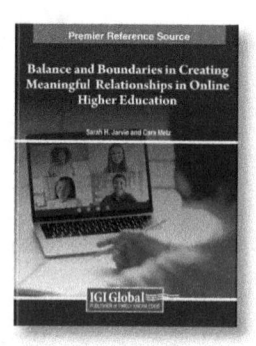

The overall success of an authored book project is dependent on quality and timely manuscript evaluations.

Applications and Inquiries may be sent to:
development@igi-global.com

Applicants must have a doctorate (or equivalent degree) as well as publishing, research, and reviewing experience. Authored Book Evaluators are appointed for one-year terms and are expected to complete at least three evaluations per term. Upon successful completion of this term, evaluators can be considered for an additional term.

If you have a colleague that may be interested in this opportunity, we encourage you to share this information with them.

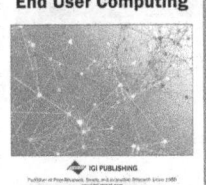

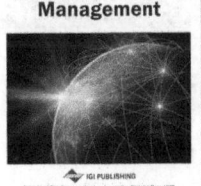

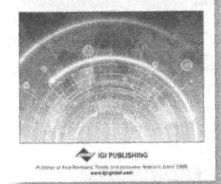

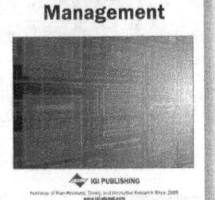

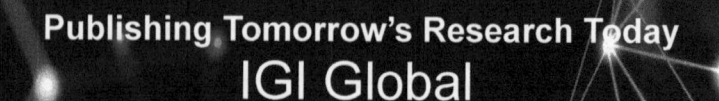

Publishing Tomorrow's Research Today
IGI Global
e-Book Collection

Including Essential Reference Books Within Three Fundamental Academic Areas

Business & Management
Scientific, Technical, & Medical (STM)
Education

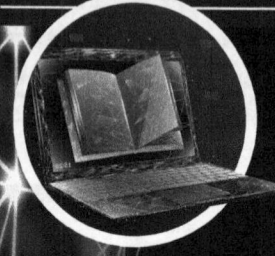

- Acquisition options include Perpetual, Subscription, and Read & Publish
- No Additional Charge for Multi-User Licensing
- No Maintenance, Hosting, or Archiving Fees
- Continually Enhanced Accessibility Compliance Features (WCAG)

| Over 150,000+ Chapters | Contributions From 200,000+ Scholars Worldwide | More Than 1,000,000+ Citations | Majority of e-Books Indexed in Web of Science & Scopus | Consists of Tomorrow's Research Available Today! |

Recommended Titles from our e-Book Collection

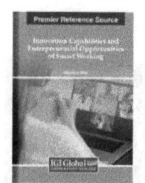

Innovation Capabilities and Entrepreneurial Opportunities of Smart Working
ISBN: 9781799887973

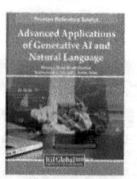

Advanced Applications of Generative AI and Natural Language Processing Models
ISBN: 9798369305027

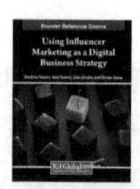

Using Influencer Marketing as a Digital Business Strategy
ISBN: 9798369305515

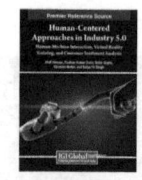

Human-Centered Approaches in Industry 5.0
ISBN: 9798369326473

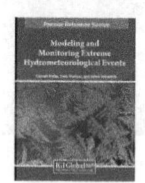

Modeling and Monitoring Extreme Hydrometeorological Events
ISBN: 9781668487716

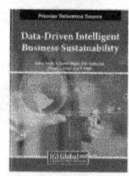

Data-Driven Intelligent Business Sustainability
ISBN: 9798369300497

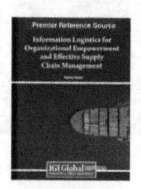

Information Logistics for Organizational Empowerment and Effective Supply Chain Management
ISBN: 9798369301593

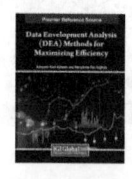

Data Envelopment Analysis (DEA) Methods for Maximizing Efficiency
ISBN: 9798369302552

Request More Information, or Recommend the IGI Global e-Book Collection to Your Institution's Librarian

For More Information or to Request a Free Trial, Contact IGI Global's e-Collections Team: eresources@igi-global.com | 1-866-342-6657 ext. 100 | 717-533-8845 ext. 100

Are You Ready to Publish Your Research?

IGI Global
Publishing Tomorrow's Research Today

IGI Global offers book authorship and editorship opportunities across three major subject areas, including Business, STM, and Education.

Benefits of Publishing with IGI Global:

- Free one-on-one editorial and promotional support.
- Expedited publishing timelines that can take your book from start to finish in less than one (1) year.
- Choose from a variety of formats, including Edited and Authored References, Handbooks of Research, Encyclopedias, and Research Insights.
- Utilize IGI Global's eEditorial Discovery® submission system in support of conducting the submission and double-blind peer review process.
- IGI Global maintains a strict adherence to ethical practices due in part to our full membership with the Committee on Publication Ethics (COPE).
- Indexing potential in prestigious indices such as Scopus®, Web of Science™, PsycINFO®, and ERIC – Education Resources Information Center.
- Ability to connect your ORCID iD to your IGI Global publications.
- Earn honorariums and royalties on your full book publications as well as complimentary content and exclusive discounts.

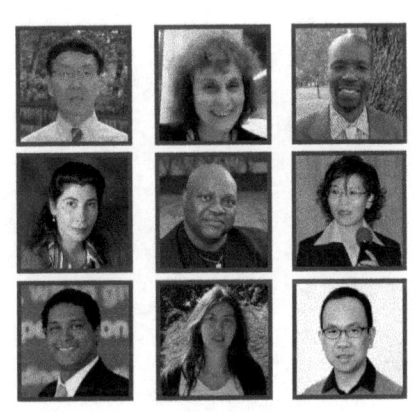

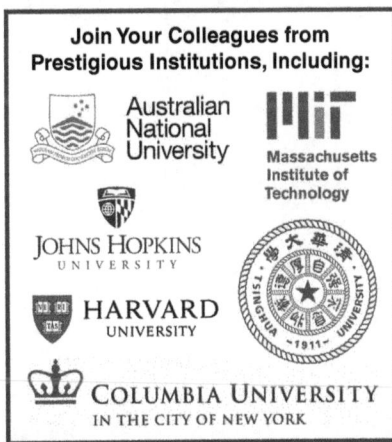

Join Your Colleagues from Prestigious Institutions, Including:

Australian National University
MIT — Massachusetts Institute of Technology
Johns Hopkins University
Harvard University
Tsinghua University
Columbia University in the City of New York

Learn More at: www.igi-global.com/publish
or by Contacting the Acquisitions Department at: acquisition@igi-global.com

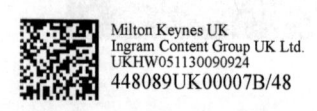

Milton Keynes UK
Ingram Content Group UK Ltd.
UKHW051130090924
448089UK00007B/48

9 798369 371572